The Changing Disability Policy System

Active Citizenship and Disability in Europe Volume 1

Edited by Rune Halvorsen, Bjørn Hvinden, Jerome Bickenbach, Delia Ferri and Ana Marta Guillén Rodriguez

Routledge
Taylor & Francis Group
LONDON AND NEW YORK

First published 2017 by Routledge

2 Park Square, Milton Park, Abingdon, Oxfordshire OX14 4RN
52 Vanderbilt Avenue, New York, NY 10017

Routledge is an imprint of the Taylor & Francis Group, an informa business

First issued in paperback 2020

British Library Cataloguing in Publication Data
A catalogue record for this book is available from the British Library

Library of Congress Cataloging in Publication Data
Names: Halvorsen, Rune, editor. | Hvinden, Bjørn, 1949- editor. | Bickenbach, Jerome Edmund, editor. | Ferri, Delia, editor. | Guillén Rodriguez, Ana, editor.
Title: Active citizenship and disability in Europe / edited by Rune Halvorsen, Bjørn Hvinden, Jerome Bickenbach, Delia Ferri, and Ana Marta Guillén Rodriguez.
Other titles: Routledge advances in disability studies.
Description: Abingdon, Oxon; New York, NY: Routledge, 2017. | Series: Routledge advances in disability studies | Includes bibliographical references and index.
Identifiers: LCCN 2016051022 | ISBN 9781138652880 (hbk) | ISBN 9781315623931 (ebk)
Subjects: LCSH: People with disabilities–Government policy–Europe. | Citizenship–Europe. | Political participation–Europe. | Social participation–Europe. | MESH: Public Policy | Disabled Persons | Human Rights | Social Welfare | Europe.
Classification: LCC HV1559.E85 A28 2017 | DDC 362.4/04561094–dc23
LC record available at https://lccn.loc.gov/2016051022

ISBN: 978-1-138-65288-0 (hbk)
ISBN: 978-0-367-59519-7 (pbk)

Typeset in Times New Roman
by Deanta Global Publishing Services, Chennai, India

The Changing Disability Policy System

Being an 'active citizen' involves exercising social rights and duties, enjoying choice and autonomy, and participating in political decision-making processes which are of importance for one's life. Amid the new challenges facing contemporary welfare states, debate over just how 'active' citizens can and ought to be has redoubled. Presenting research from the first major comparative and cross-national study of active citizenship and disability in Europe, this book analyses the consequences of on-going changes in Europe – what opportunities do persons with disabilities have to exercise Active Citizenship?

The Changing Disability Policy System: Active Citizenship and Disability in Europe Volume 1 approaches the conditions for Active Citizenship from a macro perspective in order to capture the impact of the overall disability policy system. This system takes diverse and changing forms in the nine European countries under study. Central to the analysis are issues of coherence and coordination between three subsystems of the disability policy system, and between levels of governance.

This book identifies the implications and policy lessons of the findings for future disability policy in Europe and beyond. It will appeal to policymakers and policy officials, as well as to researchers and students of disability studies, comparative social policy, international disability law and qualitative research methods.

Rune Halvorsen is Associate Professor in Social Policy in the Department of Social Work, Child Welfare and Social Policy, Oslo and Akershus University College of Applied Sciences, Norway. His research focuses on comparative social policy, disability policy, social movements, social citizenship and recognition politics.

Bjørn Hvinden is Professor in Sociology and Head of Research at Norwegian Social Research (NOVA), an institution at Oslo and Akershus University College of Applied Sciences, Norway. His main research interests are comparative and European social policies, social citizenship, climate change and welfare, disability, poverty and youth job insecurity.

Jerome Bickenbach is Permanent Visiting Professor at the Department of Health Sciences and Health Policy, University of Lucerne, Switzerland, Professor Emeritus at Queen's University, Canada and Head of the Disability Policy Unit at Swiss Paraplegic Research (SPF), Nottwil, Switzerland. His research focuses on disability epidemiology, definition and conceptual analysis, as well as issues in disability policy and law.

Delia Ferri is a Lecturer in Law at Maynooth University and member of the Maynooth Centre for European and Eurasian Studies, Ireland. She is also affiliated researcher at the Dirpolis Institute of Scuola Superiore Sant'Anna, Italy. Her research interests include EU Law, European Constitutional Law and International and Comparative Disability Law.

Ana Marta Guillén Rodriguez is full Professor of Sociology and Head of Department at the University of Oviedo, Spain. Her research interests include comparative social and labour policy, Europeanization and European integration.

Routledge Advances in Disability Studies

Towards a Contextual Psychology of Disablism
Brian Watermeyer

Disability, Hate Crime and Violence
Edited by Alan Roulstone and Hannah Mason-Bish

Branding and Designing Disability
Reconceptualising Disability Studies
Elizabeth DePoy and Stephen Gilson

Crises, Conflict and Disability
Ensuring Equality
Edited by David Mitchell and Valerie Karr

Disability, Spaces and Places of Policy Exclusion
Edited by Karen Soldatic, Hannah Morgan and Alan Roulstone

Changing Social Attitudes Toward Disability
Perspectives from historical, cultural, and educational studies
Edited by David Bolt

Disability, Avoidance and the Academy
Challenging Resistance
Edited by David Bolt and Claire Penketh

Autism in a De-centered World
Alice Wexler

Disabled Childhoods
Monitoring Differences and Emerging Identities
Janice McLaughlin, Edmund Coleman-Fountain and Emma Clavering

Intellectual Disability and Being Human
A Care Ethics Model
Chrissie Rogers

Contents

List of figures

List of tables

List of contributors

Jerome Bickenbach is Permanent Visiting Professor at the Department of Health Sciences and Health Policy, University of Lucerne, Switzerland; Professor Emeritus at Queen's University, Canada; and Head of the Disability Policy Unit at Swiss Paraplegic Research (SPF), Nottwil, Switzerland. His research focuses on disability epidemiology, definition and conceptual analysis, and issues in disability policy and law.

Julie Beadle-Brown is Professor in Intellectual and Developmental Disabilities at the Tizard Centre, University of Kent, UK and Professor in Disability Studies at the Living with Disability Research Centre, La Trobe University, Australia. Her research, teaching and consultancy have particularly focused on de-institutionalisation and the development of community-based services, and on the implementation of person-centred approaches such as person-centred active support to improve quality of life.

Kjetil Klette Bøhler is a Senior Researcher at Norwegian Social Research (NOVA), an institution at Oslo and Akershus University College of Applied Sciences, Norway. Recently he has worked with research on Active Citizenship for persons with disabilities and research on the consequences of unemployment among young adults in Europe. In addition, Bøhler works with research dealing with the intersection between aesthetics and politics, and in particular the relationship between music and politics in a changing Latin America.

Edmund Coleman-Fountain is Research Fellow in Social Policy Research Unit at the University of York, UK. His interests are in narrative identities and social transformations.

Timo Dins is Junior Researcher at the Institute for Pedagogy and Rehabilitation for Persons with Intellectual and Severe Disabilities at the University of Cologne, Germany. His research interests include disability studies, disability ethics, and capability theory.

Delia Ferri is a Lecturer in Law at Maynooth University and member of the Maynooth Centre for European and Eurasian Studies, Ireland. She is also affiliated researcher at the Dirpolis Institute of Scuola Superiore Sant'Anna, Italy.

Her research interests include EU Law, European Constitutional Law and International and Comparative Disability Law.

Eilionóir Flynn is Deputy Director of the Centre for Disability Law and Policy and Senior Lecturer with the School of Law, National University of Ireland, Galway, Ireland. Her interest in disability law include assisted and supported decision-making, rights-enforcement mechanisms and access to justice.

Rune Halvorsen is Associate Professor in Social Policy in the Department of Social Work, Child Welfare and Social Policy, Oslo and Akershus University College of Applied Sciences, Norway. His research focuses on comparative social policy, disability policy, social movements, social citizenship and recognition politics.

Bjørn Hvinden is Professor in Sociology and Head of Research at Norwegian Social Research (NOVA), an institution at Oslo and Akershus University College of Applied Sciences, Norway. His main research interests are comparative and European social policies, social citizenship, climate change and welfare, disability, poverty and youth job insecurity.

Šárka Káňová is Researcher in Department of Special Education, Charles University in Prague and a senior lecturer at the Faculty of Education, University of West Bohemia in Pilsen, Czech Republic. Her research interests include the issue of the life course of people with disabilities and exploring the possibilities of fulfilling the roles associated with their Active Citizenship.

Anemari Karačić is Junior Researcher at the International Research Unit in Disability Studies (iDiS), University of Cologne, Germany. Her research interests include disability studies, the cultural and political sociologies of 'dis/ability' and biopolitics.

Sinéad Keogh is a post-doctoral researcher at the Centre for Disability Law and Policy (CDLP) at National University of Ireland, Galway, Ireland. She has previously worked as a lecturer in Economics and researched time-use patterns of farm household members in the West of Ireland.

Jennifer Kline is a post-doctoral researcher at the Centre for Disability Law and Policy (CDLP) at National University of Ireland, Galway, Ireland. She has expertise in immigration, human rights, and disability law.

Rafael Lindqvist is Senior Professor in the Department of Sociology, Uppsala University, Sweden. His main research interests are the emergence of the Nordic welfare states, with an emphasis on reforms and organisation in sickness insurance, vocational rehabilitation and disability policy.

Gerard Quinn is Professor of Law and the Director of the Centre for Disability Law and Policy, the School of Law National University of Ireland, Galway, Ireland. His main expertise is in international and comparative disability law and policy.

Ana Marta Guillén Rodriguez is Professor of Sociology and Head of Department at the University of Oviedo, Spain. Her research interests include comparative social and labour policy, Europeanization and European integration.

Roy Sainsbury is Professor of Social Policy in the Department of Social Policy and Social Work at the University of York, UK. His main research interests are reforms in social security systems, administration and delivery of benefits, and the relationship between social security, disability and the labour market.

Victoria Schuller is a PhD student in Health Sciences and Health Policy, University of Lucerne, Lucerne, Switzerland. Her research interests include gender and disability, Active Citizenship and social inclusion of persons with disabilities.

Marie Sépulchre is a PhD Candidate in the Department of Sociology, Uppsala University, Sweden. Her research interests centre on citizenship, disability, activism and digital media.

Jan Šiška is Associate Professor at the Faculty of Education, Charles University, and West Bohemia University, Pilsen, Czech Republic. His main research interests are disability policies, special and inclusive education, de-institutionalisation and community living.

Andreas Sturm is Junior Researcher at the International Research Unit in Disability Studies (iDiS), University of Cologne, Germany. His research focuses on biopolitics, the cultural and political sociologies of 'dis/ability', the disability rights movement and interest representation of persons with disabilities.

Jan Tøssebro is Professor of Social Work and Director of NTNU Social Research, Trondheim, Norway. His primary research interests are disability policy—notably de-institutionalisation—inclusive education, families with disabled children, standards of living and working life experience.

Bruno Trezzini is Group Leader in the Empowerment, Participation and Social Integration Unit, Swiss Paraplegic Research, Nottwil, Switzerland. His research interests include work and employment across the life course of persons with disabilities, vocational rehabilitation of persons with spinal cord injury, welfare regimes and social insurance reforms, and disability studies.

Lisa Waddington is Professor at the Faculty of Law, Maastricht University, the Netherlands. She holds the European Disability Forum Chair in European Disability Law. Her principal areas of research are European and comparative disability law, the UN Convention on the Rights of Persons with Disabilities, and European and comparative equality law in general.

Anne Waldschmidt is Professor of Sociology and Politics of Rehabilitation, Disability Studies, and Director of the International Research Unit in Disability

Studies (iDiS) at the University of Cologne, Germany. Her research focuses on the cultural and political sociologies of 'dis/ability', body sociology, contemporary disability history, the political participation of persons with disabilities and transnational disability policies.

Preface

This book is the result of the collective effort of a team of European researchers working together within a project co-funded by the European Union's Seventh Framework Programme for research, technological development and demonstration (FP7). The full title of the project is 'Making persons with disabilities full citizens – New knowledge for an inclusive and sustainable European social model (DISCIT)' (grant agreement number 320079). Jerome Bickenbach, Bruno Trezzini and Victoria Schuller gratefully acknowledge additional financial support from the Swiss National Science Foundation (grant agreement no. 150229). The project was coordinated by Bjørn Hvinden, Bettina Uhrig and Rune Halvorsen of the Norwegian Social Research (NOVA), an institution at Oslo and Akershus University College of Applied Sciences.

We would like to thank the contributors to this book for their enthusiasm in writing their chapters. During our work with the book, we have benefited from encouragement and support from a number of people. In particular we would like to mention Carlotta Besozzi, Peter Blanck, Mary Ann Kenny, Monica Menapace, Jan Monsbakken, Catherine Naughton, Inmaculada Placencia Porrero, Robert Salais, Marta Szebehely and Jenny Williams. In preparing this book we have benefited enormously from the participation of the European Disability Forum and the Mental Disability Rights Initiative, Serbia as consortium members in the project. The European and national stakeholder committees in the DISCIT project have provided invaluable support and advice in all stages of the preparation of this book. We would also like to extend our thanks to all interviewees who have shared their views and experiences with the researchers in Czech Republic, Germany, Ireland, Italy, Norway, Serbia, Sweden, Switzerland and UK.

Rune Halvorsen, Bjørn Hvinden, Jerome Bickenbach,
Delia Ferri and Ana Marta Guillén Rodriguez
Oslo/ Lausanne/ Dublin/ Oviedo, March, 2017

1 Introduction

Is public policy in Europe promoting the Active Citizenship of persons with disabilities?

Bjørn Hvinden, Rune Halvorsen, Jerome Bickenbach, Delia Ferri and Ana Marta Guillén

In this book we ask whether European and national polices are enhancing the Active Citizenship of persons with disabilities. More specifically, we investigate whether such policies include explicit goals, appropriate means and coordinated efforts. To the extent that the answer is no, we consider what kinds of changes are called for in the design and implementation of these policies. The investigation builds on the collective efforts of researchers from nine European countries within the context of the project 'DISCIT—Making persons with disabilities full citizens'. This project received funding from 2013 to 2016 from the European Union's Seventh Framework Programme for research, technological development and demonstration under grant agreement no. 320079.

This chapter introduces the major issues discussed in the book and presents the key perspectives, concepts and methods adopted to produce new and relevant knowledge about these issues. At the centre of our research is the concept of Active Citizenship. As a backdrop for the empirical analyses that make up most of the chapters of the book, the second part of this chapter will outline some factors and mechanisms that may explain why actual developments towards accomplishing Active Citizenship for persons with disabilities are likely to be uneven and variable.

What do we mean by Active Citizenship?

While existing scholarship provides a number of conceptualisations of social citizenship in broad terms, precise concepts of Active Citizenship are rare. To the extent that we find such conceptualisations, they tend to focus on one particular and rather narrow aspect, for instance linked to the 'active social policy' discourse, privatisation of social risk protection, encouragement of charitable work, political activism and 'citizen education' to promote socially responsible political participation (see Johansson & Hvinden, 2007; Halvorsen & Hvinden, 2013 for overviews).

By contrast, the research behind this book has adopted a multi-dimensional concept of Active Citizenship. So far, scholars have seldom discussed the Active

Citizenship of persons with disabilities and if they have, they usually only mention it in passing (e.g. Barnes & Mercer, 2003: 20–2; Priestley, 2003: 116–142; Dwyer, 2004: 116–117; Annetts et al., 2009: 12, 20–28; Roulstone & Prideaux, 2012: 34–35). This book presents the first extensive, systematic, theoretically informed and empirically based comparative analysis of the scope and prospects for the Active Citizenship of women and men with disabilities in Europe.

Our conceptualisation of 'Active Citizenship' focuses on three forms or dimensions of Active Citizenship (while acknowledging that there may also be others):

- A first dimension is whether public policy (largely) through redistributive measures enables citizens to maintain a sense of security by making effective use of the social rights meant to protect them against major risks and contingencies.
- A second dimension is whether public policy by a mix of redistributive and regulatory measures allows citizens to be capable of exercising autonomy, defining their needs, making their own choices and pursuing the kind of life they have reasons to value.
- A third dimension is whether public policy creates the conditions for citizens' participation in deliberation and decision-making, related to the services or other provisions to which they are entitled and may claim, or to the direction of public policy more broadly.

While seeing these three dimensions as analytically distinct, we expect them to be overlapping in practice, that is, in the lives and practices of people. Moreover, we assume that the three dimensions may be interacting and mutually supporting each other. For instance, we find it improbable that citizens would be able to enjoy real possibilities for exercising independence and influence on matters of importance for their lives unless they can make use of social rights to a predictable and adequate income and have access to necessary and high-quality services. For the same reasons, the understanding of Active Citizenship presented here is very close to the meaning of 'full and effective participation in society on an equal basis with others' of the UN Convention on the Rights of Persons with Disabilities (UN CRPD 2006, Preamble, item e; cf. Art. 1 & 3).

Obviously, the design of public policy may be oriented towards securing or improving the situation of persons with disabilities along one or more of these dimensions *without* framing policies in terms of promoting 'Active Citizenship'. Yet, the common element of all three dimensions is whether public policy embodies an aim of enhancing citizens' sense of their own agency, their ability to act, participate in and be in charge of their own lives (Lister, 2003: 39). A basic issue is therefore to what extent public policy of relevance for the lives of persons with disabilities succeeds in creating and sustaining the necessary conditions for such active agency and if it does not, what are the considerations, mechanisms or factors that lie behind this absence.

Hence, in this book, our interest centres on whether public policy has an explicitly stated goal to promote the agency of persons with disabilities, as well as on the extent to which the design and implementation of public policy de facto enables persons with disabilities to exercise agency along the three dimensions of Active Citizenship. The chapters of this book review relevant policy at European and national levels and seek to clarify whether persons with disabilities in nine European countries actually are in a position to exercise Active Citizenship. The book also examines the role of public policy in shaping the conditions in which persons with disabilities can become active citizens, and discusses potential improvements of this role. The nine countries involved are the Czech Republic, Germany, Ireland, Italy, Norway, Serbia, Sweden, Switzerland and the United Kingdom.

To provide the necessary information to answer the key research questions, the researchers in DISCIT have:

- Reviewed and summarised the main aspects of relevant European and national policies and the situation of persons with disabilities, based on existing research, available statistics and official publications.
- Carried out coordinated life-course interviews with equal numbers of women and men with four types of disabilities and belonging to three different birth cohorts in nine countries.
- Undertaken a coordinated series of expert interviews in the same countries and at EU-level.

While national teams of researchers have had the main responsibilities for different arenas and specific aspects of Active Citizenship, the researchers have in many cases worked together on the analyses and the writing of chapters for this and the accompanying volume. An overall model of the conditions for social change towards Active Citizenship for persons with disabilities has informed the more detailed analyses presented in the two volumes (see Figure 1.1).

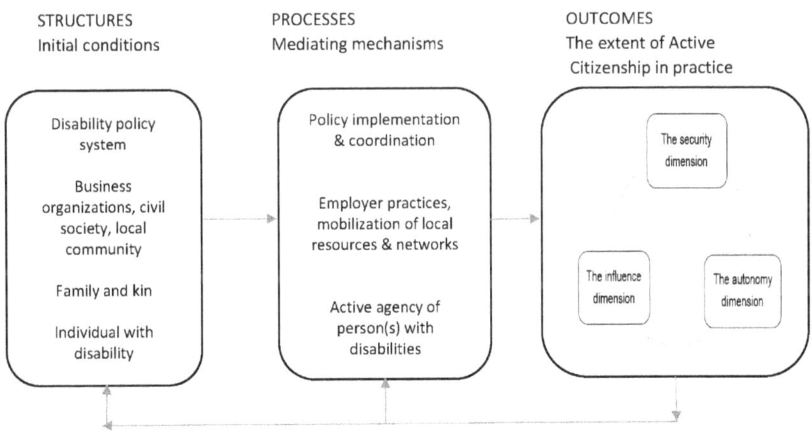

Figure 1.1 The DISCIT model for change towards Active Citizenship for persons with disabilities.

What role does public policy play in promoting Active Citizenship?

Evidently, many and diverse aspects of supranational and national policy may affect the actual possibilities open to persons with disabilities to exercise Active Citizenship, but only as an *unintended effect*. Therefore, in the rest of this chapter we will limit the discussion to whether public policy *explicitly and clearly* aims to promote such Active Citizenship (or at least a sense of and capability for active agency), and if it does, whether it improves disabled people's scope for exercising Active Citizenship in practice.

The empirical chapters of this book (and the accompanying volume) analyse in detail the existing policies and achievements towards the realisation of Active Citizenship in the nine DISCIT countries. Not surprisingly, these policies and achievements have been uneven and variable across the nine countries. In this introductory chapter we concentrate on some aspects of supranational policy.

First, the United Nations has played an important role in codifying legal and other requirements for enabling persons with disabilities to exercise active agency and also Active Citizenship. In December 1993, the United Nations General Assembly adopted *The Standard Rules on the Equalization of Opportunities for Persons with Disabilities* (UN Standard Rules, 1993). Even if these rules were not a legally binding instrument, they represented a strong commitment by national governments to take action to attain equalization of opportunities for persons with disabilities. However, the international community made a great step forward with the 2006 adoption of the UN Convention on the Rights of Persons with Disabilities (UN CRDP, 2006). We have already referred to the great emphasis the UN CRPD gives to the notion of full and effective participation on an equal basis with others. The EU is a party to the Convention and it has as such taken on the responsibility to support and monitor its implementation in member states (see European Commission, 2014).

Second, at EU level, Article 26 of the 2000 Charter of Fundamental Rights of the European Union (European Union Charter, 2012) comes very close to committing the EU to a general goal of Active Citizenship for persons with disabilities:

> The Union recognises and respects the right of persons with disabilities to benefit from measures designed to ensure their independence, social and occupational integration and participation in the life of the community.
>
> (European Union Charter, 2012: 400)

More specifically, Article 21 of the Charter prohibits discrimination based on disability. According to the Treaty on the Functioning of the EU (European Union, 2012), the Union shall combat discrimination based on disability when defining and implementing its policies and activities (Article 10). Moreover, it has the power to adopt legislation to address such discrimination (Article 19).

The European Disability Strategy 2010–2020 (European Commission, 2010b) covers a number of aspects of and instruments for accomplishing the dimensions of Active Citizenship, although to an uneven extent. On the one hand, substantial parts of the Strategy confirm the EU's commitment to enhancing disabled people's full and effective *participation* on an equal basis with others (European Commission, 2010b: 1, 3–4, 5–6, 11). More briefly, it mentions *disabled people's organisations and involvement in these* (10), *empowering* people with disabilities a couple of times (4, 11), *independence*, including economic independence (3, 7), and *choice* (4, 7). On the other hand, the strategy does not make explicit references to disabled people's *political participation* or to clear and enforceable *rights to social benefits or services*, although it stresses the adequacy of social protection to protect against economic hardship and disabled people's need to be able to benefit from social protection (European Commission, 2010b: 4). The Strategy's uneven coverage of the areas of the UN Convention (and the dimensions of Active Citizenship) reflects the fact that many areas of the Convention fall within the competence of the member states.

To what extent is it fair to say that a systematic consideration of disabled people's Active Citizenship is incorporated in the more general and ambitious Europe 2020 strategy for smart, sustainable and inclusive growth? This question is difficult to answer in a definitive way.

On the one hand, we find two references to the situation of persons with disabilities in the Commission Communication that initiated the Europe 2020 strategy in 2010 and then under the flagship initiative: *European Platform against Poverty* (European Commission, 2010: 19). According to the European Disability Strategy, the Commission intends to 'tackle the situation of people with disabilities through the Europe 2020 strategy, its flagship initiatives and the relaunch of the single market' (European Commission, 2010b: 4). The Strategy even asserts that 'full economic and social participation of people with disabilities is essential if the EU's Europe 2020 strategy is to succeed in creating smart, sustainable and inclusive growth' (European Commission, 2010b: 4) and promises 'to make full use of Europe 2020 and its instruments' (11).

On the other hand, one may ask whether the EU has been able to follow up on this assertion, and if so, to what effect. For instance, in November 2015, a draft report from the Commission noted that the gap between the activity rates of persons with and without disabilities had not diminished (European Commission, 2015: 12). Similarly, the gap between the proportion of people with and without disabilities who were at risk of poverty was also unchanged (European Commission, 2015: 29). At the same time, the report pointed to a number of initiatives in some member states that seem to offer persons with disabilities better possibilities for independent living. However, it also referred to the fact that some member states had reduced the compensation level ('generosity') of disability-related benefits in order to enhance incentives to work. Evidently, the overall implications of these examples for the actual scope available to disabled people to exercise Active Citizenship in contemporary Europe are mixed and ambiguous.

The mixed picture we get from the above-mentioned examples and similar statistical indicators emphasise that we in European countries are likely to find varying and contradictory developments and uneven achievements regarding the Active Citizenship of persons with disabilities. The final part of this chapter will therefore present some possible explanations for such variation and unevenness.

What factors can prevent, undermine or erode the political pursuit of Active Citizenship for persons with disabilities?

We find it fruitful to distinguish between three levels of factors or mechanisms that can prevent, undermine or erode consistent efforts to create the necessary conditions for enabling persons with disabilities to exercise Active Citizenship (see Table 1.1)

- Meta- or pre-political factors
- Factors related to institutional or policy design
- Factors related to the implementation or enforcement of relevant policy

Meta- or pre-political factors

The most fundamental set of factors are the processes that may prevent or allow the situation, needs and demands of people with disabilities more broadly, and issues of Active Citizenship more specifically, from entering the political agenda. Two rather different strands of theorisation inspire our thinking about such processes.

First, feminist and social philosopher Nancy Fraser has developed a normative theory of social justice where she initially contrasted the socio-economic redistribution of resources and the socio-cultural recognition of status as two complementary and mutually supporting ways of promoting social justice. Based on dialogue with a great number of scholars who engaged with and criticised her theory, she saw the need for adding a third process, political representation, that she now sees as equally important as redistribution and recognition. She refers here to 'political' in a specific and constitutive sense of the mechanisms and decision-rules that structure public processes of contestation and determine whose claims for redistribution and recognition will be discussed and decided upon (Fraser, 2013: 195). In other words, she focuses on the factors that include some people's claims as well as the factors that exclude other claims from consideration and adjudication. Moreover, she distinguishes between two levels of misrepresentation. The most obvious and well known, 'ordinary-political misrepresentation', is when a particular decision-rule means that some people find it difficult to participate fully (or elect representatives for taking part) in political decision-making. The other level of misrepresentation, which she calls 'misframing', is when the boundary-setting aspect of the political process means that some people are excluded completely from participation or consideration in decision-making forums (Fraser, 2013: 196–197).

Second, the political scientists Anne Schneider and Helen Ingram (1993, 2005; see also Schneider & Sidney, 2009) have formulated a general framework for understanding how various categories of citizens and potential target groups of public policy are perceived or 'constructed' differently by policymakers. For instance, one dimension is whether political elites regard a certain category of citizens as 'strong' or 'weak' in terms of power and access to political resources, while another dimension is whether political elites tend to regard a category of citizens

Table 1.1 Factors and mechanisms potentially preventing, undermining or eroding effective public policy to enhance the Active Citizenship of persons with disabilities

Analytic level–how basic barriers are	*Possible factors and mechanisms*
Meta- or pre-political factors	Issues related to the situation of persons with disabilities in general and, more specifically, to the Active Citizenship (or more generally, the agency) of people with disabilities, are absent from the political agenda, for instance because: • Established ways of defining what are 'political issues', combined with the power struggle, competition and settlement between dominant actors, mean that consideration for the needs and demands of people with disabilities never enters their agenda (see Fraser, 2008: 18–20 & 2013: 195–296 on the boundary-setting aspect of the political and 'misframing') • Cultural representations, prejudices and stereotypes of persons with disabilities define them as less able to exercise agency, autonomy or Active Citizenship (see Schneider & Ingram, 1993, 2005; Schneider & Sidney, 2009 on policymakers' 'social construction' of target groups).
Factors related to institutional or policy design	Even if consideration for the needs and demands of people with disabilities does enter the agenda and goals of policymaking bodies, they may not receive sufficient attention or priority when decision-makers decide on general goals as well as on the operational aims and instruments to reach them, including budget allocations. Goals related to promoting the active agency or even Active Citizenship of persons with disabilities may remain marginal and insufficiently integrated with other goals. Alternatively, such goals may become invisible because of policy integration ('mainstreaming'): • In practice, there may be gaps between the stated emphases of sector-responsibility and inter-sector coordination on the one hand and, on the other, the organisational design of the apparatus for implementation and the specific tasks and mandates of the different parts of this apparatus (see Hvinden, 1994; Goodin et al., 1999; & Halvorsen & Hvinden, 2016 on institutional and policy design) • Insufficient representation of persons with disabilities in policymaking bodies may make it difficult to ensure the prioritisation of the goal of enhancing the Active Citizenship of persons with disabilities or the development of appropriate instruments to make this a reality (see Phillips, 1995 on the politics of presence and Fraser, 2008:18–20 & 2013: 197 on (concrete) forms of misrepresentation).
Factors related to the implementation or enforcement of relevant policy	Deficient practical coordination by actors involved in the implementation of disability-relevant policy, for instance: • Actors at subordinate levels of governance resist or evade the requirements of superordinate levels to collaborate and coordinate their efforts in order to protect their own operational autonomy (Hvinden, 1994; Halvorsen & Hvinden, 2016)

in positive or negative terms. The authors argue that the various combinations of such constructions or attributions are important for what political elites will expect of members of a category in terms of capacity, participation and contribution to society, or conversely, in terms of demands, lack of participation and burden on society. To the extent that political elites build on such constructions in the direction of policy and allocation of resources vis-à-vis categories of citizens, the constructions are evidently to some extent self-confirming, reinforcing the relative and differentiated positions of persons belonging to these categories. Based on this conceptual framework, Schneider and Ingram suggest how one can imagine that some groups within the population of persons with disabilities risk being seen as less able to exercise active agency and, consequently, that political elites will be less concerned to create conditions for members of these groups to exercise Active Citizenship.

One can object to the Fraser and Schneider-Ingram frameworks on the grounds that they both tend to be somewhat static and do not take into account the possibility of transformational social change. For instance, even members of marginalised and apparently politically weak groups may turn out to be able to exercise active agency, both on individual and collective levels. Through social mobilisation and organising in social movements, people with disabilities have been able to make a considerable political impact, on a national as well as a supranational level. The strong international mobilisation among people with disabilities and their organisations in the process leading up to the UN Convention on the Rights of Persons with Disabilities is one important example of such active participation and its potential.

More generally, one may argue that the representatives of disabled people's organisations control resources or events that are of interest or value for politicians and government officials, that is, resources and events that they cannot access in other ways than through the involvement of civil society representatives. Obviously, politicians and officials are in control of resources and events of value for the organisations and their members or constituencies (e.g. change of access to financial resources, services and housing or rules and regulations.). Yet, there are reasons to assume that disabled people's organisations and their leaders may control three types of resources and events of considerable interest to politicians and officials:

a Detailed and first-hand knowledge of the situation, needs and world-view of the citizens they speak on behalf of,
b Ideas and proposals for more relevant and appropriate policies and instruments to reach them, given (a), and
c Possibilities to question or even undermine the legitimacy of politicians and officials, and potentially threaten or undermine their ability to uphold current positions.

Obviously all three types of resources depend on the existence of a fairly well-functioning mass democracy, including the freedom of expression and critical media as well as a political culture where politicians need to demonstrate commitment and the ability to improve the situation of the least well-off in society. Given that these conditions exist, they may lead to a greater dispersion of power than a simple understanding of power as residing at the top of political hierarchies would suggest.

Factors related to institutional and policy design

Even if consideration for the needs and demands of people with disabilities does enter the agenda and goals of policymaking bodies, they may not receive sufficient attention or priority when decision-makers decide on general goals as well as on the operational aims and instruments to reach them, including budget allocations. Goals related to promoting the active agency or Active Citizenship of persons with disabilities may remain marginal and insufficiently integrated with other goals. Alternatively, such goals may risk becoming invisible because of policy integration ('mainstreaming'). The literature on policy design suggests that in practice there may be a mismatch between the official emphasis on sector-responsibility and inter-sector coordination on the one hand and, on the other hand, the organisational design of the apparatus for implementation and the mandates of the different parts of this apparatus (Hvinden, 1994; Goodin et al., 1999; Halvorsen & Hvinden, 2016).

The risk of such a mismatch is probably greater because people with disabilities have weak or no representation in the significant policymaking bodies (government cabinets, parliaments and key committees within these). The absence or insufficient representation or lack of voice of persons with disabilities in policymaking bodies may make it difficult to ensure the prioritisation of the goal of enhancing the Active Citizenship of persons with disabilities or provision of appropriate instruments to make this a reality. Especially, feminist scholars have emphasised the significance of having representatives or being present when the details of policies and instruments are decided. For instance, Anne Phillips (1995) in her work on the politics of presence has pointed to the importance of being present and participating in the right arenas or in the relevant bodies at the right time, to prevent your cause or interest being excluded from the premises underlying political decisions. In the vocabulary of Fraser, there may be political obstacles to participatory parity, denying people with disabilities 'equal voice in public deliberations and fair representation in public decision-making' (Fraser, 2013: 195–196). According to Fraser,

> misrepresentation occurs when political boundaries and/or the decision rules function to wrongly deny some people the possibility of participating on a par with others in social interaction — including, but not only, in political arenas.
> (Fraser, 2013: 196)

The result of not being present and participating in decision-making bodies may be 'political invisibility'. Your cause is left out, forgotten or implicitly defined as less relevant or important.

Factors related to the implementation or enforcement of relevant policy

Finally, a large body of research on policy implementation has demonstrated gaps between the general aims and procedures decided by policymakers on the one hand, and, on the other, the practices and results as we find them at local level or in the direct interaction with members of the target groups of public policy. Hence, there are reasons to expect deficient or insufficient practical coordination by actors involved in the implementation of disability-relevant policy. For instance, actual coordination may be limited because actors at subordinate levels of governance resist or evade the requirements of superordinate levels to collaborate and coordinate their efforts in order to protect their own operational autonomy (Hvinden, 1994; Halvorsen & Hvinden, 2016)

The empirical chapters in this and the accompanying volume will discuss to what extent there are indications of progress towards the practical achievement of Active Citizenship for persons with disabilities in Europe. If we find only mixed or limited evidence of such progress, this will lead us to examine possible implementation deficits in disability policy in general and, more specifically, in policy that promises to enhance the active agency and Active Citizenship of persons with disabilities.

References

Annetts, J., Law, A., McNeish, W. & Mooney, G. (2009). *Understanding Social Welfare Movements*. Bristol: The Policy Press.

Barnes, C. & Mercer, G. (2003). *Disability*. Cambridge: Polity.

Dwyer, P. (2004). *Understanding Social Citizenship*. Bristol: The Policy Press.

European Commission (2010). *European Platform against Poverty*.

European Commission (2010b). Communication from the Commission to the European Parliament, the Council, the European Economic and Social Committee and the Committee of the Regions: *European Disability Strategy 2010–2020: A Renewed Commitment to a Barrier-Free Europe. European Commission*, 15.11.2010 COM(2010) 636 Final.

European Commission (2014). Commission Staff Working Document: *Report on the implementation of the UN Convention on the Rights of Persons with Disabilities (CRPD) by the European Union*. 5.6.2014. SWD (2014) 182 final.

European Commission (2015). Draft Joint Employment Report from the Commission and the Council accompanying the Communication from the Commission on the Annual Growth Survey 2016, European Commission, 26.11.2015, COM (2015) 700 Final.

European Union (2012). Consolidated version of the Treaty of the Functioning of the European Union, *Official Journal of the European Union*, 26.10.2012, C 326 / 47.

European Union Charter (2012). Charter of Fundamental Rights of the European Union (2012/C 325/02), *Official Journal of the European Union*. 26.10.2012 C 326. 391–407.

Fraser, N. (2008). *Scales of Justice: Reimagining Political Space in a Globalising World*. Cambridge: Polity.

Fraser, N. (2013). *Fortunes of Feminism: From State-Managed Capitalism to Neoliberal Crisis*. London: Verso.

Goodin, R. E., Headey, B., Muffels, B. & Dirven, H.-J. (1999). *The Real Worlds of Welfare Capitalism*. Cambridge: Cambridge University Press.

Halvorsen, R. & Hvinden, B. (Eds.). (2013) *Active Citizenship for Persons with Disabilities — Current Knowledge and Analytical Framework: A Working Paper.* DISCIT Deliverable 2.1., 31.08.2013. Retrieved 28 January 2015 from https://blogg.hioa.no/discit/publications

Halvorsen, R. & Hvinden, B. (2016). How to achieve Active Inclusion in a multi-layered context. In R. Halvorsen & B. Hvinden (Eds.). *Combating Poverty in Europe: Active Inclusion in a Multi-Level and Multi-Actor Context* (3–24). Cheltenham, UK: Edward Elgar.

Hvinden, B. (1994). *Divided Against itself: Integration in Welfare Bureaucracy.* Oslo: Scandinavian University Press.

Johansson, H. & Hvinden, B. (2007). What do we mean by active citizenship? In B. Hvinden & H. Johansson (Eds.), *Citizenship in Nordic Welfare States: Dynamics of Choice, Duties and Participation in a Changing Europe* (33–49). London: Routledge.

Lister, R. (2003). *Citizenship: Feminist Perspectives.* Basingstoke: Palgrave Macmillan.

Phillips, A. (1995). *The Politics of Presence.* Oxford: Oxford University Press.

Priestley, M. (2003). *Disability: A Life Course Approach.* Cambridge: Polity.

Roulstone, A. & Prideaux, S. (2012). *Understanding Disability Policy.* Bristol: The Policy Press.

Schneider, A. & Ingram, H. (1993). Social construction of target populations: Implications for politics and policy. *American Political Science Review*, 87, 334–347.

Schneider, A. & Ingram, H. (2005). *Deserving and Entitled: Social Construction and Public Policy.* Albany, NY: SUNY Press.

Schneider, A. & Sidney, M. (2009). What is next for policy design and social construction theory? *The Policy Studies Journal*, 37, 103–119.

United Nations Convention on the Rights of Persons with Disabilities (UN CRDP) (2006). *United Nations Convention on the Rights of Persons with Disabilities.* Retrieved 15 December 2015, from: http://www.un.org/disabilities/documents/convention/convopt-prot-e.pdf

United Nations Standard Rules (1993). *The Standard Rules on the Equalization of Opportunities for Persons with Disabilities.* Adopted by the United Nations General Assembly, forty-eighth session, resolution 48/96, annex, of 20 December 1993. Retrieved 2 May 2016, from: http://www.un.org/esa/socdev/enable/dissre00.htm

2 Diversity and dynamics of disability policy in Europe

An analytical framework

Rune Halvorsen, Anne Waldschmidt, Bjørn Hvinden and Kjetil Klette Bøhler

In this chapter, we set ourselves two tasks. First, we ask what perspectives, concepts and models can help us to capture the complexity and the development of public policy and legislation of significance for exercising Active Citizenship by persons with disabilities. We discuss how such policy and legislation build upon, as well as structure, the roles of the market, families and the voluntary sector in relation to providing the conditions, opportunities and resources for persons with disabilities to exercise Active Citizenship. Second, we ask what overall picture of this complexity and development we obtain if we use the available comparative statistics of the working of disability policy in Europe. We will use two currently dominating discourses on social policy, on austerity and social investment, to discuss the emerging patterns of similarities and differences between the nine countries covered in the research project DISCIT - Making persons with disabilities full citizens (Czech Republic, Germany, Ireland, Italy, Norway, Serbia, Sweden, Switzerland and United Kingdom). Finally, we will outline a possible typology of the redistributive disability policy systems we find in European countries.

How to capture the diversity of relevant public policy?

In comparative welfare research in general we find well-established typologies of different welfare 'models' or 'regimes' (e.g. Esping-Andersen, 1990, 1999; Leibfried, 1993; Ferrera, 1998; Hall & Soskice, 2001; Goodin et al., 1999; Korpi & Palme, 1998). These typologies provide macro-level and simplified images of the similarities and differences in the overall arrangements of welfare provision and the relationships between various providers of well-being and protection against adversity. While the state dominates as such a provider in some countries, in other countries the family, civil society (the voluntary sector) or the market have substantial and important provider roles. An overarching issue is, therefore, how the scope of public versus market-, family-based or civil-society risk protection varies between countries. To the extent that one focuses on the role of public authorities, key issues are to what extent they protect citizens against loss of market income (or bereavement of the family provider) and give them access to basic services for health, care and education. As providers of social security, through cash transfers or services provision, public authorities may target specific groups or aim to cover the needs of the whole population, be more (or less) generous, and offer provision that is more (or less) rights-based. Yet, there are reasons to assume that individual countries not only differ in their approaches to these aspects but also in how they go about ensuring citizens' opportunities for participation and Active Citizenship in society.

There are different opinions on how helpful established general welfare typologies are for understanding the specific similarities and differences in countries' disability policies, including the forces and factors lying behind these similarities and differences (e.g. Hvinden, 2003; 2004). Yet, general as well as specific strands of social theory (e.g. varieties of institutional theory) lead us to expect that national policy legacies, the overall affluence or scarcity of resources in a country, and the relative power and participation of different societal actors, including organisations of and for persons with disabilities, have shaped nation states' disability policies. More specifically, during recent decades, legal and political developments at the supranational level have given important impulses for changes in this policy field domestically. Consequently, our analysis will stress that disability policy develops in a multi-layered context and faces the general challenges of multi-level governance (e.g. Halvorsen & Hvinden, 2016). Later chapters in this volume will show how the United Nations (e.g. through the UN Standard Rules, 1993, and more recently the UN Convention on the Rights of Persons with Disabilities (CRPD), 2006) has had important implications for reforms in national disability policy. Similarly, the Council of Europe and the European Union (EU) have influenced national disability policy (Hvinden & Halvorsen, 2003; Whittle & Halvorsen, 2007; Waldschmidt, 2009; Hvinden, 2009; Halvorsen & Hvinden, 2009; Halvorsen, 2010; Hvinden, 2016; Waldschmidt, 2016).

Our analysis of the challenges faced by European countries and the European Union in promoting Active Citizenship for persons with disabilities builds on a theoretical understanding of disability as a social construction (e.g. Waldschmidt, 2005). As a starting point we adopt a rather broad and functional concept of 'disability policy'. We use this term to refer to the totality of policy measures, with intended or unintended consequences, for the welfare, living conditions, autonomy, participation and dignity of persons with disabilities (Halvorsen & Hvinden, 2009). We see disability policy as covering broad areas of policy and sectors of society that may or may not have 'disability' or similar terms in their names (Bickenbach & Cieza, 2011). For practical reasons, however, we have to restrict much of the review of existing data about relevant dimensions of public policy presented in this chapter to policies or provisions that explicitly refer to 'disability' or similar terms. In these cases, disability policy refers to a plurality of different measures or programmes in a country and/or cross-nationally or across political levels. Since there are reasons to expect that measures or programmes in practice will interact with each other or even depend on each other if they are to achieve their stated aims, we use the term 'disability policy system' to refer to this plurality.

The interactions between cash transfer, service delivery and social regulation

To start with, we see a country's disability policy system as consisting of three analytically different but in practice overlapping subsystems involving the following efforts (Figure. 2.1).

- *a cash transfer system*: to provide income security for persons out of paid work, to redistribute monetary resources, and to compensate for higher expenses due to special needs (e.g. diet, transportation, heating),
- *a service delivery system:* to enhance the capabilities of persons with disabilities to lead active lives and be part of the community, to enjoy independence and participate in the major arenas of society (e.g. through health and social services, rehabilitation, education and vocational training, assistive technology, personal assistance, and related provisions), and
- *a social regulation subsystem*: to influence the functioning of markets and the behaviour of non-governmental actors, with the goal of promoting welfare policy objectives or human rights.

Both the cash transfer and service delivery subsystems aim at *redistributing resources* among differing population groups and equalising their life chances. The funding may come from general taxes, mandatory or private social insurance or contributions from the protected persons and employers. By contrast, social regulation will in many instances aim at *remedying market failures*. Governments seek to influence the markets and their functioning as well as the behaviour of non-governmental actors, for example, by setting legal standards for health, security and labour protection or by stimulating the development of industry standards for the accessibility and usability of products and services (Majone, 1993; Ogus, 2000: 83; Jordana & Levi-Faur, 2004: 3).

As mentioned above and as Figure 2.1 suggests, we regard disability policy as a system in the sense that the three subsystems are interconnected and interdependent with the effect that changes in one part are likely to have consequences in the other two, whether by design (with intent) or default (without intent). From this first perspective, a key issue is whether governments have designed the three subsystems of public policy of relevance for promoting the Active Citizenship of persons with disabilities to mutually support each other, and if so, whether

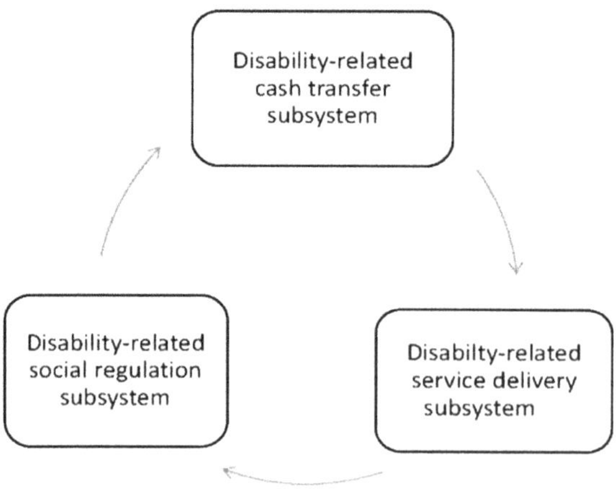

Figure 2.1 The disability policy system as consisting of three interdependent subsystems.

interdependence and mutual support are achieved in practice. Later chapters of this book will deal with the issue of whether the EU, its member states and other European countries have found the right balance between the different subsystems to effectively promote Active Citizenship and achieve an inclusive and sustainable European social model. While subsystem-specific analyses are numerous and offer important insights, the broader picture has often been missing. The amount of cross-national and comparative research on the interactions between the three disability subsystems and their impact is still limited (Halvorsen & Hvinden, 2009; Waldschmidt, 2007, 2009; Hvinden, 2009). This is unfortunate, since there are strong reasons to expect that redistributive and regulatory provisions to a certain extent can substitute for each other, for example, in the area of employment policy for disabled people (see Levi-Faur 2014: 606, and Chapter 5).

Concerning the two subsystems of cash transfer and service delivery, there are considerable differences in the levels of public spending in the nine DISCIT countries, and the relative spending on cash benefits versus services. Table 2.1 shows the empirical situation in the year 2013.

One often views the proportion of the Gross Domestic Product (GDP) spent on a particular area as a rough indicator of policy effort, that is, of how strongly the government of a country gives this area political priority. Interpreted in this way, Sweden and Norway seem to give relatively higher priority to redistributive disability provisions, while Ireland and Italy give relatively lower priority to such provision (see the middle column of Table 2.1). Sweden and Germany appear to have the strongest orientation towards service-provision, whereas Italy and Serbia have the weakest orientation towards the provision of services (right column in Table 2.1). Overall, these two sets of figures are among several indicators that the empirical diversity in European disability policy systems does not necessarily correspond very well to established welfare typologies.

Considering the social regulatory subsystem, policy measures take different forms. We can classify many of them as either legislative means, financial

Table 2.1 Levels of redistributive disability-related public spending and profiles of spending in the DISCIT countries for 2013

	Total spending on disability benefits as % of GDP (2013)	*Spending on disability-related services as % of total spending on disability benefits (2013)*
Czech Republic	1.3	10.3
Germany	2.2	34.9
Ireland	1.2	11.2
Italy	0.7	6.1
Norway	4.0	12.4
Serbia	1.8	9.4
Sweden	3.6	60.0
Switzerland	2.3	27.8
United Kingdom	1.7	28.1
(Average)	*(2.1)*	*(22.2)*

Source: Eurostat Database, Social protection expenditure by function (Retrieved 7 September 2016) (10 September 2016).

incentives or persuasion through information and appeals to actors' social conscience (Etzioni, 1961; Bemelmans-Videc et al., 1998). Each type of policy measure depends on different assumptions about how one may influence non-governmental actors. *Legislation* presumes that it is possible to force actors to behave in certain ways, or at least prevent them from behaving in unwanted ways, given the prospect of sanctions if they do not comply with the rules. *Financial incentives* presuppose that it is possible to encourage actors to act in certain ways, even if they do not have to, because the desired measures are cost-effective or profitable. *Persuasion through information and appeals* presupposes that one may motivate actors to behave in certain ways by convincing them of what is morally and normatively right to do. In other words, the assumption is that it would affect adversely their conscience, self-respect, or at least, reputation if they do not comply with the moral standards of society ('name and shame'); thus, there are supposed to be intrinsic benefits deriving from compliance.

Some forms of social regulatory policies have gained a particular significance in the European multi-level context:

- The Council Directive 2000/78/EC on equal treatment in employment and occupation ('Employment Equality Directive') has been implemented in all member states. The Court of Justice of the European Union has developed the interpretation of the directive through case law. Norway has introduced related shadow legislation and bodies for awareness-raising, monitoring, supervision, and enforcement. Serbia has yet to adopt similar disability employment legislation (UN, 2016). According to an assessment report on the implementation of the directive in 2014, a main challenge still is to raise public awareness of the protection provided and to ensure better practical application of the directive. The European Commission continues to monitor developments in member states and instigates infringement proceedings if necessary (European Commission, 2014; see also Quinn, 2005).
- The EU has signed and ratified the UN Convention on the Rights of Persons with Disabilities (United Nations, 2006) as a party to the Convention (European Union, 2009), as have all the DISCIT countries at the time of writing except for Ireland, which has only signed the CRPD (UN, 2015). The full implementation of the CRPD within the EU system is still on-going (see Chapter 11).
- In the autumn of 2015, the Commission proposed a directive on accessibility (European Commission, 2015). The EU has also sought to promote accessibility though legislation for the internal market (see Whittle & Halvorsen, 2007; Waddington, 2009; Halvorsen, 2010, and Chapter 8).

These are a few examples of the ways in which bodies at supranational level influence—to a growing extent—the disability policy system by creating, monitoring and enforcing duties for both public and non-public actors at national and subnational levels. They illustrate the significance of our first perspective on disability policy as a multi-layered system of social redistribution and regulation.

Currently, there is a lack of systematic and cross-national data about the working of social regulatory systems and their impact on the lives of persons with disabilities that could match the richness of such data for the working of redistributive systems and their impact. Yet, considerable progress has been made in establishing indicator sets on the operation of social regulatory systems in practice, for instance indicators related to different dimensions of accessibility for persons with different kinds of disabilities (e.g. Kubitschke et al., 2013; Dion et al., 2015).

Interrelated disability provisions at different levels of governance

Further, we regard the disability policy system as a multilayered system of governance, reaching from the global via the European, national and subnational levels, down to the local level interacting directly with individuals with disabilities and their families (Figure 2.2). From this perspective, the critical issue is whether entities, actors and efforts at different levels of governance operate together in a coordinated way to enhance the Active Citizenship of persons with disabilities in Europe.

In general, governance has a vertical as well as a horizontal dimension. Here we focus on the vertical dimension—the discussion and negotiation to achieve consensus as well as coordinated efforts, synergies or collaboration of actors (entities) across different territorial levels (Halvorsen & Hvinden, 2016). The concept of multi-level governance is quite recent and research based on it is still under rapid development. While the analysis of multi-level governance has been widening out to include issues of global policy coordination as well as intra-national policy integration and coherence, studies related to the evolving relationships between the supranational level—represented by the EU—and national and subnational levels have so far dominated the field (see Stephenson, 2013 for a review).

As indicated by Figure 2.2, the growing significance of the UN Convention on the Rights of Persons with Disabilities (UN CRPD, 2006) makes it essential to include the global level in our analytical framework. All the DISCIT countries are 'States Parties' to the CRPD; however, Ireland has only signed but not ratified the Convention (UN, 2015). The EU has signed and ratified the Convention as a 'regional integration organisation' (European Union, 2009). Since the EU is a party to the Convention, a successful implementation of the Convention is an important obligation for the supranational level as such and not only an issue for the governments of the member states that have ratified it. The full implementation of the CRPD within the EU system and beyond is still on-going (see Chapters 10 and 11).

Public disability provision interacting with the market, family and civil society

Finally, we regard the disability policy system as interacting with, seeking to influence and itself being dependent on processes taking place not only inside,

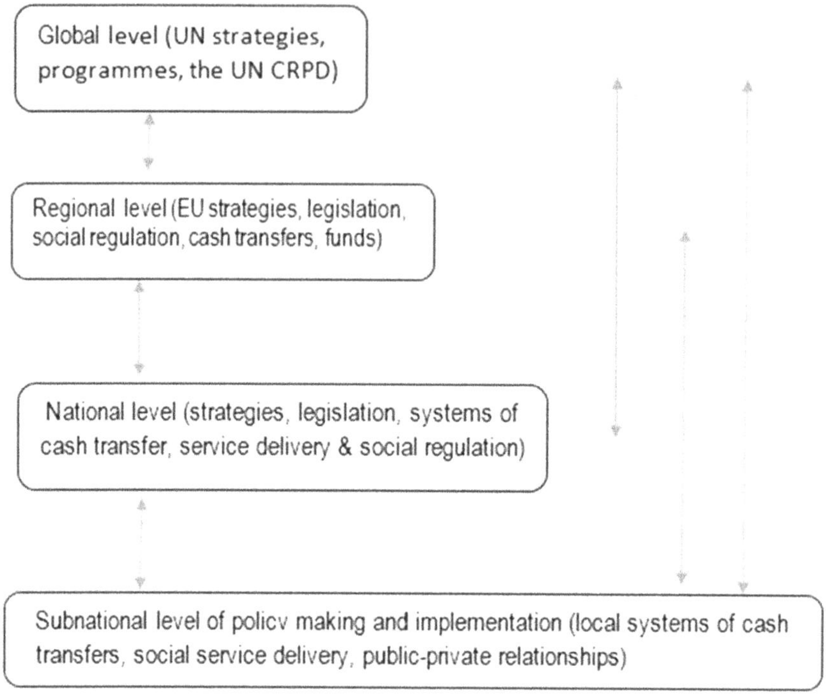

Figure 2.2 The disability policy system as multi-level system of governance.

but also outside the government. This chapter has already dealt with the role of public authorities as policy makers and service providers. Here, we are concerned in particular with processes within the market, in the family and in organised civil society (see Figure 2.3).

Employers as decision-makers in *the market* largely determine whether persons with disabilities will be able to find and retain paid jobs and whether workplaces are accessible and accommodated to a diverse workforce, including women and men, younger and older employees, with different ethnicities and, last but not least, different kinds of disabilities. As producers of goods and services, private business determines to a great extent whether principles of universal design, accessibility and usability for all are the basis for the development of new products (Chapter 8). In some countries one also finds market-based and commercial providers of services for persons with personal assistance needs.

However, the market is also an arena where non-governmental actors can act as complements to public providers, either building on a mandate from public authorities or on a voluntary basis. Examples are fringe benefits, services provided as part of an employment contract ('occupational welfare') or private insurance that people take out voluntarily to complement public provision. Estimates by the OECD (Adema et al., 2011) suggest that non-public forms of social protection make up different shares of the total social protection across countries. For instance, among

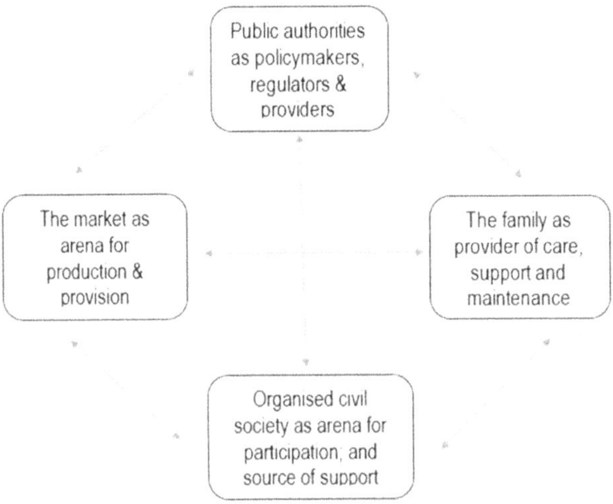

Figure 2.3 The disability policy system regarded as partly shaped by processes in an intersection of the market, the family and organised civil society, and partly itself shaping processes in the market, the family and organised civil society.

the six DISCIT countries covered by these estimates, spending on mandated private social protection ranged from 3 to 23 per cent of total social spending, while expenditure on voluntary private protection varied from 1 to 18 per cent of total social protection expenditure (not shown here). The variation for 'incapacity-related' (i.e., a category somewhat wider than disability-related) social spending was even greater. Here the mandated private social spending ranged from 1 per cent (Czech Republic) to 36 per cent of all spending (Germany), whereas expenditure on voluntary private protection ranged from 1 per cent (Switzerland) to 14 per cent of all incapacity-related social expenditure (United Kingdom). These data illustrate that we are likely to find different forms of 'welfare mix' (Ascoli & Ranci, 2002) in the disability policy systems of the DISCIT countries.

In the case of *the family*, parents (and their social background or status) influence to a substantial degree whether children born with or acquiring a disability in early life receive the care, training and stimulation they need to enable them to flourish as they grow up. Parents are in many cases a major source of care, support and maintenance over the first life phases of the disabled person. Yet, especially when appropriate public provision for children with disabilities is absent or weak, young persons may become excessively dependent on their parents and meet obstacles in the ordinary transition from childhood and youth to adulthood (Biggeri et al. forthcoming).

Last but not least, *organised civil society*—that is the whole range of voluntary associations of various kinds but in our context in particular self-governed organisations of and for persons with disabilities—is for many a source of (peer) support complementing public provision or family support. In countries where public authorities offer only limited or basic support, the role of organised self-help is likely to be more essential than in countries with more ample public provision, both in terms of economic resources and services. In addition, organised civil society offers an arena for social participation and voluntary engagement, while organisations representing persons with disabilities in particular enable participation and influence related to political issues (see Karačić et al., forthcoming).

In general, we expect a country's disability policy system to be shaped by processes in the market, the family and organised civil society, for instance as a result of active efforts by actors in these sectors to influence the direction, scope or generosity of public policy. Conversely, we also assume that expansion or contraction of public policy and provision for persons with disabilities contributes to shaping the extent to which—and the ways in which—actors in the three institutional systems deal with or respond to the situation and needs of persons with disabilities. In other words, we expect to see examples of interdependence and mutual influence between all four institutional systems illustrated in Figure 2.3. From this third perspective, a critical issue is whether the four institutional subsystems tend to operate based on narrow sectorial considerations or tend to work together to remove barriers to the Active Citizenship of person with disabilities.

A crosscutting criterion for assessing the achievements of the different aspects of disability policy systems we have reviewed here might be whether they enable persons with disabilities to make effectively use of access to resources into well-being, agency and control over their own lives, as proposed in the Capability Approach.

The disability system from the perspective of the Capability Approach

From a *Capability Approach* perspective, the key question is whether the disability policy system provides the conditions for transforming or 'converting" the resources into effective capacities that allow people to act freely, to participate in society and pursue the kind of life they have reasons to want (Sen, 2009; Nussbaum, 2000, 2011). In other words, this approach asks whether the disability policy system provides the facilitators that allow persons with disabilities to convert resources and commodities into those 'beings and doings' that individuals value (Robeyns, 2005). Combining ethics with economic principles, the Capability Approach has provided the raison d'être for including participation and empowerment as central features of human developmental processes (Deneulin & Shahani, 2009; Trani et al., 2011). In our context, a capability-oriented approach adds innovative value to disability policy research by asking about the effective abilities that someone has in order to participate in society.

Sen (1999) has pointed out that overcoming the passive receipt of social benefits and situations of social exclusion depends on the possibilities of converting resources like cash benefits into effective capabilities such as realising ordinary social roles and participating on an equal basis with others. Equal forms of economic, social, political and cultural participation cannot be achieved alone by providing more resources and better services, it is also necessary to take into account the specific circumstances of individuals with disabilities and their freedom of choice: 'Without the substantive freedom and capability to do something, a person cannot be responsible for doing it' (Sen, 1999: 88). Thus, transforming redistribution resources into Active Citizenship requires the active participation of disabled citizens in decisions concerning the benefits and services provided to them (Sen, 1993).

The criticism by a number of scholars and disability policy advocates of the function of income transfers in many disability policy systems echoes the Capability perspective (see Hvinden, 2009, for a review of the criticism). For instance, it has been argued that the main function of such transfers is to exclude persons with disabilities from participation in the mainstream labour market, and hence to contribute to their societal segregation (and social control). Quinn (2004: 8, 2005: 279) maintains that redistributive provisions entrap rather than liberate and that 'they purchase the absence of the other'. Kemp (2006, 2008) and the OECD (2010) argue that having to claim and receive benefits through redistributive arrangements implies categorization, passivity and dependence for citizens with disabilities.

In the last part of this chapter, we raise the following questions:

1 Have the financial crises starting in 2008 and the fiscal consolidation measures adopted in DISCIT countries involved a shift towards *austerity* in national disability policy systems, weakening their capacity to support persons with disabilities in exercising Active Citizenship?
2 Has disability policy in the DISCIT countries moved in the direction of the kind of *social investment* strategy promoted by the European Union? Have we seen a shift of emphasis from income protection and economic security for persons with disabilities towards service delivery, especially of services promoting their capacity and autonomy ('capability')?

Shifts towards austerity in disability policies in the DISCIT countries?

A prominent strand in current scholarship on the welfare state suggests that a combination of maturing welfare provision (pension systems based on social insurance models of the pay-as-you-go version), demographic changes and the transition to service-oriented provision (health and care services in particular) has caused unsustainable levels of public deficit in many European countries (Pierson, 2001; Schäfer & Streeck, 2013; Hvinden, 2016). A volatile international economy has resulted in lower tax revenues and a higher demand for income protection. These challenges are said to have forced governments to make substantial and lasting cuts in public spending to consolidate public finances, for instance by tightening eligibility rules, excluding some recipient groups and reducing the levels and duration of benefits in cash and kind. The result is claimed to be a situation of *austerity*, or, according to some analysts, a state of 'permanent austerity', and downward retrenchment. Some observers have argued that the impact of the austerity state is likely to be particularly severe for persons with disabilities in Europe (e.g. Hauben et al., 2012).

Available statistical evidence about trends in the spending on social benefits of relevance for persons with disabilities is limited and gives a mixed and somewhat ambiguous picture. For instance, according to the OECD, government consolidation measures have most frequently focused on 'working age transfers' for savings, including benefits for persons with disabilities, Yet, in the period 2007–2010, overall there has been a minor increase in the spending on disability pensions in OECD countries (OECD, 2014).

Whether one can find evidence of a trend towards permanent austerity depends on exactly what period and which countries one considers and what indicators one adopts. For instance, many analysts, statistical agencies and international organisations use the percentage of the gross domestic product (GDP) spent on social benefits as the sole indicator of public policy effort. As already mentioned, this indicator is presumed to tell how much of the hypothetically 'available resources' a government allocates for a particular purpose. However, we also need an indicator of what happens in 'real terms', that is, spending measured in purchase power standards per inhabitant (and, hence, in actual living standards and in the scope for exercising Active Citizenship or capability more generally).

Based on the most up-to-date statistics at the time of writing, in the period from 2004 to 2013, 14 of 30 European countries reduced their total spending on disability-related provisions (both cash transfers and services) in terms of per cent of GDP. However, the scale of reductions varied considerably. Two DISCIT countries, the United Kingdom and Switzerland were, together with Malta, among those with largest cuts in spending levels, measured in this way (Eurostat Database).

If we use the other indicator, we find that only five of the 30 countries reduced their spending in terms of purchase power standards per inhabitant. Sweden and the United Kingdom were among these five countries. However, while United Kingdom and Malta had major cuts (up to a quarter of the 2004 level), other countries (including Sweden) had smaller cuts around plus or minus five per cent of the 2004 level. Among the other DISCIT countries, especially Ireland and Germany had substantial growth in real terms spending.

As summarised in Table 2.2, the other five DISCIT countries where we have sufficiently long times series give a more mixed picture, but not one that suggests a strong and consistent shift towards austerity. Whether national levels of spending are sufficient and available provisions adequate in the DISCIT countries is a different issue that cannot be answered on the basis of these aggregated data. The thematic chapters below give some insights on this issue.

Another possible indicator of a turn towards austerity might be whether some European countries have adopted, to a greater extent than others, means-testing as a way to regulate and potentially limit access to disability benefits by deterring potential claimants (Table 2.3). However, in general we find that European

Table 2.2 A shift towards austerity in DISCIT countries? Changes in the levels of total spending on disability benefits between 2004 and 2013

		Change in total spending on disability benefits as share of GDP 2004–2013	
		Decrease	*Stability or increase*
Change in total spending on disability benefits in real terms (purchase power* parities per inhabitant)	Decrease	Sweden United Kingdom	
	Stability or increase	Czech Republic Germany Norway Switzerland	Ireland Italy

Source: Eurostat Database (2016).

*'The Purchase Power Standard (PPS) is an artificial reference currency unit that eliminates price level differences between countries. Thus, one PSS buys the same volume of goods and services in all countries. This unit allows meaningful comparisons of economic indicators across countries' (Eurostat, 2015: 6).

Table 2.3 A shift towards austerity in DISCIT countries? Changes in the share on total spending on disability benefits provided as means-tested benefits between 2004 and 2013

	2004	*2013*	*Difference*
Czech Republic	0	0	0
Germany	23.7	27.9	4.2
Ireland	45.3	55.5	10.2
Italy	24.3	22.3	–2.0
Norway	1.7	1.8	–0.1
Serbia	–	11	–
Sweden	0.1	0.3	0.2
Switzerland	6.9	11.4	4.5
United Kingdom	35.1	41.3	6.2

Source: Eurostat Database (2016).

countries that had a fairly high share of means-tested spending on disability benefits in 2013 tended also to have that in 2004, suggesting a fairly strong path dependency. Among the DISCIT countries, the share of means-tested disability benefits showed the clearest increase in Ireland, United Kingdom, Germany and Switzerland.

Overall, for the DISCIT countries, based on the macro indicators used here, we do not find evidence of a general shift toward an austerity state for persons with disabilities in Europe since the onset of the great recession in 2008. This indicates that austerity has played only a limited role in weakening social provision of relevance for the Active Citizenship of persons with disabilities. At the same time austerity is likely to have had negative effects on the security and autonomy of many persons with disabilities, probably most so in the United Kingdom (see Hauben et al., 2012; Room, 2015).

Shifts towards disability policy based on social investment?

When Esping-Andersen (1996), as one of the first, referred to social investment in a European context, it was in cautious and rather uncommitted language, arguing that

> Rather than draconian roll-backs, the idea is to redirect social policy from its current bias in favour of passive income maintenance towards active labour market programmes that 'put people back to work', help households harmonize work and family obligations and train the population in the kinds of skills that post-industrial society demands.
>
> (Esping-Andersen, 1996: 3)

As suggested by this statement, one core meaning of social investment is a shift towards active measures to improve people's skills or 'human capital', as opposed to a one-sided focus on providing income maintenance benefits ('passive benefits'). At the same time, Esping-Andersen expressed concern that this approach's longer-term viability was 'doubly uncertain' and in particular when 'very high unemployment rates seem to contradict the validity of an active "social investment"' approach (Esping-Andersen, 1996: 14–15).

Almost two decades later, a number of scholars have whole-heartedly embraced the social investment approach, albeit based on different understandings and emphases (e.g. Esping-Andersen, 2002; Hemerijck, 2013; Morel et al., 2012, Vandenbroucke et al., 2011). Others scholars have adopted a more critical stance to the approach and its practical uses (e.g. Jenson, 2009; Sipilä, 2012). One of the critics, Cantillon (2014: 307–309), uses the situation of persons with disabilities to argue that the social investment approach tends to have a narrow employment-promotion focus and lacks a consideration of how social spending can enhance people's independence and autonomy. Yet, in most of the existing literature on social investment we find a relative neglect or lack of explicit attention to the situation of persons with disabilities. There are good reasons to be concerned about this. One can doubt whether governments and policymakers will see persons with disabilities as citizens in whom it is worth investing. Still, the European Commission suggests that a social investment approach might offer a renewal of and boost for disability policy in Europe.

There is hardly any explicit use of the term 'social investment' in the available comparative welfare statistics of Eurostat or the OECD. Pragmatically we will therefore interpret a relative shift from 'pure' income protection for persons with disabilities to an emphasis on the provision of disability-related services as compatible with a turn towards 'social investment'. First, we consider whether the DISCIT countries have reduced their funding of disability-related cash benefits and increased their funding of disability-related services. We find that among the eight countries where time series data are available, Germany, Sweden and the United Kingdom had made this shift if we use 'share of GDP' as measure of spending levels (see Table 2.4). If we look at spending levels in real terms, only Sweden and the United Kingdom made this shift between 2004 and 2013 (see Table 2.4).

Second, we compare spending allocated to disability services as share of total spending on disability-related social provisions in 2004 and 2013 (Table 2.5). Sweden had the largest increase in the share of services-spending, and the United Kingdom with second largest increase. While Germany had a smaller increase in this share, the five other countries under consideration showed no substantial difference or even decrease in the share allocated to disability-services.

Overall, these findings indicate that the DISCIT countries only to a very limited extent had changed the profiles of their disability-related social spending in a way that is compatible with a de facto turn towards a social investment approach to

Table 2.4 A shift towards social investment in DISCIT countries?—Changes in spending on disability-related cash benefits and disability services respectively between 2004 and 2013

		Change in spending on disability cash transfers as share of GDP 2004–2013	
		Decrease	*Stability or increase*
Change in spending on disability services as share of GDP 2004–2013	Decrease	Norway Switzerland	Czech Republic
	Stability or increase	Germany Sweden United Kingdom	Ireland Italy
		Change in spending on disability cash transfers in real terms (purchase power parities per inhabitant) 2004–2013*	
		Decrease	*Stability or increase*
Change in spending on disability services in real terms (purchase power* parities per inhabitant) 2004–2013	Decrease		Norway
	Stability or increase	Sweden United Kingdom	Czech Republic Germany Ireland Italy Switzerland

Source: Eurostat Database (2016).

*See Table 2.2 for explanation.

Table 2.5 A shift towards social investment in DISCIT countries?—Changes in the share of total spending on disability benefits provided as services between 2004 and 2013

	2004	*2013*	*Difference*
Czech Republic	12.6	10.3	–2.3
Germany	31.3	34.9	3.6
Ireland	10.4	11.2	0.8
Italy	6.3	6.1	–0.2
Norway	17.8	12.4	–5.4
Serbia	–	9.4	–
Sweden	40.0	60.0	20.0
Switzerland	27.8	27.0	0
United Kingdom	17.4	28.1	10.7

Source: Eurostat Database (2016).

disability policy. At the same time there has been a remarkable diversity between these profiles and also in how this diversity developed over time. This is clearly an issue that calls for more research.

Do policy traditions matter? Towards a typology of disability policy systems

The data presented in this and subsequent chapters confirm that European countries do not only use different policy instruments, but their efforts to enhance the opportunities for exercising Active Citizenship for persons with disabilities also have distinct overall profiles. Earlier analyses of the diverse institutional contexts demonstrate how these distinct policy profiles have been influenced by different national policy traditions, public-private divisions of labour and roles of social partners and disabled people's organisations in the design and implementation of the policy (Halvorsen & Hvinden, 2009; Waldschmidt, 2009; Halvorsen, 2010; Halvorsen & Hvinden, 2011).

We have earlier in this chapter commented that the diversity we can observe in the profiles of countries' redistributive disability policy does not fit neatly with existing general typologies of welfare models or regimes. Therefore, we will conclude by outlining a new typology of the disability policy systems of 30 European countries, including eight of the DISCIT countries (Table 2.6). For practical reasons, we use only combinations of three variables related to redistributive provisions, each dichotomised in high and low values, to construct the typology.

By doing this, we end up with three main groups or clusters of redistributive disability policies, which we give the labels 'High Spenders', 'Mixed Spenders' and 'Low Spenders'. We dichotomize each group according to how strong a role means-testing plays, and achieve six groups.

To illustrate the potential value of a new typology of disability policies, Table 2.6 also includes unweighted means of the values that the countries in each

Table 2.6 Tentative typology of disability policy systems: European countries' disability policy systems in six groups according to the level and profile of disability-related social spending and three indicators of relevance for Active Citizenship of persons with disabilities. Unweighted means for each group. Per cent. 2012

High spenders		*Mixed spenders*		*Low spenders*	
(1) High: cash High: services Weak: means-testing	(2) High: cash High: services Strong: means-testing	(3) High: cash Low: services Strong: means-testing	(4) Low: cash High: services Strong or Weak: means-testing	(5) Low: cash Low: services Weak: means-testing	(6) Low: cash Low: services Strong: means-testing
Finland, Luxembourg, Netherlands, Norway, Sweden	Austria, Belgium, Denmark, France, Germany, Iceland, Spain, Switzerland	Croatia, Italy, Portugal	Slovakia, Slovenia, United Kingdom	Bulgaria, Cyprus, Czech Republic, Estonia, Hungary, Latvia, Lithuania, Poland, Romania	Greece, Ireland, Malta
Low work intensity *21.6* Material deprivation *5.7* Poverty risk *16.4*	Low work intensity *23.3* Material deprivation *8.8* Poverty risk *18.6*	Low work intensity *24.3* Material deprivation *19.0* Poverty risk *23.1*	Low work intensity *21.7* Material deprivation *15.4* Poverty risk *18.8*	Low work intensity *24.9* Material deprivation *30.6* Poverty risk *22.1*	Low work intensity *40.3* Material deprivation *23.2* Poverty risk *23.5*

Source: Eurostat Database (2016).

Explanations

The profiles are based on whether countries have rankings over (High) or under (Low) the median on spending on disability-related cash transfers, on disability-related services-provision and on the proportion of cash spending provided as means-tested benefits (Strong or Weak). The three indicators of relevance for Active Citizenship of persons with disabilities include the risk of poverty in (2012), the risk of material deprivation in (2012) and the employment rate in (2011) of persons with disabilities.

of the six groups have on three indicators of missing conditions for exercising Active Citizenship

- *People living in households with very low work intensity:* 'The indicator persons living in households with low work intensity is defined as the number of persons living in a household having a work intensity below a threshold set at 0.20. The work intensity of a household is the ratio of the total number of months that all working-age household members have worked during the income reference year and the total number of months the same household members theoretically could have worked in the same period,(Eurostat, 2016).
- *Material deprivation risk:* Percent of persons with disabilities aged 16 to 64 reporting to lack at least 3 of 9 items considered by most people to be desirable or even necessary to lead an adequate life (Eurostat Database, 2016).
- *Relative poverty risk:* Percent of people with disabilities aged 16 to 64 who had an (equivalised) disposable income (after social transfers) below 60 per cent of the national median equivalised disposable income after social transfers (Eurostat Database, 2016).

To summarize the emerging pattern, we see that the High Spenders tend to have lower mean values on these indicators than the Mixed and Low Spenders have, and the Mixed Spenders tend to have lower mean values than the Low Spenders. Evidently one needs to be careful not to interpret these findings as evidence of casual relationships. Chapter 4 will discuss in detail some of the reasons for being cautious with making such inferences, for instance the possible confounding effects of the strongly divergent shares of people saying they have a disability across Europe.

Yet, the patterns presented in Table 2.6 do suggest that it is meaningful to go forward with developing more comprehensive typologies of disability policy systems and do only partly reflect earlier welfare regime typologies. One task for future research is to develop a broader set of relevant indicators and longer and more consistent time series of the characteristics of the regulatory disability subsystems of the countries we compare. When such indicators are available, we will be able to improve the tentative typology presented here.

Concluding remarks

In this chapter, we first asked what perspectives, concepts and models can help us to capture the complexity and the development of public policy and legislation of significance for exercising Active Citizenship by persons with disabilities. We have discussed how such policy and legislation build upon, and structure, the roles of the market, families and the voluntary sector in relation to providing the conditions, opportunities and resources for persons with disabilities to exercise Active Citizenship.

Second, we asked what overall picture of this complexity and development we obtain if we use the available comparative statistics and indicators of the working of disability policy in Europe. We used two currently dominating discourses on social policy, austerity and social investment, to highlight emerging patterns of similarities and differences between the nine DISCIT countries.

We also discussed whether disability systems in the DISCIT countries have moved towards austerity, cuts and more meagre disability-related provision, and whether the same countries have introduced reforms that bring them closer to a social investment rationale for disability policy. Based on the limited comparative European data that exists for the last decade or so, there seems not to be clear evidence for a general change either way. However, we can observe some striking changes in some countries, for instance in Germany, Ireland, Sweden and the United Kingdom, that give reason to monitor more closely the on-going and future developments in national disability policy. The empirical chapters in this book and in the accompanying volume on the lived experiences of persons with disabilities offer more detailed, nuanced and multi faceted evidence of changes that have taken place in the nine countries under study.

References

Adema, W., Fron, P. & Ladaique, M. (2011). Is the European Welfare State Really More Expensive? Indicators on Social Spending, 1980–2012; and a Manual to the OECD Social Expenditure Database (SOCX). *OECD Social, Employment and Migration Working Papers* No. 124. OECD Publishing, Paris. Retrieved 17 September 2016 from http://dx.doi.org/10.1787/5kg2d2d4pbf0-en

Ascoli, U. & Ranci, C. (Eds.) (2002). *Dilemmas of the Welfare Mix: The New Structure of Welfare in an Era of Privatization.* New York: Kluwer Academic.

Bemelmans-Videc, M. -L., Rist, R. C. & Vedung, E. O. (Eds.) (1998). *Carrots, Sticks, and Sermons: Policy Instruments and Their Evaluation.* New Jersey: Transaction Books.

Bickenbach, J. E. & Cieza, A. (2011). The prospects for universal disability law and social law. *Journal of Accessibility and Design for All*, 1, 23–37. Retrieved 20 February 2017 from: http://dx.doi.org/10.17411/jacces.v1i1.79

Biggeri, M., Arciprete, C., Barbuto, R., Ciani, F. and Griffo, G. (forthcoming). The Role of the Family in structuring the Opportunities for exercising Active Citizenship among Persons with Disabilities, in Halvorsen, R., Hvinden, B. Beadle-Brown, J., Biggeri, M., Tøssebro, J., Waldschmidt, A. (Eds.). *Lived Experiences of Persons with Disabilities: Active Citizenship and Disability in Europe Volume 2.* London: Routledge.

Cantillon, B. (2014). Beyond social investment. In B. Cantillon & F. Vandenbroucke (Eds.). *Reconciling Work and Poverty Reduction* (286–318). Oxford: Oxford University Press.

Deneulin, S. & Shahani, L. (2009). *An Introduction to the Human Development and Capability Approach: Freedom and Agency.* London: Earthscan.

Dion, B., Pineda, V. & Ginnerup, S. (2015). *Toolkit: Key indicators of accessibility: Reporting on the UN CRPD for The Delta Centre, Norwegian Directorate for Children, Youth and Family Affairs.* Prepared by The Global Alliance on Accessible Technologies and Environments (GAATS). Retrieved from: http://gaates.org/wp-content/uploads/2014/07/FINAL-Toolkit_-UN-CRPD-KEY-INDICATORS-OF-ACCESSIBILITY-2015-06-29.pdf

Equal treatment in employment and occupation. (2000). Council Directive 2000/78/EC. Retrieved from: http://eur-lex.europa.eu/legal-content/EN/TXT/HTML/?uri=URISERV:c10823&from=EN

Esping-Andersen, G. (1990). *The Three Worlds of Welfare Capitalism*. Oxford: Polity.

Esping-Andersen, G. (1996). After the golden age? In G. Esping-Andersen (Ed.). *Welfare States in Transition: National Adaptations in Global Economies* (1–31). London: Sage.

Esping-Andersen, G. (1999). *Social Foundations of Postindustrial Economics*. Oxford: Oxford University Press.

Esping-Andersen, G. (2002). A child-centred social investment strategy. In G. Esping-Andersen (Ed.). *Why We Need a New Welfare State* (26–67). Oxford: Oxford University Press.

Etzioni, A. (1961). *Comparative Analysis of Complex Organizations: On Power, Involvement, and Their Correlates*. New York: Free Press.

European Commission (2014). Report from the Commission to the European Parliament and the Council. Joint Report on the application of Council Directive 2000/43/EC of 29 June 2000 implementing the principle of equal treatment between persons irrespective of racial or ethnic origin ('Racial Equality Directive') and of Council Directive 2000/78/EC of 27 November 2000 establishing a general framework for equal treatment in employment and occupation ('Employment Equality Directive') COM(2014) 2 final. Retrieved 20 February 2017 from: http://ec.europa.eu/justice/discrimination/files/com_2014_2_en.pdf

European Commission (2015). Proposal for a Directive of the European Parliament and of the Council on the approximation of the laws, regulations and administrative provisions of the Member States as regards the accessibility requirements for products and services. COM (2015) 615 final 2015/0278 (COD). Retrieved from: http://eur-lex.europa.eu/resource.html?uri=cellar:202aa1e4-99a0-11e5-b3b7-01aa75ed71a1.0021.02/DOC_1&format=PDF

European Union (2009). Council Decision of 26 November 2009 concerning the conclusion, by the European Community, of the United Nations Convention on the Rights of Persons with Disabilities (2010/48/EC), *Official Journal of the European Union*, 27.1.2010, L 23/35

Eurostat (2015). *Social protection*. Reference metadata in the Euro SDMX metadata. Retrieved from: http://ec.europa.eu/eurostat

Eurostat (2016). *Glossary: Persons Living in Households with Low Work Intensity*. Retrieved from http://ec.europa.eu/eurostat/statistics-explained/index.php/Glossary:Persons_living_in_households_with_low_work_intensity

Eurostat Database (2016). Retrieved 7 September 2016 from http://ec.europa.eu/eurostat/data/database

Ferrera, M. (1998). The four 'social Europes': Between universalism and selectivity. In M. Rhodes and Y. Mény (Eds.). *The Future of European Welfare* (81–96), Basingstoke: Macmillan.

Goodin, R. E., Headey, B., Muffels, R. & Dirven, H.-J. (1999). *The Real Worlds of Welfare Capitalism*. Cambridge: Cambridge University Press.

Hall, P. A. & Soskice, D. (2001). An introduction to varieties of capitalism. In P. A. Hall & D. Soskice (Eds.). *Varieties of Capitalism: The Institutional Foundations of Comparative Advantage* (1–68). Oxford: Oxford University Press.

Halvorsen. R. (2010). Digital freedom for persons with disabilities: Are policies to enhance eAcessbility and eInclusion becoming more similar in the Nordic countries and the US? In L. Waddington & G. Quinn (Eds.). *European Yearbook of Disability Law*, Vol. 2 (77–102). Antwerp: Intersentia.

Halvorsen, R. & Hvinden, B. (2009). Nordic disability protection meeting supranational equal treatment policy: A boost for the human rights of persons with disabilities? In

H. Sinding Aasen, R. Halvorsen & B. da Silva (Eds.). *Human Rights, Dignity and Autonomy in Health* Care and *Social Services* (177–202). Mortsel: Intersentia.

Halvorsen, R. & Hvinden, B. (2011). *Andre lands modeller for å fremme sysselsetting blant personer med nedsatt funksjonsevne*. NOVA report 14/2011. Oslo: NOVA Norwegian Social Research.

Halvorsen, R. & Hvinden, B. (2016). How to achieve Active Inclusion in a multi-layered context. In R. Halvorsen & B. Hvinden (Eds.). *Combating Poverty in Europe: Active Inclusion in a Multi-Level and Multi-Actor Context* (3–24). Cheltenham, UK: Edward Elgar.

Hauben, H., Coucheir, M., Spooren, J., McAnaney, D. & Delfosse, C. (2012). *Assessing the Impact of European Governments' Austerity Plans on the Rights of People with Disabilities*. Brussels: European Foundation Centre (EFC).

Hemerijck, A. (2013). *Changing Welfare States*. Oxford: Oxford University Press.

Hvinden, B. (2003). The uncertain convergence of disability policies in Western Europe. *Social Policy and Administration*, 37, 609–624.

Hvinden, B. (2004). Nordic disability policies in a changing Europe: Is there still a distinct Nordic model? *Social Policy and Administration*, 38, 170–189.

Hvinden, B. (2009). Redistributive and regulatory disability provisions: Incompatibility or synergy? In G. Quinn & L. Waddington (Eds.). *European Yearbook of Disability Law*, Vol. 1 (5–27). Mortsel: Intersentia.

Hvinden, B. (2016). Beyond the welfare state: What next for the European social model? In P. Blanck & E. Flynn (Eds.). *Routledge Handbook of Disability Law and Human Rights* (16–30). London: Routledge,

Hvinden, B. & Halvorsen, R. (2003). Which way for European disability policy? *Scandinavian Journal of Disability Research*, 5, 296–312.

Jenson, J. (2009). Lost in translation: The social investment perspective and gender equality. *Social Politics*, 15, 446–483.

Jordana, J. & Levi-Faur, D. (2004). The politics of regulation in the age of governance. In J. Jordana and D. Levi-Faur (Eds.). *The Politics of Regulation: Institutions and Regulatory Reforms for the Age of Governance* (1–28). Cheltenham, UK: Edward Elgar.

Karačić, A., Sturm, A., Waldschmidt, A. and Dins, T.(forthcoming). Identity and political participation throughout the life course – the experiences of persons with disabilities in European countries, in Halvorsen, R., Hvinden, B., Beadle-Brown, J., Biggeri, M., Tøssebro, J. , Waldschmidt, A. (Eds.). *Lived Experiences of Persons with Disabilities: Active Citizenship and Disability in Europe Volume 2*. London: Routledge.

Kemp, P. A. (2006). Comparing trends in disability benefit recipiency. In P. A. Kemp, A. Sunden & B. B. Tauritz (Eds.). *Sick Societies? Trends in Disability Benefits in Post-Industrial Societies* (7–22). Geneva: International Social Security Association.

Kemp, P. A. (2008). The transformation of incapacity benefits. In M. Seeleib-Kaiser (Ed.). *Welfare State Transformations* (164–181). Basingstoke: Palgrave Macmillan.

Korpi, W. & Palme, J. (1998). The paradox of redistribution and strategies of quality: Welfare state institutions, inequality, and poverty in the Western countries. *American Sociological Review*, 63, 661–687.

Kubitschke, L., Cullen, K., Dolphin, C., Laurin, S. & Cederbom, A. (Eds.) (2013). *Study on Accessing and Promoting E-Accessibility*, Final Report, Brussels: European Union. Retrieved 20 February 2017 from https://ec.europa.eu/digital-single-market/en/news/study-assessing-and-promoting-e-accessibility

Leibfried, S. (1993). Towards a European welfare state? In C. Jones (Ed.). *New Perspectives on the Welfare State in Europe* (133–154). London: Routledge.

Levi-Faur, D. (2014). The welfare state: A regulatory perspective. *Public Administration*, 92, 599–614.

Majone, G. (1993). The European Community between social policy and social regulation. *JCMS: Journal of Common Market Studies*, 31, 153–170.

Morel, N., Palier, B. & Palme, J. (2012). Beyond the welfare state as we knew it? In N. Morel, B. Palier & J. Palme (Eds.) *Towards a Social Investment State? Ideas, Policies and Challenges* (1–30). Bristol: The Policy Press.

Nussbaum, M. C. (2000). *Women and Human Development: The Capabilities Approach*. Cambridge: Cambridge University Press.

Nussbaum, M. C. (2011). *Creating Capabilities: The Human Development Approach*. Cambridge, Mass.: The Belknap Press of the Harvard University Press.

OECD (2010). *Sickness, Disability and Work: Breaking the Barriers*. Paris: OECD.

OECD (2014). *Society at a Glance 2014: OECD Social Indicators*. Paris: OECD.

Ogus, A. (2000). New techniques for social regulation: Decentralisation and diversity. In H. Collins, P, Davies & R. Rideou (Eds.). *Legal Regulation of the Employment Relation* (83–93). New York: Kluwer Law International.

Pierson, P. (2001). Coping with permanent austerity: Welfare state restructuring in affluent democracies. In P. Pierson (Ed.). *The New Politics of the Welfare State* (410–456). Oxford: Oxford University Press.

Quinn, G. (2004). *Disability Rights – An American Invention*. 11th Annual Valerie Gordon Human Rights Lecture, Galway: National University of Ireland, Galway, Faculty of Law.

Quinn, G. (2005). The European social charter and the EU anti-discrimination law in the field of disability: Two gravitational fields with one common purpose. In G. de Burca & B. de Witte (Eds.). *Social Rights in Europe* (279–304). Oxford: Oxford University Press.

Robeyns, I. (2005). The capability approach: A theoretical survey. *Journal of Human Development*, 1, 93–114.

Room, G. (Ed.) (2015). *Alternatives to Austerity*. IRR Spotlight. University of Bath. Retrieved 21 February 2017 from http://www.bath.ac.uk/ipr/pdf/policy-briefs/alternatives-to-austerity.pdf

Schäfer, A. & Streeck, W. (Eds.) (2013). *Politics in the Age of Austerity*. Cambridge: Polity.

Sen, A. (1993). Capability and well-being. In M. C. Nussbaum & A. Sen (Eds.). *The Quality of Life* (30–53). Oxford: Clarendon Press.

Sen, A. (1999). *Development as Freedom*. Oxford: Oxford University Press.

Sen, A. (2009). *The Idea of Justice*. London: Penguin.

Sipilä, J. (2012). The social investment state: A new trend in social expenditure or merely a popular political discourse? In G. B. Cohen, B. W. Ansell, R. H. Fox & J. Gingrich (Eds.). *Social Policy in the Smaller European Union States* (81–104). New York: Berghahn Books.

Stephenson, P. (2013). Twenty years of multilevel governance: 'Where does it come from? Where is it? Where is it going?' *Journal of European Public Policy*, 20, 817–837.

Trani, J-F., Bakhshi, P. Bellanca, N., Biggeri, M. & Marchetta, F. (2011). Disabilities through the capability approach lens: Implications for public policies. *Alter*, 5, 143–157.

United Nations (2015). *Convention and Optional Protocol Signatures and Ratifications: Countries and Regional Integration Organizations*. Retrieved from: https://www.un.org/development/desa/disabilities/convention-on-the-rights-of-persons-with-disabilities.html

United Nations (2016). Concluding observations on the initial report of Serbia. CRPD/C/SRB/CO/1, Committee on the Rights of Persons with Disabilities, Geneva: United Nations

United Nations (2006). Convention on the Rights of Persons with Disabilities. Retrieved 27 February 2017 from: http://www.un.org/disabilities/documents/convention/convopt-prot-e.pdf

Vandenbroucke, F., Hemerijck, A. & Palier, B. (2011). The EU needs a social investment pact. *OSE Paper Series*, no. 5, May. Retrieved 27 February 2017 from: http://www.ose.be/files/OpinionPaper5_Vandenbroucke-Hemerijk-Palier_2011.pdf

Waddington, L. (2009). A disabled market: Free movement of goods and services in the EU and disability accessibility. *European Law Journal*, 15(5), 575–598.

Waldschmidt, A. (2005). Disability studies: Individuelles, soziales und / oder kulturelles Modell von Behinderung? *Psychologie und Gesellschaftskritik*, 29(1), 9–31. Retrieved 20 February 2017 from: http://bidok.uibk.ac.at/library/waldschmidt-modell.html

Waldschmidt, A. (2007). Disability as social problem. In G. Ritzer (Ed.), *The Blackwell Encyclopedia of Sociology* Vol. III. (1168–1170). Oxford: Blackwell Publishing.

Waldschmidt, A. (2009). Disability policy of the European Union: The supranational level. ALTER: *European Journal of Disability Research / Revue Européenne de Recherche sur le Handicap*, 3, 8–23.

Waldschmidt, A. (2016). Europäische und Internationale Behindertenpolitik. In M. Dederich, I. Beck, G. Antor & U. Bleidick (Eds.). *Handlexikon der Behindertenpädagogik. Schlüsselbegriffe aus Theorie und Praxis* (440–445). Stuttgart, Weimar: Kohlhammer.

Whittle, R. & Halvorsen, R. (2007). From disabling barriers to participation: The opportunities created by the EU equality strategy. In B. Hvinden & H. Johansson (Eds.). *Citizenship in Nordic Welfare States: Dynamics of Choice, Duties and Participation* (183–199), London: Routledge.

3 How do we know whether changes in public policy and legislation improve the conditions for exercising Active Citizenship by persons with disabilities?

Jerome Bickenbach

DISCIT's aim has been to produce new knowledge for achieving full and effective participation of persons with disabilities in Europe, in terms of a multifaceted concept of Active Citizenship designed to operationalise the 'full and effective participation' outlined in the United Nations Convention on the Rights of Persons with Disabilities (CRPD) (UN, 2007). While, compared to other conceptualisations of Active Citizenship, DISCIT's approach provides a robust theoretical foundation, it also creates operationalisation and measurement challenges in practice. This chapter examines these challenges and develops a framework for data harmonisation in light of the available European data, as well as an analytical strategy for socio-economic, process and outcome indicators to measure the impact of policy changes mandated by the implementation of Active Citizenship in European policy. An 'indicator' is something that can be quantified or measured that 'indicates' a trend or state of interest. Social indicators (such as the unemployment rate of persons with disabilities, the percentage of women attending medical school, or the number of voting booths that are accessible to wheelchairs) are important because they allow us to use available information to show the extent to which a social goal, like Active Citizenship, has been achieved. This chapter therefore looks at ways of developing indicators, whether quantitative or qualitative, for measuring the effects of public policy and legislation on the conditions for exercising Active Citizenship by persons with disabilities (see Chapters 1 and 2 in this volume for more details about DISCIT's conception of Active Citizenship).

More specifically, in this chapter we construct a set of Active Citizenship indicators that:

1. identify and quantify the strengths and weaknesses of existing policy strategies;
2. isolate the right balance between redistributive and regulatory policies;
3. locate the effective governance level, as well as the appropriate public, private and civil-society stakeholders, for effective policy implementation and monitoring; and finally
4. align the preconditions of Active Citizenship with the legal obligations of the CRPD and other relevant European human rights documents.

This task depends primarily on the technical exercise—explained below—of 'harmonising' data across different European surveys, censuses and other sources of information. In particular this requires a decision about what definition of 'disability' (of the many used in European surveys) should be adopted for our purposes (see Chapter 4) and it also entails identifying a set of indicators that are precise enough to align with the details of DISCIT's conception of Active Citizenship, yet are general enough to be practical.

This chapter begins by identifying DISCIT Active Citizenship indicators and integrating them with human rights indicators for the CRPD. As we develop these indicators ('AC/CRPD indicators'), we discover methodological and conceptual challenges to obtaining reliable and usable data. Without such data, indicators are of little use. Specifically, the indicator development component of DISCIT research showed that obtaining the evidence we need to demonstrate whether true social change for persons with disabilities has taken place depends on answers to the following questions:

1. What is the balance between fidelity to the conceptualisation of Active Citizenship and the feasibility of using these indicators to measure changes in policy?
2. What is the best way to find a definition of disability that makes it possible to harmonise data collected from different sources?
3. Should we create the best indicators and then try to find for them, or should we develop our indicators in light of the data that we already have?
4. What are the prospects of improving the quality and availability of European disability data for the purposes of social change?

As with all forms of action-oriented social science research, the point is not merely to describe social facts about the situation of persons with disabilities in Europe, it is also about finding a programme for changing those facts to achieve social progress, where progress is assessed by recognised ideals and human rights. If there is one lesson that social reformers have learned over the years it is that real social change requires some indicators, and a measurement strategy needs to be found and used in order to demonstrate that change has occurred.

Developing AC/CRPD indicators

Active Citizenship is intrinsically a 'rights-imbued' concept and the chapters of these volumes demonstrate in detail that the underlying values of Active Citizenship are variants of the values of the CRPD as stated in Article 3, namely, respect for human dignity and individual autonomy, non-discrimination, full and effective participation and inclusion, respect for difference, equality of opportunity and accessibility. In Articles 31 and 33 the CRPD sets out the obligations of states with respect to data collection and statistical tools, including indicators 'to promote, protect and monitor implementation' of the Convention. It is therefore a natural step to try to find common ground between the indicators of Active Citizenship and proposed indicators for the CRPD. In this manner we could show that our indicators are consistent with the general values and specific human rights of the CRPD.

Unfortunately, there is currently no agreement about how best to develop indicators that can be useful for human rights in general, or more specifically for a notion like Active Citizenship. It is worth reviewing two recent attempts to develop indicators, one for a theory of active citizenship that is different than DISCIT's and the other for CRPD monitoring. Both attempts provide us with important lessons.

Developing indicators for Active Citizenship: The CRELL experience

As a component of the 2001 Lisbon Agenda (European Commission, 2001), a project was initiated by the European Commission's Centre for Research on Lifelong Learning (CRELL) to develop indicators to measure 'active citizenship', understood primarily as political involvement or 'civil competence' (De Weerd et al., 2005). Specifically, the group defined active citizenship as: '[p]articipation in civil society, community and/or political life, characterised by mutual respect and non-violence and in accordance with human rights and democracy' (Hoskins, 2006b, 7).

Rather than trying to develop a full conceptualisation of active citizenship, Hoskins and colleagues proceeded in a much more pragmatic fashion. They first distinguished active citizenship from two related notions—social capital and social cohesion. They then followed other trends in the background literature and identified four 'operational dimensions' of active citizenship:

- Protest and Social Change: action-oriented participation and direct influence in political and civil life;
- Community Life: membership within a community, exemplifying the inherent values of solidarity and participation;
- Representative Democracy: 'conventional' political participation by proxy;
- Democratic Values: beyond mere involvement in social and political life, participation in the values typically used to characterize 'good citizenship'. (Hoskins, 2006b)

Each of these dimensions of Active Citizenship is then divided into subcomponents, and each subcomponent is linked to between one and five indicators. Thus Protest and Social Change is broken down into Protest, Engagement in Trade Union Organisations, Engagement in Environmental Organisations and Engagement in Human Rights Organisations. Each of these subcomponents is then associated with indicators. Thus, Protest is associated with five indicators: signing a petition, taking part in a lawful demonstration, boycotting products, ethical consumption and contacting a politician. The three other dimensions are similarly divided into subcomponents and each of these is linked to a collection of indicators. The end result is a list of 61 indicators of (their notion of) active citizenship.

Data-led and Indicator-led approaches

The first lesson learned from the CRELL experience was that, in the absence of a fully elaborated theory, it is difficult to avoid the impression that the four dimensions, their components and the associated indicators have all been somewhat arbitrarily selected. In the end, Hoskins and Mascherini (2009) had little choice in the matter since, as they acknowledge at the outset of their study:

> The greatest difficulty we faced has been the limitation of existing international data sources on citizenship practices and values which at this current moment in time do not cover the breadth or the depth of the concept of active citizenship … Due to these limitations, this research should be considered exploratory and to be a first step towards measuring active citizenship (460).

In the end, they decided to use the European Social Survey (ESS) as their single source of European data, and the indicators selected correspond to the questions in this survey. This choice of using only one data source obviously maximises the comparability of their 61 indicators, but it also explains why their methodological decisions appear arbitrary and lacking any empirical basis.

At the risk of over-simplifying a substantial body of literature on indicator development, there are two strategies for developing indicators: One can start with actual sources of information (such as surveys and questionnaires) that are intuitively relevant to the phenomenon of interest and then create (or find existing) indicators to link to these data. This data-led approach presumes a linking between questions in the survey and the intuitive subcomponents of the phenomena, or underlying concepts, for which indicators are desired. The opposite strategy is to develop indicators that are directly linked to an existing theoretical operationalisation and then look for sources of information or data relevant to these indicators. This indicator-led approach requires an operationalisation that is unambiguous and precise enough to use for indicator creation, but it is a far riskier strategy since there simply may be no relevant sources of information to use.

Evidently, the CRELL researchers believed that only a data-led approach was available to them. They are certainly not alone in this view. The seminal work done on equality indicators by the United Kingdom's Equality and Human Rights Commission in 2009–2011, including indicators for political participation, were also developed using a 'data-led' strategy, based on the results of the Office for National Statistics (UK ONS) Equality Data Audit (Alkire, et al., 2009; UK ONS, 2007).

The highly influential work on CRPD indicators carried out since 2009 by the Academic Network of European Disability experts (ANED) began with an indicator-led approach (given that it was grounded in the concepts of the CRPD), but it was soon confronted with the fact that there were no plausible data sources to serve those indicators (Van Oorschot, 2009; Grammenos, 2009).

This in turn led to an attempt to create a novel collection of indicators based on three European data sources—Eurostat's EU-SILC and EQLS and the three waves of the SHARE study (Grammenos, 2010)—which in turn led to a much shortened and simplified list of indicators suitable for the European survey EU-SILC (Grammenos, 2011). This was coordinated with the European Agency for Fundamental Rights (FRA) study on the right to political participation for persons with disabilities in which the indicators were developed as a data-led exercise relying on the European Social Survey and the European Quality of Life Survey (FRA, 2014).

In light of this previous work, it was perhaps inevitable that the DISCIT study would proceed in a similar, data-led fashion, since it was clearly extremely challenging to develop indicators for a complex concept such as that of Active Citizenship using a standard 'top-down' process of conceptualisation, operationalisation and specification of the concept, selection of indicators appropriate to the specification and identification of relevant and longitudinal datasets to serve those indicators. Because of this—and the need to use a functional definition of 'disability' for closer alignment with European data sources—we ended up using the following European data sources: European Statistics of Income and Living Condition (EU-SILC), the European Labour Force Survey (EU LFS), the European Health and Social Integration Survey (EHSIS), the European Social Survey (ESS), the European Quality of Life Survey (EQLS), Eurobarometer and selected National Disability Surveys.

The Composite Indicator

The second lesson learned from the CRELL experience concerns the ultimate aim of that project to develop a single Active Citizenship Composite Indicator (ACCI) for comparing levels of active citizenship across Europe. Unlike the fairly rough and intuitive process that led to the 61 indicators, the steps to constructing and validating the ACCI were highly technical and grounded in solid statistical methods (see Nardo et al., 2005). In the end, the composite indicator could be used in more or less the same way as socio-economic indices, such as GDP and the Human Development Index.

For our purpose, the decision was not to take the step of developing a composite indicator or Active Citizenship index, despite the seductive attraction of being able to use such a measure to represent in one number the extent of a country's recognition of Active Citizenship for persons with disabilities, and rank countries accordingly. We took this decision because of the statistical need, whenever dealing with a multi-dimensional phenomenon, to rank the significance of potential impacts of each of the dimensions. This is often done by asking a panel of experts to reach a consensus about the relative importance of each dimension or element of the notion.

Although reliance on expert consensus weighting can be methodologically justified for relatively objective and descriptive notions such as health (compare Murray et al., 2002) or even gender empowerment (compare World Economic Forum (WEF), 2013), DISCIT's conceptualisation of Active Citizenship is very different. Although composed in part of objectively measureable components,

Active Citizenship is ultimately a prescriptive or normative notion in which the relative significance or weight of the component parts, represented by indicators, will of necessity shift over time and place. More importantly, the relative importance of each element should not be a matter of some academic 'expertise' but instead reflect a democratic consensus, politically negotiated. (Much the same can be said for the indicators relevant for monitoring the implementation of the CRPD.) Finally, and most importantly, the composite indicator—and the 'expert consensus' methodology for creating it—is inconsistent with the necessity for experience-based indicators, a feature of the DISCIT approach to which we now turn.

The essential experiential perspective: qualitative indicators

The third lesson learned from CRELL was that in order to capture the notion of Active Citizenship both quantitative socio-economic indicators and qualitative experience indicators were required. This was the primary failing of the CRELL study. The DISCIT methodology involved two steps. First, quantitative (socio-economic) indicators were constructed in terms of a Specification Matrix in which salient aspects of the Active Citizenship conceptualisation were operationalised in terms of social practices and external outcomes; secondly, indicators operationalised by contextual and experiential aspects of the Specification Matrix were developed in parallel with the questions used in the Life Course interviews. Although the DISCIT qualitative and quantitative indicators were integrated they could not be aggregated to create a composite measure.

Is the experiential qualitative perspective on Active Citizenship essential? Serge Ebersold has forcefully argued that social participation—of which security, autonomy and influence are dimensions—is fundamental to Active Citizenship because it secures a bond (which he calls 'social belonging') between the individual and the social institutions that provide the essential social resources of citizenship (Ebersold, 2007). Active Citizenship, in other words, is not merely a criterion of integration in which persons with disabilities have access to the same resources, opportunities and sources of social recognition and respect that others do; it is also a matter of the active recognition of interdependency.

Sometimes expressed more simply as 'a sense of belonging' (Edwards, et al., 2015), the recognition of the 'lived experience' of Active Citizenship accords with the modern understanding of the experience of disability as interactive between the individual and the environment at large, and in particular the social environment (Hästbacka & Nygård, 2013). While participation stresses the value of interdependence and involvement in the shared social existence of others, it needs to be supplemented with autonomy, which tends to emphasise the independence and detachment of the individual from others.

DISCIT Indicators for Active Citizenship

The DISCIT methodology began with operationalising the DISCIT conceptualisation into aspects and attributes for which indicators are required (see Chapters 1 and 2 for clarification of these terms). We first distinguish three meta-attitudes: *Structures*: external or internal structures that impact, positively or negatively on the achievement of Active Citizenship; *Practices*: routine or reflexive actions, experiences and reactions, practices and engagements either at the social level ('Outside') or individual level ('Inside') that are relevant to achieving Active Citizenship; and *Outcomes*. According to the DISCIT conceptualisation, *Outcomes* are the results or consequences of the impact of Outside Practices on the Internal and External Structures that constitute the Conditions of Active Citizenship. These results may either be collective results of Active Citizenship across the three dimensions of Security, Autonomy and Influence (that is, the 'Outside' results) or person-level results such as greater effective freedom, improved well-being, self-respect and the sense of being respected by others (that is, the 'Inside' results). Table 3.1 summarises these distinctions for each of the three dimensions of Autonomy, Security and Influence.

Three varieties of indicators were developed; quantitative: *Socio-economic Indicators* and two varieties of qualitative indicators: *Contextual Indicators* and *Experience Indicators.* Contextual and Experience indicators both rely on first-person narratives. Contextual Indicators identify information about what has been experienced, while Experience Indicators identify subjective appraisal, evaluation or judgments about what was experienced. Both indicators are valuable and equally reliable, but it is important to distinguish between, for example, information that a social benefit has been received (Contextual) and information that the benefit was inadequate or that the process was humiliating or degrading (Experience).

Unlike quantitative indicators in which there is a clear need to link indicators to specific data sources (e.g. linking indicators to data collected from responses to specific questions in a self-report population survey) this is not the case for most qualitative indicators. Qualitative data is more narrative in nature and interpretative skills will always be required to link the indicator to information arising from an analysis of the responses given to the questions.

Table 3.2 sets out the combined list of 47 Socio-economic, Contextual and Experience Indicators for the DISCIT conceptualisation of Active Citizenship (see Bickenbach, 2014 for more details).

Integrated AC/CRPD Indicators

How do the Active Citizenship indicators in Table 3.2 fit with existing CRPD indicators? In 2008, the United Nations High Commissioner for Human Rights (UNHCHR) published a highly influential methodological report on the development of human rights indicators (UN, 2008). The analytical distinctions presented there have become standard and have provided guidance for responding to Articles 31 and 33 of the CRPD for monitoring the implementation of the Convention. Unfortunately, at present there is no consensus on an indicator set for any of the Articles of the CRPD, although there is much academic literature being produced (UNDP, 2014).

Table 3.1 Specification Matrix

DIMENSION	*EXTERNAL STRUCTURES*	*INTERNAL STRUCTURES*	*PRACTICES*		*OUTCOMES*	
	Outside	*Inside*	*Outside*	*Inside*	*Outside*	*Inside*
	Cultural, social and political forces, institutional and organizational arrangement: global, regional, national, local	Personal features of enduring or temporary dispositions, experience, knowledge, competences, perceptions and judgments	Social arrangements, behaviours and practices	Individual arrangements, behaviours and practices *as perceived by the individual*	Structures of policies, social conditions and participation rates	Social structures, conditions and participation rates *as perceived by the individual*

Table 3.2 Complete list of proposed indicators for Active Citizenship

	SOCIO-ECONOMIC INDICATORS (Social practices and external outcomes)
1	Annual spending on cash and in-kind benefits programmes
2	Rate of non-take-up of benefits in cash and kind
3	Rate of poverty before and after transfers
4	Prevalence difference between disposable income for persons with disabilities
5	Prevalence of severe material deprivation
6	Rate of use of different living arrangements
7	Rate of use of in-home, residential or community support services
8	Rate of use of personal mobility and communication supports
9	Rates of distinct employment patterns
10	Rates of participation in organisations and campaigns
11	Rates of participation in conventional politics
12	Prevalence of discrimination
	CONTEXTUAL INDICATORS (External structures)
1	Structure of social benefit system
2	Structure of social services system
3	Structure of social regulation system
4	Structure of legal and practical provisions for effective and full participation in public, political and organizational life
5	Structure for co-determination in personalised services
6	Accessibility system
7	Anti-discrimination system
	EXPERIENCE INDICATORS (Internal structures, practices and outcomes)
1	Health condition and coping styles
2	Dispositions
3	Perceptions and judgments of self and others
4	Knowledge
5	Reaction
6	Critical awareness
7	Accessibility
8	Discrimination
9	Availability, adequacy and relevance of benefits
10	Participation in efforts to achieve security improvements
11	Social accept or stigma
12	Poverty traps
13	Conditions for receiving cash or services
14	Change in benefits
15	Change in standard of living
16	Degree of economic freedom
17	Previous and current living arrangements
18	Participation in efforts to achieve autonomy improvements
19	Stigma related to living arrangements
20	Accessibility, availability, adequacy, quality of supports

Table 3.2 (Continued)

1	Shift towards independent living
2	Accessibility, availability, quality of in-home, personal mobility, communication supports
3	Employment prospects, related supports
4	Participation in campaigns, advocacy groups, organisations (Disabled Persons' Organizations (DPOs) and others)
5	Participation in conventional politics
6	Participation in provider discussions, organisations, campaigns and conventional politics
7	Effective influence (or co-influence) at individual level and collective level
8	Participation in discussion with service providers

Given the state of the art of CRPD indicator development, it would not be possible to directly align DISCIT Active Citizenship indicators with CRPD indicators. Following the guidance of the UNHCHR Report, however, an important first step can be taken. We propose here to identify CRPD attributes for the Articles relevant to the specifications derived from the DISCIT conceptualisation of Active Citizenship given above. These CRPD attributes are then linked to the most appropriate Socio-economic, Contextual or Experience Indicators listed in Table 3.2 above. The result is a combined—and aligned—set of indicators relevant both to the operationalisation of Active Citizenship and the monitoring of CRPD human rights that are conceptually linked to Active Citizenship (for details see Bickenbach, 2015).

Broadly speaking, the DISCIT conception of Active Citizenship aligns with the human rights expressed in the CRPD, but diverges from the CRPD in adding the dimension of individual obligations to, in effect, take up the freedoms guaranteed by CRPD. While highlighting essential human rights, the CRPD does not include individual obligations to take up and exercise these rights. The only duty-bearer is the state. The individual is guaranteed the effective, positive freedom to, for example, participate in political and community life, but not the obligation to do so. It should be emphasised, however, that the DISCIT Frame is merely DISCIT's theoretical starting point, and it is quite possible to envisage other conceptualisations of Active Citizenship that are fully compliant with the CRPD.

The challenge of data harmonisation

The development of qualitative and quantitative indicators for Active Citizenship demonstrates how the DISCIT conceptualisation of Active Citizenship can be effectively used to monitor the reform of disability policy. Yet, though a major step to meeting the measurement challenge of Active Citizenship, indicators are only useful if there is relevant data available as input. This requires not only content-relevant data disaggregated for disability, but also, when several data sources are being used, the complex task of data harmonisation.

In general terms, data harmonisation requires procedures for standardising the inputs and outputs of surveys to ensure the comparability of the data collected

(University of Michigan, 2011). Input harmonisation engages processes that standardise the wording of questions, response options to questions and questionnaire design, primarily the sampling frame, data coding and documentation. As the name implies, input harmonisation can only be done prior to data collection and typically only during the development, or amendment, of a survey.

When national statistical offices engage in input harmonisation they select a set of questions that provide information about a population of interest and ensure that these questions are included in existing surveys that investigate specialised domains such as economic activity, health, housing, transportation and so on (see, for example, UK ONS, 2008). This is especially important where there is an underlying common focus, such as equality, and a need to review a range of impact areas, such as age, gender, disability and so on, with the result that several survey instruments are required. Input harmonisation makes it possible to compare across populations by means of a common set of harmonised variables (see UK ONS, 2007). The end result is essentially a data dictionary applicable across all national surveys (see UK ONS, 2013).

When, as is the case with DISCIT, a novel conceptualisation is proposed, the input approach to harmonisation is not possible (at least in the short term) and output harmonisation is the only option. Output harmonisation, except when the indicators used are widely accepted, involves *ex post* harmonisation of the concepts used in the questions, the response options to questions (through a process called 'conversion'), the data coding rules and other procedures. Although a complete output harmonisation is a laborious task, the benefits are considerable since it makes it possible for a head-to-head direct comparison of data from a wide variety of surveys and questionnaires, or even other data sources such as administrative records.

During the course of DISCIT research the most widely available and relevant data sources for disability indicators in Europe were identified and a fairly standard data harmonisation protocol and plan—focusing primarily on concept and response option harmonisation—was developed. In this section our primary focus is not these specific technical results, rather we want to highlight and comment on the challenges of data harmonisation. These challenges are in fact unresolved issues that need to be addressed, not only for the DISCIT approach to Active Citizenship, but more broadly for any systematic and effective implementation of human rights treaties, such as the CRPD.

Definition of disability

How can fidelity to the DISCIT conceptualisation be balanced against the feasibility of dealing with the challenges of developing indicators to measure changes in policy and meet the objectives of the study? Perhaps the most dramatic example of this is the on-going issue of how best to standardise the definition of disability for data collection purposes.

The received conceptualisation of disability for research, policy, and measurement understands disability as a multi-dimensional experience that arises out of an interaction between intrinsic, essentially biomedical features of the person and the physical, human-built, interpersonal, attitudinal, social, cultural, legal and political environment in which the person lives and acts. This is the 'biopsychosocial' model found in the World Health Organization's (WHO) *International Classification of Functioning, Disability and Health* (ICF) (WHO, 2001), in disability scholarship and advocacy (e.g. Shakespeare, 2013), and the CRPD itself: 'Persons with disabilities include those who have long-term physical, mental, intellectual or sensory impairments which in interaction with various barriers may hinder their full and effective participation in society on an equal basis with others.'

Although terminological suggestions in this area are fraught with controversy, for convenience 'disability' will represent the full, lived experience of a person in context, that is the full outcome of the person–environment interaction. The experience of disability is the person's experience, not a determinant of it—such as a health problem or impairment—but the actual holistic experience. For policy purposes it is not enough to identify a group who, because of their state of health or impairments, are at risk of experiencing disability—we need to know those who actually do experience disability.

The person side of the person–environment interaction includes all 'under the skin' or intrinsic 'capacity' determinants of disabilities—especially a person's health conditions, impairments of body function and structure as well as all directly resulting decrements in functioning in basic and complex activities—from simple activities such as walking, listening, concentrating, dressing, engaging in discussion with others to ever more complex activities, behaviours and roles such as having intimate relationships, participating in educational activities, working and participating in politics. In short 'capacity' represents measureable phenomena that the person, in the person–environment interaction, contributes. Following the ICF model, the environment side of the interaction contributes either in the form of a facilitator (making it possible for the person to actually perform the activity at a level or extent beyond what a person's capacity would predict) or a barrier (reducing, limiting, or preventing a person from performing the activity at the level or extent the person's capacity would predict). A person with a problem of capacity in some functioning domain may have a disability, if the environment does not facilitate him or her (or makes the problem worse), but may not have a disability if the environment (e.g. an assistive device or accommodating workplace) ensures that the problem of capacity does not determine what the person actually can do.

With this distinction it is possible to distinguish two basic approaches to the characterisation of 'disability' found in surveys, questionnaires, and indeed all disability assessment instrumentation. One can use a *capacity approach* by characterising disability in the survey instrument in terms of underlying health conditions, impairments of body function and structure or the resulting level of capacity to perform all activities, from simple to complex. Alternatively, one can use a *disability approach* by using questions that elicit the actual, person–environment interactive, lived experience of disability: that is, what the person's life actually is like, what the person can actually do or not do, by way of activities, simple and complex.

The difference in these two approaches is obvious: the capacity approach identifies a population at risk of disability; the disability approach identifies a population that actually experiences disability.

A capacity question in a survey would ask either: what health condition, disease, symptom, or sign the person exhibits; what impairments of body function or structure they have; or what limits they experience because (and only because) of their health condition or impairments. As the focus of a capacity question is the person, so the question will, in one way or another, ask the respondent to identify the limitation to the health condition, impairment or capacity limitation. An example of a capacity question is the following (from Continuous Labour Force Survey, ad hoc module 'Employment of people with longstanding health problems', DG Statistics and Economic Information, 2011):

> Are there certain tasks you cannot carry out such as carrying heavy loads, working outdoors, sitting for a long time?
>
> —yes, because of a health condition or disease
> —yes, because of a basic activity difficulty
> —yes, because of both
> —no.

An influential example of the capacity approach for identifying disabilities, principally for insertion into censuses for a rough determination of overall prevalence, is the United Nations Washington Group Short Set:

> The next questions ask about difficulties you may have doing certain activities because of a *health problem.*
>
> 1 Do you have difficulty seeing, even if wearing glasses?
> 2 Do you have difficulty hearing, even if using a hearing aid?
> 3 Do you have difficulty walking or climbing steps?
> 4 Do you have difficulty remembering or concentrating?
> 5 Do you have difficulty (with self-care such as) washing all over or dressing?
> 6 Using your usual (customary) language, do you have difficulty communicating, (for example understanding or being understood by others)? (Washington Group on Disability Statistics, 2009)

The Washington Group Short Set uses four response options: (1) No, no difficulty, (2) Yes, some difficulty, (3) Yes, a lot of difficulty and (4) Cannot do it at all (Washington Group on Disability Statistics, 2009). The work of the Washington Group was strongly motivated by the argument that since disability prevalence between countries is a function of how disability is characterised rather than real differences in the numbers of people with a disability (see, among others, WHO, 2001; Ravaud et al., 2002, Tøssebro & Kittelsaa, 2004; Weathers, 2009), standardising data collection in terms of a preferred characterisation of disability would improve world disability statistics. The choice of the capacity approach, however, is rarely defended, merely asserted without reasons (see, e.g. Mont, 2007, p. 9). Yet the intended purpose of using these questions is clear: '... the WG short set was designed to identify a population which, due to difficulty functioning in core domains, *is at risk of restricted participation in a non-accommodating environment*' (Madans et al., 2015: 2, emphasis added).

A disability question, by contrast, asks about what the person actually does, is limited in doing, or cannot do in his or her actual environment, taking full account of all facilitators (e.g. assistive devices, personal assistants, environmental modifications such as a ramp, elevators and self-opening doors, helpful and supportive attitudes of others, accommodations at school or work, or laws, regulations or policies that enhance ability to perform activities. From the same employment module in the Continuous Labour Force Survey quoted above, here is an example of a disability question:

> Are there any other reasons, not related to health conditions or difficulties that limit you in your employment?
>
> —Lack of qualifications/experience
> —Lack of appropriate job opportunities
> —Lack or poor transportation to and from workplace
> —Employers' lack of flexibility
> —Employment influences social allowance
> —Family/caring responsibilities
> —Personal reasons
> —Other reasons. (DG, 2011)

In terms of survey design, the capacity strategy lends itself to the common pattern of beginning with a set of capacity questions (about health conditions, impairments or, as with the Washington Group Short Set, capacity to perform simple actions) that are used to define, or 'screen' a population of respondents. The rest of the survey, depending on its focus, will continue with questions about healthcare, education, employment, family relationships or whatever. Results are analysed by comparing results for the screened 'disabled' population with those of the non-disabled population. Such surveys as there are that use disability questions tend, as the examples above show, to include mention of specific environmental factors that, positively or negatively, impact the person's actions and social roles.

The WHO is currently engaged in piloting a Model Disability Survey (MDS) that uses the disability strategy (WHO, n.d.). The MDS employs both capacity questions and disability questions in a general population survey.

> *Capacity*: How much difficulty do you have doing household tasks because of your health?
> *Disability*: How much of a problem is using public or private transportation?

The MDS was designed to avoid the traditional disability data collection strategy of identifying a population of individuals labelled 'disabled' in terms of their health conditions or impairment and then probing for difficulties in life. Instead, MDS asks people—not previously identified in terms of the health conditions—what they do, or do not do, in their lives. These are questions about how people actually function in multiple domains given the environmental barriers and facilitators that constitute their real life situation. The MDS also includes, in separate sections, general questions about the person's health and a range of questions about the respondent's physical environment and use of specific assistive technology and personal assistants. Disability information, on this approach, is statistically derived from the data collected rather than based on predetermined impairments or medical categories.

In the DISCIT research, the decision was made to use the capacity approach for defining disability. The argument for this decision had two parts. The first was grounded in considerations of feasibility: the DISCIT study should use a definition of disability that minimises the likelihood of variation in results across different European and national data sources. It was also suggested that the capacity approach is easier to implement for DISCIT indicators inasmuch as the two major European surveys that provide the bulk of available comparative data on education and employment (the 2011 module of the European Commission Labour Force Survey) and on social exclusion, risk of poverty, severe material deprivation, receipt of social transfers and living conditions (the European Commission, Statistics of Income and Living Condition (EU-SILC)), both use capacity questions to screen for the 'disabled' subpopulation. It is noteworthy that both the CRELL operationalisation of Active Citizenship and the entire indicator work of The Academic Network of European Experts (ANED) also presumed the capacity approach to disability definition.

It is important to remind ourselves that overcoming obstacles to measurement is important because the DISCIT concept of Active Citizenship is only of interest if it can positively affect the 'full inclusion and participation' of persons with disabilities in Europe. In this sense the DISCIT study was meant to have the same impact as the CRPD itself; however, that kind of impact requires Active Citizenship to be operationalised and measured. To be effective, disability human rights activists need to develop tools that demonstrate the complex causal links between poor human rights outcomes and shortcomings in states' policy efforts, shortcomings that may be invisible because they are systemic and entrenched. Pragmatic considerations about the form in which available European data is expressed are obviously important, but they should not be allowed to undermine the point of the research.

The second part of the argument was more methodological. It was claimed that the full person–environment, or disability approach combines in one concept issues related both to the identification of the group and the barriers and social consequences experienced by that group. Yet, it was argued, the point of research like DISCIT is to determine whether, and to what effect, persons with disabilities experience environmental barriers that limit their full inclusion and participation in society. If such barriers are made part of the definition of disability itself, then the study of social consequences approaches a tautological nature. Therefore, a study like DISCIT should stick to a definition of the group under investigation and then empirically demonstrate the barriers that are experienced, and the social consequences thereof.

Although at first glance this seems a reasonable point of methodology, a second look reveals that it is at odds with the DISCIT conceptualisation of Active Citizenship, and certainly the spirit of any research aimed at social reform. Active Citizenship, at least as it is conceptualised in DISCIT, is not a social role that applies abstractly to impairments or health conditions; it only applies to people who experience impairments or health conditions in their actual lives—that is, in their actual environments. DISCIT is an investigation into the lived experience of disability, not health conditions or impairments. Although the severity and nature of impairment has an impact on the range of activities that a person can accomplish, decrements in functioning are not barriers to Active Citizenship (nor are they barriers to the enjoyment of human rights). Only environmental factors, and in particular those factors amenable to social change, are barriers to Active Citizenship. Persons with impairments or health conditions, in the abstract, are not the study population of DISCIT; people with disabilities are.

In short, policy shortcomings and disability human rights violations are located in the social environment of persons with disabilities, not in their bodies. In statistical terms, the difference between the lived experience of disability in a country with good human rights protections and one without will never be a matter of differences in the prevalence of capacity problems. According to the *World Report on Disability* (WHO, 2011), ignoring short-term shifts in prevalence caused by natural and man-made disasters, the prevalence of capacity problems associated with disability is stable at between 10 to 20 per cent of the world population, through time and across geography. The difference in prevalence of the enjoyment of human rights, Active Citizenship, and 'full inclusion and participation' among persons with disabilities is, however, highly variable across both time and geography. As far as human rights and the quality of the lived experience of disability are concerned, capacity is irrelevant.

So why focus our attention on capacity when we should be focusing on disability? Although public health prevention measures and better access to healthcare services have an impact on capacity rates, and although people with disabilities obviously have a human right to these services, as a general matter the human rights agenda is not primarily concerned about comparing capacity rates across countries. These rates tell us very little about the extent to which human rights are implemented or how the basic parameters of Active Citizenship are empowered by policy reform. By contrast, we should be very much concerned about differences in rates of disability across countries, as these rates demonstrate the impact of the environment on the lives of people with limitations in capacity. Differences in the rates of disability, across time and geography, provide information that is directly relevant to the fundamental issue of what difference reforms in social policy, or CRPD implementation, could make, if only we had the evidence to document that impact.

Defining disability in terms of the disability approach—which takes into account the impact of the physical, social and attitudinal environment on the lives of persons with health problems, impairments and capacity limitations—is consistent with the conceptualisation of Active Citizenship in DISCIT. In contrast, it is not clear that defining disability by the capacity approach is consistent with this conceptualisation, either in detail or in principle. That the capacity is more feasible cannot be doubted, but that it is irrelevant to the aspirations of DISCIT, and the CRPD, is equally certain.

Data-led or indicator-led approaches

A related challenge for data harmonisation concerns the general strategic decision whether to measure a complex social phenomenon or human rights value by developing only those indicators for which secure, preferably longitudinal data sources exist or rather to use a 'top-down' approach and begin with a conceptualisation and develop indicators in light of the operationalisation, without any consideration of whether there are stable data sources to serve the indicators. In short, are we more likely to know whether public policy reforms will improve the conditions for exercising Active Citizenship by prioritising indicators in light of actual social data collected, or by leading with indicators and seeking to influence data collection practices to collect relevant data?

The decision in DISCIT was to rely on the 'data-led' procedure since DISCIT, of necessity, has to take the definitions in national and European survey datasets as its point of departure. This is indeed a powerful motivation for proceeding as we have in the development of DISCIT indicators. Nonetheless, it raises the question whether innovative social research should be content to continue to reproduce results that embody either a definition of disability or a method of indicator development that ignores the starting point of critical disability research: that the lived experience of disability is not shaped entirely by a person's health condition, impairments and limitations in capacity, but by environmental barriers and facilitators, most of which are modifiable by social action.

European data: quality and availability

In the end, surprisingly, the challenge of data harmonisation for the DISCIT study seems to come down to the issue of existing European data and the question: what are the prospects of improving the quality and availability of European disability data for the purposes of social change?

We have already seen that many disability researchers acknowledge that the lack of availability of European data relevant to disability and useful for indicators of Active Citizenship and CRPD human rights implementation is a serious obstacle to better research and positive social change (e.g. Landman, 2004; Hoskins, 2006a; UK ONS, 2007; Van Oorschot, 2009). Given the enormous effort—at both the level of the United Nations system and at the national level—to solve the technical problems of monitoring the implementation of the CRPD, the question of data must eventually be addressed. There may well be sophisticated statistical methods to transform existing data, based on a capacity approach, into data that truly applies to the phenomenon of disability as a lived experience. Nonetheless, chances are that the only available route is to find better evidence, solidly grounded in the interactive person–environment conception of disability that underwrites not only the DISCIT study, but the CRPD as well.

Conclusion

What the effort to develop Active Citizenship–CRPD indicators has shown is that, given the large number of attributes linked to the CRPD Articles, most of the proposed DISCIT indicators are relevant to the most general statements of the CRPD, rather than to the many subprovisions of these rights. Indeed, several CRPD rights (Article 8 Awareness-raising; Article 9 Accessibility; Article 19 Living independently and being included in the community; Article 20 Personal mobility; Article 21 Freedom of expression and opinion, and access to information; Article 25 Health; Article 27 Work and employment; Article 28 Adequate standard of living and social protection and Article 29 Participation in political and public life—UN, 2007) essentially provide instructions to states parties about what specific measures they can take in order to implement the human right.

Besides revealing on-going issues of conceptualisation, definition and operationalisation, the DISCIT harmonisation exercise also exposed some open interpretative questions, both for research on Active Citizenship and how we understand CRPD. First, although the notion of Active Citizenship intuitively aligns with human rights involving personhood, political participation and social supports, the DISCIT research suggests it does not clearly align itself with education or participation in cultural life. Does this mean that the DISCIT approach was inadequate or that human rights to personhood and political participation are conceptually unrelated to education? Second, although CRPD firmly reinforces the DISCIT dimensions of Autonomy and Influence it conceives of them as positive freedoms rather than individual obligations. Is this a notable feature of human rights discourse in general, or merely a misinterpretation of Active Citizenship?

DISCIT research about how and when we can know that changes in policy and legislation improve the conditions for exercising Active Citizenship by persons with disabilities has merely scratched the surface. Certainly it has raised more questions and challenges than it has solved or resolved. But the fact that this chapter focuses almost entirely on challenges and obstacles to effective monitoring of change through socio-economic and experiential indicators should not be taken to mean that monitoring social change is not feasible. It is rather a recognition that only by pinpointing specific questions that need answers will it be possible to move forward towards innovations in our governance systems that can create not only stakeholder collaborations, but also coordinated policy instruments that can promote opportunities for persons with disabilities to participate.

References

Alkire, S., Bastagli, F., Burchardt, T., Clark, D., Holder, H., Ibrahim, S., Munoz, M., Terrazas, P., Tsang, T., and Vizard, P. (2009). *Developing the Equality Measurement Framework: Selecting the Indicators* (Researchreport: 31). Equality and Human Rights Commission. Retrieved 11 February 2017 from: http://eprints.lse.ac.uk/43745/

Bickenbach, Jerome. (2014). DISCIT: Making persons with disabilities full citizens: New knowledge for an inclusive and sustainable European social model. Deliverable 3.2. *Proposal for a Set of Indicators for Active Citizenship*. Retrieved 11 February 2017 from: https://blogg.hioa.no/discit

Bickenbach, Jerome. (2015). DISCIT: Making persons with disabilities full citizens: New knowledge for an inclusive and sustainable European social model. Deliverable 3.4 (D3.4) *Harmonization of Indicators for Active Citizenship and Proposed Indicators for Monitoring the Implementation of the CRPD in Europe*. Retrieved 11 February 2017 from: https://blogg.hioa.no/discit

De Weerd, M., Gemmeke, M., Rigter, J. & van Rij, C. (2005). *Indicators for Monitoring Active Citizenship and Citizenship Education*. Amsterdam: Regioplan Beleidsonderzoek.

DG Statistics and economic Information. Continuous Labour Force Survey. 2011. Retrieved 11 February 2017 from http://www.gesis.org/missy/files/documents/EU-LFS/BE_ahm2011_questionnaire_EN.pdf

Ebersold, S. (2007). Affiliating participation for Active Citizenship. *Scandinavian Journal of Disability Research*. 9(3–4), 237–253.

Edwards, M., Onyx, J., Maxwell, H., Darcy, S., Bullen, P., and Sherker, S. (2015). A conceptual model of social impact as Active Citizenship. *VOLUNTAS*. 26(4), 1529–1549.

European Agency for Fundamental Rights (FRA) (2014). *The Right to Political Participation for Persons with Disabilities: Human Rights Indicators*. Vienna: FRA. Retrieved 11 February 2017 from: http://fra.europa.eu/en/publication/2014/right-political-participation-persons-disabilities-summary

European Commission (2001). *Lisbon Strategy for Growth*. Retrieved 11 February 2017 from:http://ec.europa.eu/archives/growthandjobs_2009/

European Commission, Eurobarometer (n.d.). Retrieved 11 February 2017 from: http://ec.europa.eu/COMMFrontOffice/publicopinion/index.cfm

European Commission, Health and Social Integration Survey (EHSIS) (n.d.). Retrieved 11 February 2017 from:http://ec.europa.eu/eurostat/web/health/disability/data

European Commission, Labour Force Survey (EU LFS) (n.d.). Retrieved 11 February 2017 from:http://ec.europa.eu/eurostat/web/microdata/european-union-labour-force-survey

European Commission, Statistics of Income and Living Condition (EU-SILC) (n.d.). Retrieved 11 February 2017 from: http://ec.europa.eu/eurostat/web/income-and-living-conditions/overview

European Quality of Life Survey (EQLS) (n.d.). Retrieved 11 February 2017 from: http://www.eurofound.europa.eu/surveys/european-quality-of-life-surveys-eqls/european-quality-of-life-survey-2012

European Social Survey (ESS) (n.d.). Retrieved 11 February 2017 from: http://www.europeansocialsurvey.org/

Grammenos, S. (2009). *Indicators of Disability Equality in Europe: An Evaluative Report on the Feasibility of Using Existing Data Sources*. Retrieved from: http://www.disability-europe.net/theme/comparative-data/reports-comparative-data

Grammenos, S. (2010). ANED Task 4. *Preliminary List of Comparative Indicator Items for Pilot. Comparative Data on a Selection of Quantitative Implementation*

Indicators. Retrieved 11 February 2017 from: http://www.disability-europe.net/theme/comparative-data/reports-comparative-data

Grammenos, S. (2011). ANED Task 4. *Update and Extend the Piloting of Quantitative Implementation Indicators. Comparative Data on a Selection of Quantitative Implementation Indicators*. Retrieved 11 February 2017 from: http://www.disability-europe.net/theme/comparative-data/reports-comparative-data

Green, M. (2001). What we talk about when we talk about indicators: Current approaches to human rights measurement. *Journal of Social Indicator Research*. 23(4), 1062–1097.

Hästbacka, E. & Nygård, M. (2013). Disability and citizenship: Politicians' views on disabled persons' citizenship in Finland. *Scandinavian Journal of Disability Research*. 15(2), 1–18.

Hoskins, B. (2006a). *A Framework for the Creation of Indicators on Active Citizenship and Education and Training for Active Citizenship*. Ispra: Joint Research Centre. Retrieved 11 February 2017 from: http://farmweb.jrc.cec.eu.int/CRELL/ActiveCitizenship/Conference/01_Hoskins%20_framework_final.pdf

Hoskins, B. (2006b). Working towards indicators for Active Citizenship. Ispra: Joint Research Centre. Retrieved 11 February 2017 from: http://crell.jrc.ec.europa.eu/ActiveCitizenship/conference%20report%20final3.pdf

Hoskins, B. L., Jesinghaus, J., Mascherini, M., Munda, G., Nardo, M., Saisana, M. Van Nijlen, D., Vidoni, D. and Villalba, E. (2006). *Measuring Active Citizenship in* Europe, *Institute for the Protection and Security of the Citizen* (CRELL Research Paper 4). Retrieved 11 February 2017 from: http://crell.jrc.ec.europa.eu/ActiveCitizenship/conference%20report%20final3.pdf

Hoskins, B. & Mascherini, M. (2009). Measuring active citizenship through the development of a composite indicator. *Journal of Social Indicator Research*. 90(3), 459–488.

Landman, T. (2004). Measuring human rights: Principle, practice and policy. *Human Rights Quarterly*. 26(4), 906–931.

Madans, J. H., Mont, D. & Loeb, M. (2015). A comment on developing statistical measures of disability. *International Journal of Environmental Research and Public Health*, 12, 1– 3.

Mont, D. (2007). *Measuring Disability Prevalence. Social Protection*. (Discussion Paper Series, No. 0706). New York: The World Bank. Retrieved 11 February 2017 from: http://siteresources.worldbank.org/DISABILITY/Resources/Data/MontPrevalence.pdf.

Murray, C. J. L, Salomon, J. A., Mathers, C. D & Lopez, A. D. (Eds.) (2002). *Summary Measures of Population Health: Concepts, Ethics, Measurement and Applications*. Geneva: WHO.

Nardo, M., Saisana, M., Saltelli, A., Tarantola, S., Hoffman, A. & Giovannini, E. (2005). *Handbook on Constructing Composite Indicators: Methodology and User Guide*. (OECD Statistics Working Papers 2005/3). OECD Statistics Directorate. Retrieved 11 February 2017 from: http://www.oecd.org/els/soc/handbookonconstructingcomposite indicatorsmethodologyanduserguide.htm

Ravaud, J-F., Letourmy, A. & Ville, I. (2002). Identifying the population with disability: The approach of an INSEE survey on daily life and health. *Population-E 2002*, 57(3), 529–552.

Shakespeare, T. (2013). *Disability Rights and Wrongs Revisited*. New York: Routledge.

Tøssebro, J. & Kittelsaa, A. (2004). Studying the living conditions of disabled people: Approaches and problems. In J. Tøssebro & A. Kittelsaa (Eds.). *Exploring the Living Conditions of Disabled People* (17–43). Lund: Studentlitteratur.

UK Office for National Statistics (ONS) (2007). *Report from the Review of Equality Data*. Newport & London: Office for National Statistics. Retrieved 11 February 2017 from: http://www.google.ch/search?q=%22Report+from+the+review+of+equality+data%22

UK Office for National Statistics (2008). *Harmonised Concepts and Questions for Social Data Sources. Introduction to Harmonised Standards*. Version 3.0. Retrieved 11 February 2017 from: http://www.google.ch/search?q=%22Introduction+to+Harmonised+Standards%22

UK Office for National Statistics (2013). *A-Z Quick Reference Guide to Harmonised Concepts and Questions for Government Social Surveys*. Retrieved 11 February 2017 from: http://www.ons.gov.uk/ons/guidemethod/harmonisation/harmonisation-index-page/index.html

United Nations (2007). *Convention on the Rights of Persons with Disabilities*. G. A. Res. 61/106. Retrieved 11 February 2017 from: http://www.un.org/esa/socdev/enable/rights/convtexte.htm

United Nations (2008). *Report on Indicators for Promoting and Monitoring the Implementation of Human Rights*. HRI/MC/2008/3. Retrieved 11 February 2017 from: http://www2.ohchr.org/english/issues/indicators/docs/HRI.MC.2008.3_en.pdf

United Nations, Partnership to Promote the Rights of Persons with Disabilities (2014). UNPRPD: Strategic and Operational Framework. Retrieved 11 February 2017 from: http://www.undp.org/content/undp/en/home/librarypage/poverty-reduction/inclusive_development/disability-rights--he-un-partnership-to-promote-the-rights-of-pe.html

United Nations, Washington City Group Short Set (WCG) (n.d.). *Washington Group on* Disability Stati*stics: Development of Internationally Comparable Disability Measure for Censuses*. Retrieved 11 February 2017 from: https://www.cdc.gov/nchs/data/washington_group/meeting8/nso_report.pdf

University of Michigan. (2011). *Guidelines for Best Practice in Cross-Cultural Survey*. Institute for Social Research, Ann Arbor: University of Michigan. Retrieved 11 February 2017 from: http://ccsg.isr.umich.edu/

van Oorschot, W. (2009). *ANED: European Comparative Data on the Situation of Disabled People: An Annotated Review*. Retrieved 11 February 2017 from: http://www.disability-urope.net/theme/comparative-data/reports-comparative-data

Washington Group on Disability Statistics (2009) Understanding and Interpreting Disability as Measured using the WG Short Set of Questions, Retrieved 7 March 2017 from http://www.washingtongroup-disability.com

Weathers, R. R. (2009). The disability data landscape. In A. Houtenville, D.C. Stapleton, R.R. Weathers and R.V. Burkhauser. (Eds.). *Counting Working-Age People with Disabilities: What current data tell us and options for improvement.* (27–68). Kalamazoo, MI: Upjohn Institute.

World Economic Forum (WEF) (2013). *The Global Gender Gap Report, 2013*. Retrieved 11 February from: http://www3.weforum.org/docs/WEF_GenderGap_Report_2013.pdf.

World Health Organization (WHO) (2001). *International Classification of Functioning, Disability and Health*. Geneva: WHO. Retrieved 11 February from: http://www.who.int/classifications/icf/en/

World Health Organization (2011). *World Report on Disability*. Geneva: WHO.

World Health Organization (n.d.). *Model Disability Survey*. Retrieved 11 February from: http://www.who.int/disabilities/data/mds/en/

4 Operational definitions of disability

Usable in comparative research on Active Citizenship?

Jan Tøssebro and Bjørn Hvinden

The aim of this book is to address the extent to which European and national policies are enhancing the Active Citizenship of disabled people. In order to inform such an endeavour, it is essential to have access to reliable data, including data that provides the opportunity to compare the situation of disabled people over time and across countries. The purpose of this and the previous chapter is to address methodological challenges. Chapter 3 discusses issues related to empirical indicators of Active Citizenship, whereas the topic of this chapter is the translation of general notions about disability into measurements for use in survey research. This chapter, however, is not a traditional methods chapter outlining the choices of the DISCIT project. The purpose is wider, namely to discuss current challenges concerning the state of the art regarding current operationalisations employed in empirical research and statistics on disabled people, and in particular to identify possible problems when comparing the situation across countries or over time.

The reason for including a chapter on the methodology of disability measurement in this book is a set of observations that gives cause for concern. One such observation is the unexpected and inexplicable variation in the proportion of the population that is classified as disabled, both within and between Western countries. The variation is from well below 10 to more than 30 per cent (Dupré & Karjalainen, 2003; Fujiura & Rutkowski-Kmitta, 2001; OECD, 2003; Purdam et al., 2008; Ravaud et al., 2002; Tøssebro & Kittelsaa, 2004; Weathers, 2009). There is little reason to believe that such variation, especially the variation within countries, can be explained by differences in health status, individual functional limitations or societal barriers. Methodological explanations are more likely and the understanding of such mechanisms is essential both for the interpretation of research findings and for the future development of disability measurement.

We will structure the discussion according to four issues:

1 *The issue of different operationalisations*: Statistical agencies and researchers have adopted a variety of measurements to identify disabled people, and differences in this respect may affect research results. In order to isolate the effect of different operationalisations and to rule out variation due to language or cultural differences, we will discuss prevalence rates and overlap between different operationalisations when controlled for time and space, that is, within single countries and a short time span.

2 *The issue of comparisons across countries*: In order to rule out possible effects of different disability measurements, we ask whether identical or seemingly identical survey questions return similar disability prevalence rates in different countries. If there is variation that appears inexplicable, comparisons across countries can only be made with substantial reservations.
3 *The issue of comparisons over time*: Similarly, we ask whether similar or identical operationalisations 'behave' the same way over time within single countries. This will suggest to what extent current operational definitions permit reliable comparisons across time.
4 *The issue of the robustness of findings*: If there is unsatisfactory consistency across measurements, space and time regarding the prevalence and composition of the group classified as disabled, there is reason to be cautious regarding comparisons of results on Active Citizenship. We will look into possible evidence on the extent to which variation in disability definitions affects findings on social indicators. This is of particular relevance since the DISCIT project uses data from different sources, based on different operationalisations, for analysing changes over time and differences between countries.

The chapter builds largely on existing research. However, only very few studies address the basis for reliable comparative statistics in disability research. Thus, we also discuss findings that have other purposes but may illuminate the questions addressed here. In reality, this is mainly data on the proportion of a population classified as disabled. Thus, this chapter reviews a small number of studies on comparability and a set of reports on prevalence, which exist in English or a Scandinavian language.

Although the main topic of this chapter is assessment of empirical definitions used in existing data sources, the issue cannot be seen in isolation from debates on the theoretical understanding of disability. There is currently international consensus on an understanding that brings in the role of the societal environment in disabling processes, which is reflected both in the UN CRPD and WHO *International Classification of Functioning, Disability and Health* (ICF) (WHO, 2001). The development of empirical definitions, however, has to a limited extent taken this theoretical understanding into account (Altman, 2001). The possible tension between the measurements addressed and theoretical developments will therefore be discussed, before we sum up with a discussion of the prospects for future developments in disability operationalisations that are usable in comparative research on Active Citizenship.

The variety of operational definitions in surveys (and censuses)

The state of the art in disability measurement is that there exists no commonly accepted operationalisation (Altman, 2001; Leonardi et al., 2006; Molden & Tøssebro, 2010; Ravaud et al., 2002). Thus, before going into the consequences of different operationalisations, we need to outline the existing variety. Grönvik (2007) has suggested a classification of current disability measurements into five groups: subjective, functional, administrative, social, and relational. Some current operationalisations use items from more than one group, but for simplicity, we will restrict the discussion to these five groups.

Subjective definitions ask respondents to classify themselves, for instance by asking 'Do you have a long-standing health problem or disability that has lasted for 6 months or more or is expected to last 6 months or more?' (the 2001 EU Labour Force Survey). This type of question exists in a number of versions. In some cases, it is shorter: 'Do you have any long-standing illness, disability or infirmity?' (UK General Household Survey, 2001) or substantially longer, such as in the Disability supplements to Labour Force Surveys in Norway and Sweden, which include long lists of examples of disabilities. It is rather common, but not universal, that the subjective self-assessment question has a follow-up, for instance: 'Are you hampered in your daily activities by this chronic physical or mental health problem, illness or disability?', with the response options: '(i) yes, severely; (ii) yes, to some extent; (iii) no' (Eurostat, 2001). Thus, subjective disability measurements build on one or a few self-assessing questions, but the questions are not identical. It is rather a family of self-assessments. This type of measurement is typical in international surveys like the EU-SILC, the European Social Survey and the European Community Household Panel, but less dominant in national surveys.

Functional definitions adopt a set of questions on specific activity limitations or functional difficulties. Typical questions include 'Can you walk up and down stairs? Is your eyesight good enough to read ordinary newspaper print?'. The OECD proposed a list of ten such items 35 years ago (McWhinnie, 1982). More recently the Washington Group on Disability Statistics has proposed a Short Set of six items, as well as an extended version (Washington Group on Disability Statistics 2009). A person is classified as disabled if they respond affirmatively to one or more items. In the language of ICF, such questions address specific activity limitations. There are, however, also examples of questions on what the ICF terms participation restrictions, such as 'Do you have a reduced ability to work', or 'Do you have difficulties using public transport?' In Grönvik's (2007) overview, activity and participation questions are seen as parts of the same family. Some may object to this but that is not our point here. The point is that functional definitions are strategically very different from general self-assessment; they employ specific questions and leave less space for subjective interpretations. However, subjective and functional definitions have one thing in common: we find a variety of versions of both types (Hahn & Pool Hegamin, 2001).

Administrative definitions are based on some kind of official recognition of disability. In some countries one can apply for a (green) card that is an explicit official recognition (Ravaud et al., 2002; the 2002 British Household Panel Survey), whereas in other countries administrative definitions classify people according to reception of benefits or services, like the work incapacity benefit. Such definitions are widely used, but often in research with a more narrow focus than disabled people in general. One example is the research on resettlement from institutions, where registers of people using the services were used to select samples. Administrative definitions occur in more general surveys as well, sometimes as the only item but more often in combination with functional questions.

Social and relational definitions are more in keeping with current theoretical definitions. They bring in the impact of the environment, with full focus on the environment in the social definitions, whereas the relational version points to the interaction between the individual and environmental barriers. There were some early attempts or outlines of how such understanding could be operationalised in empirical research (e.g., Abberley, 1992; Oliver, 1990) but until recently there have been few examples of real use. The few recent examples build on the logic of the ICF and consequently a relational definition: the 2012 European Health and Social Integration Survey (EHSIS) (Eurostat, 2015a) and surveys in developing countries by Loeb and Eide (2006). Results from those surveys are to some extent introduced into the discussion below, but since there are few results to draw upon, such definitions will mainly be addressed in the later section on theoretical validity.

Different operationalisations within countries

Reports using different operationalisations of disability tend to show substantial variation in disability prevalence rates, and this appears to occur across the board, in a number of countries. It is, among others, reported from France, the US and Norway (Ravaud et al., 2002; Tøssebro & Kittelsaa, 2004; Weathers, 2009). Weathers (2009) shows that in five data sources from 2002–2003 using different methodologies and definitions, the prevalence rates in the US vary from 5.5 to 18.7 per cent of the population. Tøssebro and Kittelsaa (2004) report variation from 7 to 30 per cent in Norway.

We will not go into detail about the variation in other countries, partly because results are so clear in the three countries, but mainly for the following reason: the variation in prevalence rates may be due to operationalisations of disability but also to sampling strategies and other methodological choices. There are, to our knowledge, only two studies that control for such possibilities. Both studies build on one national dataset, thus ruling out the possibility that methodological aspects other than operationalisation cause the variation (Molden & Tøssebro, 2010, 2012; Ravaud et al., 2002). These studies provide the opportunity to isolate the effects of measurements, and present data on prevalence rates and also on the extent to which the populations identified by different operationalisations overlap.

The study by Ravaud et al. (2002) built on a short screening questionnaire administered to 0.67 per cent of the French population during the 1999 census. It consisted of 18 items on disability that provided the opportunity to construct five different disability definitions: a functional definition (seven items), self-assessment (one item), official recognition/administrative definition (one item), services/assistive technology (also administrative, three items), and restrictions in everyday life activities for six months or more (also self-assessment, one item). The variation in disability prevalence was from 5.2 to 21.1 per cent of the population.

The most interesting part of the results is, however, the findings on overlap of people across definitions. One could expect that people classified by the low prevalence definitions were subsets of the high prevalence definitions. This appeared only partly to be the case. The authors tested overlap for three definitions: the functional, the administrative (services), and self-assessment (restrictions) definitions. Among people aged 17 to 59 years, only 10 per cent of those classified by one of the definitions were disabled by all three; 74 per cent were classified as disabled by only one of the three definitions. Thus, the study concluded that not only did different operationalisations return very different prevalence rates, the groups of people categorized as disabled by different definitions were only partly overlapping. One was simply dealing with different groups of people.

The 2010 report by Molden and Tøssebro built on a 2007 dataset on the living conditions of disabled people in Norway. The dataset provided the opportunity to test prevalence rates, overlap and results on dependent variables for ten disability operationalisations in use in Norway and other countries. It included functional, administrative, and self-assessment definitions, as well as existing definitions combining the three strategies in Norway, the US and Australia. The Washington Group Short Set was among the definitions. Molden and Tøssebro found prevalence rates ranging from 9.7 to 27.8 per cent. Self-assessment led to the highest disability prevalence rate in Norway, whereas in France the functional definition returned the highest rates (Ravaud et al., 2002). Thus, it was not the same type of definition that returned the higher disability rates in the two countries.

Molden and Tøssebro (2010) reported a degree of agreement between all pairs of definitions according to the Cohen's Kappa statistic (which measures consistency taking the skewedness of distributions into account, which is necessary when addressing small or medium-sized groups). They excluded pairs with a substantial overlap in items. Of the remaining 43 pairs, seven had an acceptable consistency (Kappa above 0.40) and only three pairs had good agreement (Kappa above 0.60). All pairs with acceptable agreement were between definitions using functional items. Neither the subjective nor the administrative definitions reached acceptable agreement with any other definition. Molden and Tøssebro also showed that if one only included people reporting severe limitations in everyday life, the agreement across definitions was higher.

In another report, the authors went into detail concerning the consequences of the lack of consistency across definitions (Molden & Tøssebro, 2012). This analysis suggested that distributions according to gender, age, marital status and when in the life course the person acquired the impairment were similar across empirical definitions. On the other hand, the type and severity of impairment varied considerably. The subjective definition classified significantly more people with chronic pain, and fewer with mental health problems and cognitive difficulties. On the other hand, the functional Washington Group definition classified more people with cognitive and mobility difficulties. There were in particular variations across definitions regarding whether people with mental health difficulties were classified as disabled or not.

The conclusion should be clear. Different definitions do not only return different prevalence rates. The people they classify as disabled constitute only partly overlapping groups. The reason is likely to be that different definitions have a different 'appeal' to people with different types and degrees of disability. We will, however, come back to this. The conclusion at this point is that existing evidence suggests caution regarding comparisons of results from reports using different operational definitions of disability. The risk of comparing 'apples and pears' is substantial.

Same operational definition: Comparing prevalence across countries

Despite a number of initiatives (Fujiura & Rutkowski-Kmitta, 2001), there appears to be little coordination across countries when it comes to operational definitions of disability. This in particular applies to the functional type of definitions, which are rarely the same or similar across countries and thus unlikely to be comparable. As for administrative definitions, these are strongly linked to national benefit or service systems and the group identified will reflect the design of these systems. Since benefit and service systems are dissimilar, such definitions are unlikely to be reliable in cross-national comparisons and will not be considered further. Thus, the main example of largely similar definitions that are used across countries is the subjective type of definitions, which has been employed in a number of European surveys. There is also one example of a European survey using a relational definition (Eurostat, 2015a).

The European surveys employing subjective definitions have returned consistent results: the same global self-assessment question does *not* operate uniformly across countries as measured by prevalence rates. The European Labour Force Survey in 2002 suggested national prevalence rates ranging from 6.6 (Italy) to 32.2 per cent (Finland) among the then 15 EU member states (Dupré & Karjalainen, 2003). This variation is consistent with results from the European Social Survey and the European Community Household Panel (Blekesaune, 2007), suggesting the lowest prevalence of 6 to 7 per cent and a highest rate of 31 to 37 per cent. The 2008 EU-SILC dataset showed variation on a question on chronic health conditions ranging from 13 (Romania, Italy) to more than 30 per cent (Finland, Slovenia). On a question on limitations in activities, prevalence varied from 9 per cent in Bulgaria to 26 per cent in Latvia. The results from the relational EHSIS data are by and large the same. The prevalence varies from 6.1 per cent in Italy to 20.1 per cent in Norway (Eurostat, 2015a).

Although functional operationalisations are rarely sufficiently similar to make it worthwhile to compare prevalence rates, there exist a few reports from studies in African countries that suggest interesting results. In general, such countries tend to report low prevalence rates (Fujiura & Rutkowski-Kmitta, 2001), but two studies (Loeb et al., 2008; Schneider et al., 2009) that use the Washington Group Short Set (functional) show prevalence rates that are not very far from figures typically reported from Western countries: 14.5 per cent in Zambia (Loeb et al., 2008) and while figures from South Africa are more problematic to extract because all ages are included, the prevalence rate there is 19.4 per cent among people aged 25 to 34 (Schneider et al., 2009). These results suggest that it may be possible to develop disability measurements based on a functional approach that can be more reliable in comparative research. This, however, is so far unknown.

Yet, the Disability supplement to the 2011 European Labour Force Survey (ELFS) also adopted functional questions (Eurostat, 2015b). The result was a variation in prevalence across countries on a par with the subjective self-assessment, from 5.3 per cent in Ireland to 23.5 per cent in Austria. However, this may be a result of how the 2011 ELFS phrased the questions about activity limitations; first asking people whether they had any activity difficulties (*yes* or *no*), and then asking a follow-up question on what kind of activity difficulty was the most and second most important. Thus, due to the very general first question, the specificity of typical functional definitions was lost.

The conclusion is that one cannot use subjective operational definitions for the purpose of comparison without strong reservations and the same applies to the one relational definition (EHSIS) we looked at. Some research using a functional approach shows results that appear more encouraging but this is yet uncertain.

Same operational definition: Comparing prevalence over time

As for comparison over time, one may expect more optimistic conclusions since sources of variation are fewer (see Discussion section below), at least in the short and medium term. The longest time series known to us is from the US (Houtenville et al., 2009). This study presents figures from the early 1980s until 2007 for four disability measurements. The prevalence rates vary considerably across measurements (from 2.3 to 8.8 per cent in 2006), but not over time. For three of the measures, variation over time is minor. The measurement with more variation is not directly a disability measurement but a question on work limitations. This varies over time from 8.3 to 11.4 per cent of the population. The variation on this measure is unsystematic but may reflect business cycles.

Similar patterns of stability are evident in the Norwegian Disability Supplement to the Labour Force Surveys (subjective definition), showing minor variation around 16 to 17 per cent of the population from 2002 to 2014 (Bø & Håland, 2014). The same consistency is also found in the Norwegian part of EU-SILC from 2003 to 2006 and the living conditions surveys of Statistics Norway in 2002 and 2005 (Normann & Rønning, 2008). The variation in prevalence across series with different operational definitions is substantial (from 15 to 28 per cent), but not over time in series using the same definition of disability. The UK censuses in 2001 and 2011 also show minor differences over time in England and Wales, although the question was slightly modified (Office for National Statistics, 2013).

Other examples of time series data show moderate changes in prevalence over time, such as the Swedish and Danish labour force surveys. In Sweden the variation from 1996 to 2013 was from 15.5 to 21.4 per cent, but with good stability since 2004 (Statistics Sweden, 2014). In Denmark, the prevalence rate varies from 15.9 to 19.8 per cent from 2002 to 2014. However, variation is minor from 2008 (Larsen & Høgelund, 2015).

Data from EU-SILC 2005–2011 also suggests reasonable stability on the question of health problems that limit activities for more than six months. This stability applies to the European level and in general also individual countries—but not without exceptions. In a few countries there were years where prevalence was more than 5 percentage points off the opposite extreme. There was for instance a drop in Italy in 2010 (but back again in 2011) and increases in Slovenia from 2009 to 2010 (Grammenos, 2013). We do not know whether countries with less stability in prevalence rates made changes to their national versions of the questionnaire in these years.

In total, the conclusion is that there are clearly fewer reservations regarding comparison over time, compared to that over space or across different measurements. Thus, research on changes in Active Citizenship over time can be done with fewer reservations, which also opens up the possibility to relate changes in Active Citizenship to policy changes.

Robustness of research results

The analysis so far suggests substantial reservations regarding comparisons across reports if the empirical definition varies and, if the same subjective definition was used, also across countries. There are fewer reservations related to comparisons within a country over time. These conclusions are, however, reached by mainly looking at prevalence rates, and partly on agreement across definitions regarding the composition of the group classified as disabled. On the other hand, some findings suggest that results on outcome variables are not necessarily very sensitive to disability definitions. The variation regarding demographic variables, such as gender and age distribution, was minor even though the variation in overall prevalence was substantial (confer section on Different operationalisations within countries; source Molden & Tøssebro, 2012). If this is the case for social indicators as well, conclusions about the dubious reliability of comparisons may be too pessimistic.

The current literature comprises few reports that are informative on this issue. We have only located one: Molden and Tøssebro's 2012 report. There are, however, indications in a few other studies, mainly related to employment rates. The Molden and Tøssebro study was constructed to look at the consequences of employing a diverse set of current disability measurements. Regarding results on social indicators, they compared seven different disability measurements, comprising administrative, subjective, functional and combined definitions. They looked at educational level, income and employment and found minor consequences of definitions regarding results on education and income. However, when it came to employment, the differences were substantial with disability employment rates varying from 32.2 to 55.8 per cent across empirical definitions. This result is not very far from equalling the top and bottom in Europe within one national dataset.

Blekesaune (2007) looked at disability employment rates in 24 European countries related to, among others, the prevalence rates of disabled people. The employment rate of disabled people was moderately correlated with the proportion of the population classified as disabled (r = 0.30). The positive correlation between disability prevalence and disability employment rates suggests that if more people are classified as disabled, it is likely that the group consists of either more people with a mild disability, or of more people with a type of impairment that has higher employment rates (for instance people with moderate hearing problems or diabetes). A similar pattern was evident in the Molden and Tøssebro (2012) study in Norway. The rank order of prevalence and disability employment rates had a full fit, if the administrative definition was excluded (to exclude this definition is reasonable, since it almost automatically includes all people out of employment (receiving the work incapacity benefit)). Thus, it appears that prevalence rates affect employment rates, and that this most likely has methodological explanations. This undermines the potential of comparisons across countries with different disability prevalence rates.

We have also looked at the published country data from the 2011 disability ad hoc module included in the European Labour Force Survey (Eurostat, 2015b and data published on web). This suggests that the correlation between the employment rate of people reporting basic activity limitations and the disability prevalence rate was between 0.63 and 0.71, depending on disability definition. It is 0.71 with the activity limitations disability measure and 0.63 with the combined activity limitations and long-standing health problems measure.

Figure 4.1 shows the relation between the disability prevalence rate and disability employment rate in a regression model that also introduces the affluence of the country and level of public spending on disability-related benefits. The disability definition employed is the proportion reporting difficulties in basic activities. It clearly suggests that the proportion of the population that reports having a disability

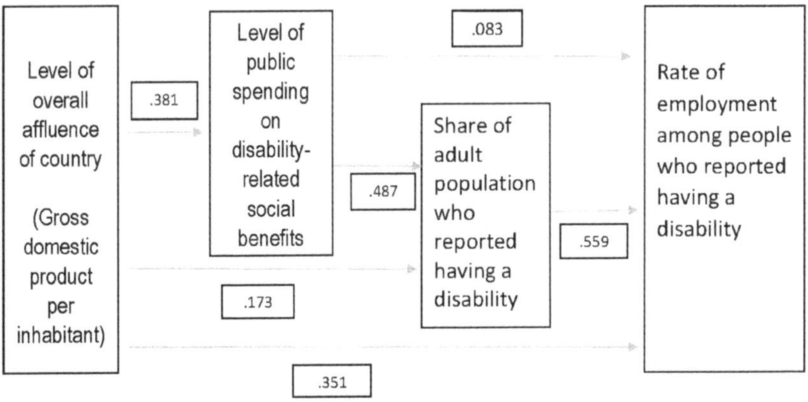

Figure 4.1 Simple linear regression analysis of variables predicting countries' rate of employment among persons who reported having a disability for 30 European countries, 2011.

Explanatory note: The small boxes show standardized linear regression coefficients for the relationships between variables at the end of each arrow (adjusted R squared = 0.618). The 30 European countries are Belgium, Bulgaria, Czech Republic, Denmark, Germany, Estonia, Ireland, Greece, Spain, France, Croatia, Italy, Cyprus, Latvia, Lithuania, Luxembourg, Hungary, Malta, Netherlands, Austria, Poland, Portugal, Romania, Slovenia, Slovakia, Finland, Sweden, United Kingdom, Iceland and Switzerland.

Source of data: Eurostat Database (2016).

affects the disability employment rate, a finding that must until proven otherwise be considered a methodological construct. On the other hand, a similar analysis of material deprivation among disabled people suggests that the disability prevalence rate does not affect the measured level of deprivation. Thus, the impact of the definition on results is *not* uniform across social indicators.

A final source of information is a US collection of papers, reporting results on employment, household income and poverty by different empirical definitions of disability. They show clear differences between four disability measurements of employment rates, but also that the differences are stable over time and that all show a slightly downward trend in disability employment rates since the late 1980s (Weathers & Wittenburg, 2009). As for median household income, two disability definitions are compared with moderately different results (ratio to the population respectively 0.58 and 0.45: Burkhauser et al., 2009). Furthermore, according to Burkhauser et al. (2009), poverty rates are clearly above that of the population in general, and vary among data sources with different disability definitions from 18.8 to 29.0 per cent.

Thus, the limited evidence we have been able to present here suggests that variation in the methodology of disability definitions does impact on results. It is, however, not so across the board. Definitions appear to have less impact on demographic variables, education and income (in Norway), and the level of material deprivation between European countries. However, the impact on disability employment rates is clear, and is also evident for poverty rates in the US. Although findings on some social indicators appear to be more robust and less sensitive to disability definitions, it will in general be too optimistic to rule out effects similar to those on employment. The general advice is that caution is required.

Current operationalisations and the theoretical understanding

Most operationalisations of disability are subjective, administrative or functional, whereas the current theoretical understanding is social or relational, which brings in the role of the environmental barriers people encounter, either fully (social) or in interaction with individual characteristics (relational). The mismatch between concept and measurement has been attributed to the fact that operational definitions tend to lag behind theoretical developments (Altman, 2001), or more strongly, that they are based on an outdated medical model of disability. Another possible interpretation is that operationalisations tend to be practical endeavours that pay little attention to the theoretical aspects of the concept. This interpretation probably described well the state of the art before 2000, but for the last 15 years substantial attention has been paid to the mismatch between theoretical and operational definitions, not least due to the international recognition of the ICF. There may be a number of reasons for the continuing mismatch, but we will argue first, that the problem is related to the logic and structure of social surveys; second, that the problem is exaggerated; and third, that there are some practical limitations related to a number of disability-specific questions in general surveys.

In social surveys, a primary aim is to compare the situation of a group with that of other groups or over time. The social groups are typically identified by individual characteristics such as gender, age, disability, and such like. However, the social and relational concepts of disability basically refer to disabling processes or individual-environment interactions rather than individual characteristics. However, on the other hand, the definitions do also refer to a specific group of people who could be identified by individual characteristics: that is, by impairments. Disabling processes are not about any kind of barriers that any kind of people may encounter. They are about factors that are barriers for *people with impairments* but not for people without impairments. The question thus arises whether such barriers need to be incorporated in the definition of disability or if this can be addressed equally well or better by separate measurements of disabling processes. If the definition of the group is separated from indicators of barriers, this means that the social group studied is not disabled people according to the theoretical concept, but people with impairments. Nevertheless, the study itself may address disability and disabling processes.

There is a set of arguments for keeping items on impairment and disabling processes separate in survey research. First, there is the risk of running into tautologies if the empirical definition identifies the group by means of the barriers or social consequences that members of the group experience. Examples of research questions in disability studies are to what extent disabled people encounter problems in the labour market or with public transport. But if disabled people are defined as people who experience barriers in the labour market or on public transport, it should be no surprise if they experience problems. This is part of the definition, as those who do not experience barriers are by definition excluded. However, it would be more interesting to know if there are mechanisms in, for instance, the labour market that disable and exclude people with impairments. This requires separation of measurements as one will want to know how typical it is that people with impairments are disabled. A partly related argument is that indicators of disabling processes have more in common with intermediate or outcome variables (social consequences) than variables identifying social groups. Barriers related to employment are better understood as part of the marginalisation processes in the labour market, and this will be impossible to address in survey research if barriers are a predefined characteristic of the social group.

This relates to what kind of research questions one can possibly address, or better, how research results can be interpreted. For example, if one makes policy innovations in order to improve accessibility to public transport, the results of a survey of people with impairments can easily evaluate whether people with reduced sight, hearing or mobility, experience fewer problems, provided adequate questions on problems with public transport are included. However, if barriers are built into the definition of the group, real changes in accessibility will not be measured with outcome variables but will come out as a reduction in the prevalence of disability. Such a result will in principle be interesting but in practice hardly of much use because it will be impossible to rule out the likelihood that the reduction is due to sampling bias or methodological issues. This problem can of course be solved by asking respondents about impairments as well as barriers, but in such a case, we do in principle separate items on impairments from items on social consequences. Such a strategy was used in the relational definitions in a survey in African countries by Loeb and Eide (2006) and the European EHSIS (Eurostat, 2015a). Both build explicitly on the relational approach of the ICF. Our argument, however, is that in such cases the relational approach is not very different from a functional one. Let us use the EHSIS as an example.

The EHSIS survey comprises, on the one hand, a subjective definition and a set of functional items and, on the other, questions on barriers related to ten life domains. Disabled people are defined as those who encounter barriers in at least one domain. In conceptualisation and arguments, the EHSIS is clearly diverging from earlier atheoretical operationalisations and takes environmental barriers into account. However, in practical use, the difference is modest. The main difference in the questionnaire itself is that the number of questions about barriers and disabling processes far exceeds that of typical social surveys. In the data analysis process, there is, furthermore, the difference that the items on barriers are made part of the definition of disability. The consequence of merging impairment and barriers questions in the definition of the group, however, is that one risks running into the problems outlined above (tautology, not being able to measure effects of policy changes). In fact, one is able to say more about disabling processes by not making barriers a part of the definition of the social group but instead using them as indicators of marginalisation processes.

There are also practical considerations, which are less important in our context. In the EHSIS and the Loeb and Eide (2006) surveys, the number of questions on disablement is large and constitutes a substantial part of the survey. This may be defended in specific disability surveys but is less likely to be accepted in general surveys. There is a need for a short set of questions that can be included in general surveys since such surveys are conducted more frequently and on a wide range of social topics. General surveys also provide the opportunity to compare disabled people (people with impairments) with other groups. The possibility of addressing disability in such surveys is lost if one opts only for empirical definitions that require a large set of questions.

Based on these arguments, it is our view that the non-theoretical and practical nature of disability operationalisations is less of a threat to validity than assumed, provided relevant social indicators are part of the survey. There may of course be good and not so good operationalisations but it is a minor problem in itself that environmental barriers are not a part of the empirical definitions. In fact, we will argue that separation of measures on impairment and disabling processes are in keeping with a relational definition of disability.

Discussion: why this fluidity?

The analyses in this chapter suggest that the current basis for comparative survey research on disability is weak and that results must be interpreted with reservations. Our findings suggest that different empirical definitions are likely to return dissimilar prevalence rates and one cannot rule out that this also affects results on social indicators and Active Citizenship variables. The findings suggest that similar subjective definitions in different countries, languages and cultures can hardly be considered to be similar after all. The potential for comparison over time with the same definition appears better. The general impression, however, is that the concept of disability (impairment) appears unexpectedly sensitive to subtle nuances when it comes to empirical definitions.

A number of points have been proposed to explain the cross-national differences in prevalence rates. The bottom line is that since 'disability cannot be measured against an objective standard' (Barnartt, 2010: 5), it is likely to be affected by a number of contextual factors. This is discussed by Barnartt (2010), amongst others. One possibility is that the same items are not similar after all when translated into national *languages*. This may be due to different choices when constructing the national versions of survey questions and/or to the fact that the terms used across languages may have the same denotation, but different connotations. This is likely to interact with *cultural differences* concerning the conception of disability. This could, amongst other factors, relate to how severe an impairment needs to be before people classify themselves disabled ('Is my vision poor enough to call it a disability?'), but also to variation regarding specific types of disabilities ('Are allergies a disability?', 'What about mental health problems?'). Cultural differences may also affect the willingness to disclose invisible impairments, possibly because of associated stigmas, but even in milder versions where people's self-image is 'I have a health problem, not a disability'.

Another point refers to *administrative systems*, such as the welfare system. It has been argued that people are less likely to feel associated with the concept if it does not have any consequences or lead to any rights. This link to support systems is probably the reason why disability prevalence tends to be low in countries with underdeveloped welfare systems (Loeb & Eide, 2004). The concept has no parallel in social structures and it is of minor practical utility. However, the impact may go well beyond core welfare provisions like incapacity benefits and assistive technology. A former student of the first author claimed that 'I never called my dyslexia a disability before entering the university and needing to apply for an extra hour at exams'. Administrative systems may also interact with language differences. Going back to before the 1960s in Norway, for instance, the current general disability notion was rarely in use. The preferred terms referred either to work incapacity or specific types of disability, such as blindness or deafness. In such a setting, general questions on disability would most likely return substantially lower prevalence rates than at present.

These explanations refer mainly to the context-dependency of the lay concept of disability, and this will obviously affect national response patterns. However, the fluidity goes beyond context-dependency, which is illustrated by the above outlined studies of Ravaud et al. (2002) and Molden and Tøssebro (2010). People with different types and degrees of disability appear to feel that they are in or out of the group, based on the wording of the empirical definition. An analysis by Tøssebro (2012) suggests that very small nuances in the wording affect responses.

He compared distribution of types of impairments in the Norwegian and Swedish supplements to the Labour Force Surveys. The definitions are intended to be the same, but there are some nuances concerning impairments that are listed as examples of disabilities. This applies to sensory impairments, diabetes, intellectual disabilities and mental health problems. The result is similar prevalence rates, but substantial differences in the distribution of types of impairments. The proportion with hearing problems and diabetes in Sweden is more than twice that in Norway, whereas more people with mental health problems are classified with impairments in Norway.

A rather different example concerns response stability. Longitudinal studies of individual self-classifications show unexpectedly low stability. In Norway (Normann & Rønning, 2008) and the UK (Burchardt, 2000) researchers have employed data spanning four to six waves to explore the issue, employing the same subjective definition across waves. The disability prevalence rates were similar over the waves in both countries, but individual movements in and out of the group were substantial. In Norway, 20 per cent classified themselves as disabled every year, but only 8 per cent in all four years of the panel. The proportion classifying themselves as disabled through all panel waves was even lower in the UK. The typical pattern was that people responded affirmatively to the disability classification only once, in a few consecutive waves, or moved in and out of the disability classification (Burchardt, 2000). The low stability may of course reflect changes in health status, and for some types of impairments, like pain or mental health problems, this is not unexpected. But by and large, the pattern of responses suggests that this is not the full explanation. The low stability may equally well be due to the uncertainty respondents feel when asked a rather general question about disability. It was shown a number of years ago that in such circumstances, response stability tends to be low, for instance regarding quality of life measures (Mastekaasa et al., 1988). Although the concept of disability has a relatively clear core related to mobility, sensory and intellectual faculties, these are parts of a very heterogeneous group of attributes with no clear line of demarcation to separate it from non-disabled people or health issues that most people are less likely to classify as disability or impairment. Disability classifications are based on dichotomisation where no such binary boundaries exist. The result is that disability, outside the core, turns out to be a fluid concept in everyday life. This fluidity is likely to make self-classifications subject to subtle nuances related to the exact phrasing of questions, and also to contextual and situational factors, even to a person's mood on the day.

The question is what consequences this fluidity has for the future development of disability or impairment measurements that will be usable in comparative research on Active Citizenship. General subjective self-classifications in particular tend to be exposed to the fluidity of the disability notion. It appears to be a better choice to employ items that are as concrete as possible and with as little context dependency as possible. This is unlikely to be possible for questions on disability in general, but may be applicable for questions on types of impairments, such as problems seeing or hearing. Thus, prospects appear to be better for functional definitions, like those proposed by the OECD in the 1980s and more recently by the Washington Group on Disability Statistics (2009). The results of the surveys from African countries by Loeb et al. (2008) and Schneider et al. (2009) are in this respect encouraging. The development of such a type of functional definition can also be made relational by adding survey items on societal barriers and disabling processes.

Our main reservations regarding empirical definitions using a set of functional items is that such a definition is likely to exclude people with impairments not explicitly specified among survey items. There may be a trade-off between possibilities for comparative research and a definition that includes the full heterogeneity of impairments. However, our intention is, in this chapter, to suggest possible routes for future developments rather than to argue for a specific solution. The current state of affairs is that we really do not know which type of measures would be more reliable in comparative research, but the results shown in this chapter indicate that there is a need for future efforts to develop more usable empirical definitions.

Finally, we need to state some reservations and shortcomings regarding the line of argument in this chapter. There are few studies that explicitly address the issues explored here and our conclusions are thus based on few reports and also on arguments based primarily on variation in prevalence rates. Although this is a reservation, the plea following from this is consistent with the general conclusion of the chapter: there is a need for more research into the methodology of empirical definitions of disability.

References

Abberley, P. (1992). Counting us out: A discussion of the OPCS disability surveys. *Disability, Handicap and Society*, 7, 139–155

Altman, B. M. (2001). Disability definitions, models, classification, schemes, and applications. In G. L. Albrecht, K. D. Seelman & M. Bury (Eds.). *Handbook of Disability Studies* (97–122). London: Sage.

Barnartt, S. (2010). Disability as a fluid state (Introduction). In S. Barnartt (Ed.). *Disability As a Fluid State* (1–22). Bingley, UK: Emerald.

Blekesaune, M. (2007). *Have some European Countries Been More Successful at Employing Disabled People Than Others?* ISER Working paper. Colchester: University of Essex.

Bø, T. P. & Håland, I. (2014). *Funksjonshemma på arbeidsmarknaden I 2014* [Disabled People in the Labour Market, 2014]. Oslo: Statistics Norway.

Burchardt, T. (2000). *The Dynamics of being Disabled.* CASE paper 36, 2000. London: London School of Economics.

Burkhauser, R., Houtenville, A. & Rovba, L. (2009). Poverty. In A. Houtenville, D. Stapleton, R. Weathers & R. Burkhauser (Eds.). *Counting Working-Age People with Disabilities* (193–226). Kalamazoo, MI: Upjohn Institute.

Burkhauser, R., Rovba, L. & Weathers, R. (2009). Household income. In A. Houtenville, D. Stapleton, R. Weathers & R. Burkhauser (Eds.). *Counting Working-Age People with Disabilities* (145–192). Kalamazoo, MI: Upjohn Institute.

Dupré, D. & Karjalainen, A. (2003). Employment of disabled people in Europe in 2002. *Eurostat, Statistics in Focus*. Population and Social Conditions, Theme 3 – 26/2003.

European Union (2001). *Labour Force Survey.*

Eurostat (2001). Disability and Social Participation in Europe. Luxembourg, Office for Official Publications of the European Communities, European Commission

Eurostat (2011). *Database, European Labour Force Survey 2011*. Retrieved 10 February 2016 from http://ec.europa.eu/eurostat/data/database.

Eurostat (2015a). *European Health and Social Integration Survey (EHSIS)*. Retrieved 29 February 2016 from: http://ec.europa.eu/eurostat/statistics-explained/index.php/Disability_statistics_-_barriers_to_social_integration

Eurostat (2015b). *Employment of Disabled People*. Luxembourg: Publications Office of the EU.

Fujiura, G. & Rutkowski-Kmitta, V. (2001). Counting disability. In G. L. Albrecht, K. D. Seelman & M. Bury (Eds.). *Handbook of Disability Studies* (69–96). London: Sage.

Grammenos, S. (2013). *European Comparative Data on Europe 2020 and People with Disabilities*. ANED report. Retrieved on 29 February 2016 from: http://www.disability-europe.net/theme/statistical-indicators/new-statistical-indicators-eu2020

Grönvik, L. (2007). *Definitions of Disability in Social Sciences. Methodological Perspectives*. Uppsala: Uppsala University.

Hahn, H., & Pool Hegamin, A. (2001). Assessing scientific measures of disability. *Journal of Disability Studies*, 12, 114–121.

Houtenville, A., Potamites, E., Erickson, W. & Ruiz-Quintanilla, A. (2009) Disability prevalence and demographics. In A. Houtenville, D. Stapleton, R. Weathers & R. Burkhauser (Eds.). *Counting Working-Age People with Disabilities* (69–100). Kalamazoo, MI: Upjohn Institute.

Larsen, M. R. & Høgelund, J. (2015). *Handicap og beskæftigelse* [Disability and Employment]. Copenhagen: SFI.

Leonardi, M., Bickenbach, J., Üstün, T., Kostanjsek, N. & Chatterji, S. (2006). The definitions of disability: What is in a name? *The Lancet*, 368, 1219–1221.

Loeb, M. & Eide, A. (2004). Exploring living conditions among people with disabilities in southern areas of Africa. In J. Tøssebro & A. Kittelsaa (Eds.). *Exploring the Living Conditions of Disabled People* (65–81). Lund: Studentlitteratur.

Loeb, M. & Eide, A. (2006). Paradigms lost: The changing face of disability in research. In B. Altman & S. N. Barnartt (Eds.). *International Views on Disability Measures: Moving Toward Comparative Measurement* (111–127). Oxford: Elsevier.

Loeb, M., Eide, A. & Mont, D. (2008). Approaching the measurement of disability prevalence: The case of Zambia. *Alter*, 2, 32–43.

McWhinnie, J. (1982). *Measuring Disability*. Paris: OECD.

Mastekaasa, A., Moum, T., Næss, S. and Sørensen, T. (1988). *Livskvalitetsforskning* [Quality of Life Research]. Oslo: ISF.

Molden, T. & Tøssebro, J. (2010). Measuring disability in survey research. *Alter*, 4, 174–189.

Molden, T. & Tøssebro, J. (2012). Disability measurements: Impact on research results. *Scandinavian Journal of Disability Research*, 14, 340–357.

Normann, T. & Rønning, E. (2008). *EU-SILC (Norge) som kilde til å avgrense gruppen av personer med nedsatt funksjonsevne* [EU-SILC (Norway) as a Source to Define People with Impairments]. Oslo: Statistics Norway.

OECD (2003). *Transforming Disability into Ability*. Paris: OECD.

Office for National Statistics (2013). *Disability in England and Wales: 2011 and Comparison with 2001*. Retrieved on 29 February 2016 from: https://www.ons.gov.uk/peoplepopulationandcommunity/healthandsocialcare/disability/articles/disabilityinenglandandwales/2013-01-30

Oliver, M. (1990). *The Politics of Disablement*. Basingstoke: Macmillan.

Purdam, K., Afkhami, R., Olsen, W. & Thornton, P. (2008). Disability in the UK: Measuring equality. *Disability and Society*, 23, 53–65.

Ravaud, J-F., Letourmy, A. & Ville, I. (2002). Identifying the population with disability: The approach of an INSEE survey on daily life and health. *Population-E 2002*, 57, 529–552.

Schneider, M., Dasappa, P., Khan, N. & Khan, A. (2009). Measuring disability in censuses: The case of South Africa. *Alter*, 3, 245–265.

Statistics Sweden (2014). *Situationen på arbtsmarknaden för personer med funtionsned-sättning 2013* [Disabled People and Employment, 2013]. Stockholm: Statistics Sweden.

Tøssebro, J. (2012). *Personer med funksjonsnedsettelser på arbeidsmarkedet* [Disabled People and the Labour Market]. Trondheim: NTNU Social Research.

Tøssebro, J. & Kittelsaa, A. (2004). Studying the living conditions of disabled people: Approaches and problems. In J. Tøssebro & A. Kittelsaa (Eds.). *Exploring the Living Conditions of Disabled People* (17–43). Lund: Studentlitteratur.

UK (2001). *General Household Survey*.

UK (2002). *British Household Panel Survey*.

Washington Group on Disability Statistics (2009) Understanding and Interpreting Disability as Measured using the WG Short Set of Questions, Retrieved 27 February 2017 from http://www.washingtongroup-disability.com

Weathers, R. (2009). The disability data landscape. In A. Houtenville, D. Stapleton, R. Weathers & R. Burkhauser (Eds.). *Counting Working-Age People with Disabilities* (27–68). Kalamazoo, MI: Upjohn Institute.

Weathers, R. & Wittenburg, D. (2009). Employment. In A. Houtenville, D. Stapleton, R. Weathers & R. Burkhauser (Eds.). *Counting Working-Age People with Disabilities* (101–144). Kalamazoo, MI: Upjohn Institute.

World Health Organisation (WHO) (2001). *International Classification of Functioning, Disability and Health: ICF*. Geneva: WHO.

5 Active Citizenship through community living

A multi-level perspective

Jan Šiška, Julie Beadle-Brown, Šárka Káňová and Jan Tøssebro

Introduction

In the last ten to fifteen years, there has been a growing recognition internationally that being an active participant in society builds on fundamental rights and that governments should provide the necessary support to enable all people to enjoy these rights, including persons with disabilities (Kozma & Petri, 2012). An important part of the shift required for this to happen is the move from institutional to community-based support for all persons with disabilities.

The UN Convention on the Rights of Persons with Disabilities (CRPD) (UN, 2006) makes the unjustified segregation of people with disabilities in congregate settings such as institutions or psychiatric long-stay hospitals a violation of human rights and calls on states to take 'effective and appropriate measures' to facilitate the full inclusion and participation of people with disabilities in society, including respect for a person's inherent autonomy and independence (Article 3). Article 19 requires that States ensure 'the equal right of all persons with disabilities to live in the community, with choices equal to others', and 'to facilitate full enjoyment by persons with disabilities of this right and their full inclusion and participation in the community'. The term 'independent' is not defined in the Convention. However, it is clear that the CRPD links the notion of independence to choice and control over daily living arrangements rather than to unsupported functional ability. Article 19 goes on to state that people with disabilities should 'have access to a range of in- home, residential and other community support services, including personal assistance necessary to support living and inclusion in the community' (UN, 2006: Article 19 (b)).

In the first section of this chapter, we explore the definition of community living and the importance of community living for achieving Active Citizenship. This will be followed by a summary of the available data on the situation of people with disabilities and how this has changed over time. Next, we examine policies, funding systems and services to facilitate and support community living from a multi-level perspective.

This chapter draws on two elements of the DISCIT research methodology. First, research teams in each country completed a template summarising the available information about community living for their country. Existing sources of data were reviewed by country teams to identify and collate literature, statistics and policies related to community living in each country. Second, semi-structured interviews were conducted with 84 disability policy and service experts across the nine countries. This chapter builds on the thematic analysis of interviews with four expert informants in each country, with a particular focus on those who had expertise related to the transition from institution to community-based services and to community living.

Community living and Active Citizenship: Conceptualisation and definitions

The concept of community living has been around for much longer than the UN Convention. Since the 1970s the ideology of normalisation and social role valorisation has been an important influence in the drive for de-institutionalisation, particularly for Nordic and Anglo-Saxon countries (Mansell & Ericsson, 1996). In contrast, in Central and Eastern European countries, the institutional, segregated model of care remained unquestioned and stable until political changes occurred in the early nineties.

One of the first definitions of 'community living' as a concept came from the Ordinary Life Initiative in the United Kingdom (Kings Fund Centre, 1980) which referred to community living as:

- Local housing with support for people of all levels of disability
- Work and work experience as an alternative to day care
- Widening participation of people with all levels of disability in community life
- Supporting people with challenging behaviour in the community.

Taylor (1991, cited in Allard, 1996) and others have given particular attention to the need for flexible housing arrangements to ensure individualised community living arrangements, including staff support when needed.

More recently, Mansell, Beadle-Brown et al. (2010) pulled together definitions from a range of sources to offer the following definition of community living:

> The aim of community living … is to enable people with intellectual disabilities to use the same range of accommodation, living arrangements and patterns of living that are available to the rest of the population, and to have a good quality of life, participating as full citizens in social, cultural and economic activities to the extent and in the ways the individual chooses.
>
> (Mansell & Beadle-Brown et al. 2010, p. 106)

They argued that this requires the following elements:

- Using accommodation located among the rest of the population, which is adequate, appropriate and accessible to the individual;

- Using the range of accommodation options ordinarily available to the wider population;
- Enabling people, to the greatest extent possible, to choose where, with whom and how they live; and
- Providing whatever help is required to enable people to participate successfully in the community.

In their view the focus has to be not just on housing and support for daily life but on developing the willingness and capacity of communities (including generic services) to support people with disabilities well. The latter point relates to the opportunities for participation in and enjoyment of a number of life domains: leisure, relationships, contributing to society (e.g. caring for others, volunteering, voting, and other forms of political participation) and work.

There is substantial overlap between community living and Active Citizenship. The three dimensions of Active Citizenship—security, autonomy and influence—have been conceptualised in different ways in different contexts and strands of social thinking. What is clear, however, is that living in the community (as opposed to an institution) is a central part of being an active citizen. Being a part of society physically as well as conceptually is critical to being able to participate in society and to being seen by others as part of that society. The segregated and isolated nature of most institutions makes this very difficult and, in many cases, impossible to achieve. Earlier research, in particular related to people with an intellectual disability, who have tended to be the last group of people to benefit from community care in almost every country, has shown that living in ordinary housing dispersed among other citizens in local communities results in a better quality of life, including better levels of participation in the community (e.g. Emerson & Hatton, 1994; Kozma et al., 2009; Mansell & Beadle-Brown, 2009).

The living situation of people with disabilities in Europe

Research has attempted to fill the gaps in the available knowledge by pulling together what information existed and where possible collecting some new data directly from institutions. For example Mansell et al. (2004) identified 2,354 institutions (defined by the European Commission as providing for more than 30 people on one site) across 29 countries. There were 175,000 people reported to be living in these institutions, with an average size of 110 and a range of 31 to 5,700 people, with variability between countries. There were no institutions reported for Sweden and Norway. For the remaining DISCIT countries covered by the report (United Kingdom, Czech Republic, Italy, Ireland) the average size of institution was between 50 and 100 people with no institutions bigger than 500 places. The exception to this was Germany where one institution was reported to be supporting over 4,000 people at that time and the average size was just over 220 places. People with intellectual disabilities made up the largest proportion of institutional residents, followed by those with mental health conditions (Mansell et al., 2004: 33).

In 2007, Mansell and colleagues (2007) reviewed available statistics on the living situation of people with disabilities across 28 European countries with the aim of identifying the number of people living in institutions of 30 places or more. The paucity, lack of completeness or inaccessibility of data meant that only estimates were possible and for some countries no data was available at all. However, approximate estimates indicated that, at the very least, 1.2 million Europeans with disabilities were living in residential services. Apart from Sweden, all countries still provided services for more than 30 people on one site.

In terms of the review of existing information conducted for our study, the lack of available data was an issue and different definitions of services types emerged in different countries (see also Townsley et al., 2010). In some countries data are collected about the number of places available in residential services but not about the number of people actually occupying them. It should also be remembered that, however services are named and classified, in reality these names might not correspond with the actual nature and quality of services provided. For example, in the Czech Republic large residential provisions were officially named institutions up to 2006. Due to legislative changes the same settings are now named 'homes for people with disabilities' but with little evidence that anything other than the name has changed. This is similar to what has been also observed in other European countries where de-institutionalisation took place through reclassification of the services rather than the services actually changing (Tøssebro et al., 2012). In Serbia, the Czech Republic, Germany and Italy, the main form of provision is still institutional at least for some groups of people. In Italy, more than 190,000 people were reported to be living in institutions. This is more than had been reported in 2007 (Mansell et al., 2007). A similar pattern was seen for Germany. For the most part, larger residential provisions are often for people with intellectual disability or mental health problems, with fewer being for people with physical or sensory impairments. This matches the findings of Townsley et al. (2010)

Although in some countries little change had been observed (e.g. Italy and Germany), in other countries there had been some movement towards de-institutionalisation and community living in the past ten years (e.g. in Ireland and to some extent in the Czech Republic). Overall, the countries were at different stages in terms of de-institutionalisation. In Serbia and the Czech Republic, de-institutionalisation has only really been happening through some EU-funded projects in the past five years. In some countries such as Italy the process is more advanced for those with mental health conditions than those with intellectual disabilities, while in Germany, for example, those with less severe disabilities have more opportunity to live in the community than those with more severe disabilities.

In Norway, Sweden and the United Kingdom the closure of the old-style institutions has been completed but with some evidence of re-institutionalisation.

For example, in Norway services for intellectually disabled people run by autonomous local governments have been, contrary to national policy guidelines, getting larger. Group homes built after 2000 are twice the size of what had been permitted in 1992 and more services are being established as 'total services' (Tøssebro et al., 2012). Similar patterns were also found in Sweden where group homes were starting to be co-located with other services such as homes for older adults or mental health services with staff shared across the settings (Tøssebro et al., 2012). In the United Kingdom, the average size of care homes has also been increasing and it is still possible for an individual or organisation to set up a service for 20, 30 or even 40 people with intellectual disabilities. In 2009, the Commission for Social Care Inspection (2009) annual report noted the average size of services for younger adults (any disability type) was 9.6 places. This was a rise from previous years. Larger residential services, with as many as 20 people, village community settings for between 50 and 100 people and private hospital settings for up to 80 people are also still found in the United Kingdom, although a campaign to close at least some of these is currently underway. However, information on the size of services is no longer published by the inspection and regulation agency—rather it comes from research (e.g. Netten et al., 2010). Even in Norway and Sweden where the citizen perspective is the strongest with rights clearly set out in the law, and in the United Kingdom which was one of the first countries to start the de-institutionalisation process for people with disabilities, there is a gap between ideology and practice.

However, a key finding from our review is again, as in previous studies, the lack of data. As such, none of the European countries are currently meeting the UN Convention Article 31 requirement for data that allows for the monitoring of the Convention, with respect to Article 19. The data that does exist is patchy and based on such varying definitions that it does not give a full picture in terms of support for community living for people with disabilities. Such data is also likely to underestimate both the numbers of those in some form of institutional provision as well as the number of those coping at home (alone or with their family) with no formal support. Only in Ireland is there any type of register that at least attempts to look at the number of people with intellectual disabilities and the number with sensory and physical disabilities and the support that they receive. The Irish register does not include those living at home with no formal support but it at least allows trends in support to be explored at a national level.

In the following sections we examine factors that may facilitate or hinder the development of community living for people with disabilities. Policies and funding systems for the existing service provision will each be considered at European and then at national level in four DISCIT countries: United Kingdom, Norway, Germany and Czech Republic. These countries are all at different stages and have followed clearly different paths in the process towards community living. They also have different disability policy systems, including different systems for providing opportunities for community living, and have different relationships with the EU.

Policy to support community living

Today the CRPD is the primary international policy driver for community living. However, even before the UN Convention, the UN Standard Rules on the Equalization of Opportunities for Persons with Disabilities set out the importance of people with a disability being able to live in their own local community (United Nations, 1993). In fact, by the late 1980s and early 1990s the issue of segregation had become a much wider human rights issue.

At European level there are a number of action plans, conventions and charters, which although pre-dating the UN convention, still have relevance to the issue of community living. First, under the European Convention on Human Rights (Council of Europe, 1953), states have an obligation to secure human rights for everyone within their jurisdiction. In particular, Article 3 prohibiting torture, 'inhuman or degrading treatment or punishment' and Article 8, which guarantees the right to respect for private and family life, can be invoked in cases where placement in an institution interferes with the person's ability to have a private life or to remain in contact with their family. Second, the Charter of Fundamental Rights of the European Union (European Union, 2000) contained specific provisions related to independent living and community participation. Article 21 prohibited any discrimination on the ground of disability and Article 26 recognised the right of persons with disabilities: '[...] to benefit from measures designed to ensure their independence, social and occupational integration and participation in the life of the community'. Both these articles were retained in the 2012 Charter (European Union, 2012).

In 2003, the European Commission adopted the EU Disability Strategy 2003–2010 (European Commission, 2003), with a focus on independent living. In 2010 the European Commission adopted a follow-up strategy for the period 2010–2020 with the objective of dismantling barriers that prevent people with disabilities from participating in society on an equal basis and to promote community living (European Commission, 2009).

In particular, since 2010 the Commission has used the Structural Funds and the Rural Development Fund to support the development of community-based services and raise awareness of the situation of people with disabilities living in residential institutions, in particular children and elderly people.

Finally, the Council of Europe Disability Action Plan 2006–2015 set up objectives to enable people with disabilities to plan their life and live as independently as possible in their community and to provide a broad range of support services at community level in order to allow for freedom of choice (Council of Europe, 2006).

However, even in the context of supportive United Nations and European-level policy, successful transition from institutions to services in the community needs to be anchored at the national and local level. At the very least there need to be local agreements between all potential service provider sectors and a plan that sets out not only when an institution would close but a detailed vision of the future care system based on robust evidence and good local knowledge.

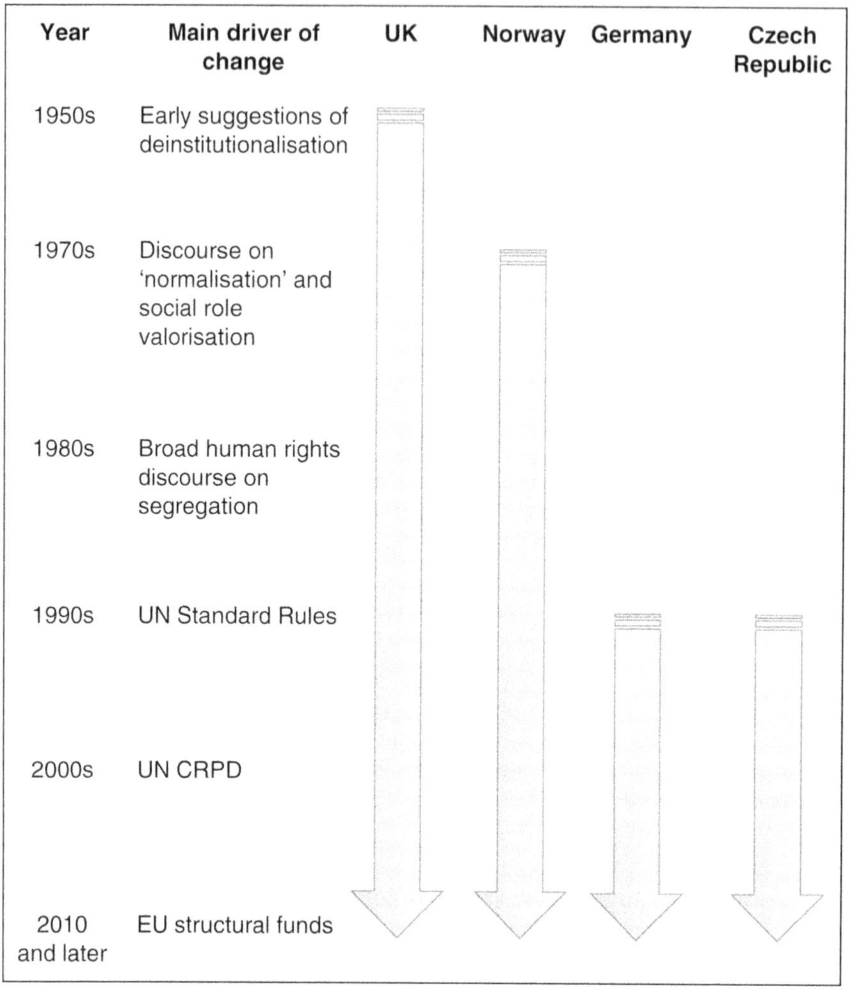

Figure 5.1 Policy trajectories in four case-study countries.

As such, Figure 5.1 traces the main policy trajectories specifically related to promoting community living in each of the four case study countries. This is by no means an exhaustive overview but brings together the key changes over time. Some countries began the process of de-institutionalisation long before the UN or EU policies existed, while for others the influence of these international bodies has played a part in starting the process. The United Kingdom started the process of de-institutionalisation earliest (at the same time as Sweden) and has had substantial policy to promote community living over the last 40 years, including policy specific to particular groups, such as people with intellectual disabilities.

In 1957 the Royal Commission on the Law relating to Mental Illness and Mental Deficiency recommended development of services outside hospitals for those with less serious problems (UK Commission, 1957). In the 1970s more places in smaller residential homes emerged for people with mental health conditions (UK Department of Health and Social Security, 1971, 1975). Yet, it was still the assumption that some people needed hospital care. In the 1980s and 1990s the United Kingdom witnessed progress towards more individualised community based services (UK Department of Health, 1989, 1998). In the 2000s and later the United Kingdom, among others, has aimed to provide more opportunities for individual choice, person-centred plans and direct payments (UK Department of Health 2001, 2006, 2007, 2009).

The overarching theme is one of promoting independence and self-determination, with personal budgets being a key route to achieving these principles (UK Department of Health, 2006). Interestingly, UK policy rarely refers to the CRPD although the United Kingdom ratified the Convention in 2009.

In Norway, the first moves towards smaller institutions and group homes appeared in the 1970s. Later the policy related to the mandatory closure of institutions (adopted in 1991) appeared to be all that was needed to achieve community living. In fact, Norway was the first country to close all institutions for people with intellectual disabilities due to a fast programme of closure between 1990 and 1995. Norway only ratified the UN Convention in 2013.

In Germany, policy related to community-based services began to emerge in the early 2000s. By 2009 Germany had ratified the CRPD. However, no more-recent policy has shifted the position further away from institutional provision. Currently people with more severe needs are still directed into institutional provision.

Finally, in the Czech Republic, national disability plans were launched in 1992, 1993 and 1998 and these served as important guides for policy-making relevant to disability and for the bodies within the central government responsible for implementation. The content of these policy documents reflected the UN Standard Rules on the Equalization of Opportunities for Persons with Disabilities (United Nations, 1993). The plans contributed to improving the awareness of governmental bodies of the impact of policy on the lives of people with disabilities and they have also raised general public awareness of disability issues (Šiška & Beadle-Brown, 2011). Like the United Kingdom and Germany, the Czech Republic ratified the CRPD in 2009 .

However, policy to promote community living in the Czech Republic is limited, although the intention to move in the direction of community living has been adopted in the national action plans. The move towards community living is still in the form of projects for the most part, rather than widespread actions.

Barriers and facilitators related to policy design

Experts across all nine DISCIT countries identified a number of barriers relating to policies to promote community living. In some countries the issue was a lack of policy altogether, while in others it was perceived that policy had the wrong focus or was not helpful in promoting community living. In Sweden, good accessibility policy was lacking while in Norway official policy to ensure community living was open to interpretation and in general still focused primarily on a more medical model of disability. Likewise in Ireland, the model in policy was still primarily the individualising medical model whereas in Italy, Serbia and Switzerland the policy that existed was not helpful in promoting community living for all. However, even where good policy existed, it was reported that there were issues of implementation.

In some countries, expert informants reported that some perverse incentives for institutional services could still be found in policy documents. For instance, it was recognised that some countries had mistranslated key terms from the UN Convention—for example in Germany the word 'integration' is used rather than the word 'inclusion'. Analysis also identified substantial variation in the definition of what constitutes community living and what is meant by 'institution' in different policy documents.

For some countries the political systems themselves were seen as barriers—for example, in Italy the lack of political stability was an issue, while in Italy and Serbia the controlling nature of government was identified as problematic.

A lack of government focus on or priority for disability issues was identified as a barrier in the Czech Republic, Norway, Italy and Germany. For example, in Norway inclusion policies (both related to school and community) were mainly off the agenda from 2000 onwards, replaced primarily by an accessibility and anti-discrimination agenda. Between 2009 and 2010, disability in general disappeared from the political agenda (Kittelsaa & Tøssebro, 2013).

Finally, in Germany and Ireland, there was an explicit barrier identified in the overriding concern of government (at different levels) regarding costs or expenditure. However, this theme was also implicit in what was said for some other countries in terms of cost cutting, cost shunting and rationing of services. In most countries, there was still a belief that there were economies of scale achieved by having bigger services; for example in Norway, this was the argument used for having larger group homes.

In terms of the facilitators, it was recognised in Sweden, Norway, the United Kingdom and Germany that strong legislation in support of community living was important, but by no means sufficient, to bring about change. It was also felt (mentioned in particular by experts in Sweden, Germany and the Czech Republic) that disability had to be seen as an important issue by politicians and that there had to be political will for change. Related to this was the need to have disability issues open for debate or discussion (in the media or in parliamentary debates), as raised by experts in Norway, the Czech Republic and Germany.

Systems to support community living

In this section we review the available information related to funding and provision of national service delivery systems. We first consider systems at national level for each of the four case-study countries. We then review barriers and facilitators identified by expert informants across all nine DISCIT countries.

Funding systems to support community living

In the four case-study countries, one of the key systems that was supportive of the development of community-based and personalised support was the availability of personal budgets, direct payments or other individualised funding (see also Townsley et al., 2010). This was true in those countries where de-institutionalisation had already been completed in the main (Norway and the United Kingdom) but it was also emerging as a supportive option in the Czech Republic and Germany. In some countries there was specific support for helping people to live in their own home (rented or bought)—for example, through housing benefit and the Supporting People Programme in the United Kingdom, and in Norway through special favourable loans and support for buying or building their own home. Special arrangements for accessible transport as well as systems to allow adaptations of housing and the purchase of equipment were available in the United Kingdom, Norway and the Czech Republic. In the United Kingdom, carers' assessments and support, the availability of respite, day provision and home help for carers has helped more people to stay in the family home.

Barriers and facilitators related to funding systems

In Norway people are supported to move out of family homes as part of normal life transitions; this is partly because of the view that young people should have this opportunity but also because parents have a right to a life without children once they are grown up. This is not the case in other countries.

The availability of funding had been seen as important in the past in Norway. Even in the United Kingdom the availability of double funding to help people move into the community without the place in the institution needing to be refilled was critical in promoting the development of early community-based supports and the closure of the hospitals. On the other hand, joint funding is seen as a barrier in the Czech Republic, as support provided in institutions is partly funded by service users and partly by the regional authorities that established them. From the perspective of a service user and his or her family, an institution guarantees long-term stability, unlike an non-government organisation (NGO) or any other provider which does not have on-going additional funding from the regional authority permanently guaranteed. Whether in reality there is equal access to funding for all service providers—large residential institutions governed by regional authorities and smaller community-based NGOs—has been seriously questioned (Šiška & Beadle-Brown, 2011), providing a perverse incentive for people to choose institutions over community-based NGOs.

In almost all nine DISCIT countries, expert informants identified the issue of insufficient spending on disability. Where people had to at least partly fund their own support (e.g. in Ireland) poverty was also an issue—with some people having to move back into institutions as they could not afford to live in the community. However, as well as insufficient spending, the issue of funding being spent on the wrong things was also raised.

Stability of funding over time was seen as very important in preventing people having to move back into congregate settings, in particular in the United Kingdom. In recent years, funding cuts have threatened this stability but expert informants were clear that stability was important. Personal budgets (where people receive their funding as a payment over which they have at least some control in terms of how to spend it) and personal assistance schemes were identified as key ways to promoting more independence, empowerment and community inclusion, although—as identified in some countries—having such a scheme did not guarantee a better life for everyone. Interestingly, none of the experts in any of the nine countries mentioned structural funds as either a facilitator or their misuse as a barrier.

Finally, as for policy, experts identified some perverse incentives for the maintenance of institutional provision. In Germany and Switzerland local government was reported as motivated to keep institutions open as they were cheaper. Mansell et al. (2007) pointed out that a lack of good cost-effective analyses (i.e. that took into account the needs and outcomes of the people supported) and the lack of a long-term view led to this misunderstanding of institutional services as being cheaper. In some countries, cost analysis showed that community living was cheaper than institutional care, whereas in the United Kingdom and Australia the cost of community living was slightly higher (Stancliffe & Lakin, 2005). In Ireland, psychiatric hospitals were still receiving funding on a per capita basis so there was no incentive for them to close. In the United Kingdom, short-term double funding had been instrumental initially in ensuring that institutions did not need to fill up beds that people had moved out of, and Norwegian expert informants also talked about the availability of the national insurance scheme as being an important source of funding for social care.

Service systems to support community living

Research teams in each country were asked to describe service types by size and nature rather than just by a label because earlier work (Mansell et al., 2007) had found that the same term could mean different things in different countries. For example, a group home in the United Kingdom normally implies accommodation for less than 6 people with shared support and shared communal areas, usually, but not always, providing 24-hour support. In Norway, a group home is usually in the form of 4 to 8 small apartments clustered together with a staff apartment attached. In Germany a group home could provide for as many as 24 people all under one roof.

In the United Kingdom and Norway the most common type of accommodation for persons with intellectual disabilities was small group homes. Although one would not normally consider services over 10 places as community living, in the United Kingdom there are still a relatively large minority of services that are between 10 and 20 places. In the United Kingdom currently larger services still exist but these are usually private hospitals, assessment and treatment units or secure units. Unlike in Norway, there has never been any requirement for services to be below a certain number of places, although work is currently being undertaken to look at having such a limitation. In both the United Kingdom and Norway some group homes for more than 10 people have been set up lately, primarily for people with intellectual disabilities but—in the United Kingdom—also some for people with physical and sensory disabilities (Emerson & Hatton, 2008; Netten et al., 2010; Norway, 2000; Söderström & Tøssebro, 2011; Commission for Social Care Inspection, 2009; Tøssebro et al., 2014).

In Germany and the Czech Republic, large residential homes are still common (Seifert, 1998; Duschek & Lemmer, 2013; Federal Republic of Germany, 2013). In the Czech Republic an interesting trend is that more people live with family as financial support has become available to family members (Czech Republic, 2015; Czech Republic Statistical Office, 2013).

In all four countries a version of personal assistance for a person with disability to live in their own house or apartment was available, including for those with intellectual disabilities. However, in all countries apart from the United Kingdom, this was primarily available mostly to those with less severe disabilities.

Apart from a few studies in the United Kingdom there was very little evidence about the quality of community-based services and how well they supported people to be active citizens, and there was just a handful of studies (in United Kingdom and Norway) that looked at issues around the choice of living situation and support. Those studies that did exist indicated that at least 50 per cent of people still had no choice of where or with whom to live. The availability of personal assistance was seen as a key determinant of whether people had choice over the support they received (but this was by no means guaranteed or available to all).

Barriers and facilitators associated with service delivery systems

One of the core themes that emerged in the analysis of the expert interviews across the nine DISCIT countries was the availability and flexibility of services and support in the community. Staff turnover and shortage of staff were reported as barriers to de-institutionalisation as well as a reason for services getting bigger or being clustered together. A lack of adequate community mental health support was raised as an issue for those with mental health problems, and experts reported that those with mental health needs in particular require a much more flexible system of funding and support so that they can have help when they are in crisis, but also have on-going support, such as self-help groups, regular counselling or advocacy, when they are well.

The severity of disability was reported as a barrier to receiving community-based support and a risk for institutionalisation across many countries. For example, in Serbia services in the community are relatively rare and children and adults are still placed in institutions according to their diagnosis—sometimes a long way away from their own community. Only those with the least severe disabilities get to live in their own home with a small level of support. A similar picture was seen in Germany, Ireland and Switzerland where only those with no or very mild intellectual disabilities get the opportunity to live in their own home with support using a personal budget or personal assistance, or even in smaller group homes. However, research has found that it is those with more severe disabilities who benefit most from moving to the community. For example, research from Norway found that those with more severe disabilities experienced the greatest change in living conditions (Tøssebro, 1996).

Even for those who could access personal budgets and/or personal assistance, the required bureaucracy was seen as a barrier to doing so and, in particular, the fact that disabled people had to be employers of personal assistants discouraged people from applying. Experts also reported discrimination against people with intellectual disability and psychosocial disabilities in terms of eligibility for personal budgets—with successful applications requiring long and difficult negotiations.

Another barrier was related to the fact that in most countries institutional services (larger scale residential care) were still being built or, at the very least, still being used for people entering the service system for the first time. This was particularly true for older people with disabilities.

Even when the main form of support was community-based and included social assistance, there were still issues identified, particularly around flexibility of support. In 6 of the 9 countries, experts raised the issue of the inflexibility of funded support—money was given to people but not necessarily for the things they wanted or needed. There was also inflexibility in terms of when support was provided and a lack of recognition that needs might differ over time and as such the level and nature of support might need to change.

There were also some issues identified with how the service system viewed people with disabilities (historically and currently). For example, in Ireland and Switzerland it was noted that systems still fostered dependency rather than independency of people with disabilities.

Finally, there were barriers identified around accessibility and availability of assistive technology. In Norway, Ireland, Italy and Sweden, issues of accessibility of the community in general were noted as problematic. In Ireland, one barrier identified to supporting people to leave institutions was the lack of accessible homes available. In the Czech Republic there was a lack of funding for assistive technology.

Conclusions

This chapter has focused on developments related to community living with a particular focus on the service subsystem. The chapter has argued that policy development at the international and European levels increasingly has become the driver of de-institutionalisation. However, it is very difficult to monitor whether progress is being made towards the realisation of Article 19 of the CRPD. Even in the four countries on which this chapter focused, there were very few sources of reliable and comprehensive data.

From the limited data available, there appeared to have been some change since 2006 but this varied from country to country in terms of both extent and direction. Although primarily project-based rather than an overall systems change, there had been some advancements in the Czech Republic. In contrast, Germany appeared to have just as many people in institutions as there had been in 2006 and there was some evidence of re-institutionalisation in Norway and the United Kingdom. Those with intellectual disabilities (and in particular those with more severe disabilities) and those with psychosocial disabilities were most likely to be institutionalised.

As mentioned in earlier sections, personal budgets were identified as one way of creating more flexible support. However, there has to be a range of good-quality services available, if people are to have choice around how to best meet their needs. There also has to be a willingness on the part of national and local governments to fund less traditional 'services' that might support people's independence and well-being and thus promote their Active Citizenship. Even without personal budgets and personal assistance schemes, small community-based services providing high-quality support that enables and empowers people can still ensure that people are active citizens (Mansell & Beadle-Brown, 2012; Beadle-Brown et al., 2015). Establishing and maintaining such high-quality services is not easy and takes time to establish, requiring staff to be well trained, motivated and supported by management (Mansell & Beadle-Brown, 2012). Skilling up the workforce and service-providing organisations to support even those with the most severe disabilities and complex needs in the community requires experience. This is another reason why it is critical to ensure that those with the most severe disabilities are included from the start in the design of community care services, for it gives providers the opportunity to hone their skills in supporting this group of people well.

Redesign of the social services subsystem from block to individualised funding was an important aspect of de-institutionalisation (Mansell et al., 2007). Since the late 1990s care package funding has become available to at least some people in most countries as a personal budget—where people have control over how to spend the money allocated to meet their care needs, either directly or through a third party who manages the funds for them. Having such a personal budget as well as being able to use it to buy personal assistance was seen in almost all countries as a facilitator for Active Citizenship through community living—and certainly facilitated more choice about where and with whom to live as well as how to receive support.

If those providing support do not do so in a way that enables and empowers the person they support, then it is unlikely that the person will experience the full benefits of community living or Active Citizenship. We know from almost four decades of research related to intellectual disabilities that living in an ordinary house, dispersed in the local community, is a necessary but not sufficient condition for improved quality of life (Mansell, and Beadle-Brown, 2010; Mansell & Beadle-Brown, 2012), especially for those with more severe disabilities. If policies, systems and processes only focus on where people live then it is highly unlikely that the majority of people with disabilities will experience substantially better outcomes than they did in the institution. Ensuring that the support people get is skilled, enabling and empowering is critical, whether this support is to enable them at home, at work, or out and about in the community. Finally, how well people are supported to participate in and contribute to their local communities (and society more generally) will influence how people are viewed by others and will increase community capacity to include people with disabilities.

References

Allard, M. A. (1996). Supported living policies and programmes in the USA. In J. Mansell & K. Ericsson (Eds.), *Deinstitutionalization and Community Living: Intellectual Disability Services in Britain, Scandinavia and the USA* (pp. 97–116). London: Chapman and Hall.

Beadle-Brown, J., Leigh, J., Whelton, B., Richardson, L., Beecham, J., Baumker, T. & Bradshaw, J. (2015). Quality of life and quality of support for people with severe intellectual disability and complex needs. *Journal of Applied Research in Intellectual Disabilities*. DOI:10.1111/jar.12200

Commission for Social Care Inspection. (2009). *The State of Social Care in England 2007–8*. London: Commission for Social Care Inspection.

Council of Europe (1953). The European Convention for the Protection of Human Rights and Fundamental Freedoms (also known as The European Convention on Human Rights) Rome, 4.XI.1950. Retrieved 15 April 2015 from: http://www.echr.coe.int/Pages/home.aspx?p=basictexts&c=

Council of Europe (2006). *Council of Europe Action Plan to Promote the Rights and Full Participation of People with Disabilities in Society: Improving the Quality of Life of People with Disabilities in Europe 2006–2015*. Retrieved 15 April 2016 from: https://rm.coe.int/CoERMPublicCommonSearchServices/DisplayDCTMContent?documentId=0900001680595206

Czech Republic. (2013). Registry of Social Service Providers. MoLSA.

Czech Republic. (2015). Proposal of Social Services Strategy 2016–2026. MoLSA.

Czech Republic Statistical Office. (2013). Disability Survey.

Duschek, K. -J. & Lemmer, A. (2013). Ergebnisse der Sozialhilfestatistik. *Wirtschaft und Statistik*, 2013(3), 199–212.

Emerson, E. & Hatton, C. (1994). *Moving Out: Relocation from Hospital to Community*. London: HMSO.

Emerson, E. & Hatton, C. (2008). *People with Learning Disabilities in England*. Lancaster: Centre for Disability Research.

European Union (2000). *Charter of Fundamental Rights of the European Union* (2000/C 364/01). Retrieved 15 April 2016 from: http://www.europarl.europa.eu/charter/pdf/text_en.pdf

European Commission (2003). *Communication from the Commission to the Council, the European Parliament, the European Economic and Social Committee and the Committee of the Regions: Equal opportunities for People with Disabilities: A European Action Plan* (COM/2003/0650 final).

European Commission (2009). *A Renewed Commitment to a Barrier-Free Europe for Disabled Persons*. (COM (2010) 636 final). Retrieved 15 April 2016 from: http://eur-lex.europa.eu/legal-content/EN/TXT/?uri=URISERV%3Aem0047

Federal Republic of Germany (2013). *Teilhabebericht der Bundesregierung über die Lebenslagen von Menschen mit Beeinträchtigungen*. Federal Ministry of Work and Social Affairs/ Bundesministerium für Arbeit und Soziales. Retrieved 16 February 2017 from: http://www.bmas.de/DE/Service/Medien/Publikationen/a125-13-teilhabebericht.html

Kings Fund (1980) *An ordinary life: Comprehensive Locally Based Residential Services for Mentally Handicapped People*. Kings Fund Centre: London.

Kittelsaa, A. & Tøssebro, J. (2013). *Kommunal praksis og personer med utviklingshemming* [*Local Government Practices and People with Intellectual Disabilities*]. Trondheim, NTNU Social Research.

Kozma, A., Mansell, J. & Beadle-Brown, J. (2009). Outcomes in different residential settings for people with intellectual disability: A systematic review. *American Journal on Intellectual and Developmental Disabilities*, 114(3), 193–222.

Kozma, A. & Petri, G. (2012). *Mapping Exclusion, Institutional and Community-based Services in the Mental Health Field in Europe*. Brussels: Mental Health Europe & Mental Health Initiative of the Open Society Foundations.

Mansell, J. & Beadle-Brown, J. (2009). Dispersed or clustered housing for adults with intellectual disabilities: A systematic review. *Journal of Intellectual and Developmental Disability*, 34(4) 313–323.

Mansell, J. & Beadle-Brown, J. (2010). Deinstitutionalisation and community living: position statement of the Comparative Policy and Practice Special Interest Research Group of the International Association for the Scientific Study of Intellectual Disabilities. *Journal of Intellectual Disability Research*, 54(2), 104–112.

Mansell, J. & Beadle-Brown, J. (2012). *Active Support: Enabling and Empowering People with Intellectual Disabilities*. London: Jessica Kingsley.

Mansell, J., Beadle-Brown, J. & Clegg, S. (2004). The situation of large residential institutions in Europe. In G. Freyhoff, C. Parker, M. Coué & N. Greig (Eds.), *Included in Society: Results and Recommendations of the European Research Initiative on Community-based Residential Alternatives for Disabled People* (28–56). Brussels: Inclusion Europe.

Mansell, J. & Ericsson, K. (Eds.) (1996). *Deinstitutionalization and Community Living: Intellectual Disability Services in Britain, Scandinavia and the USA*. London: Chapman and Hall.

Mansell, J., Knapp, M. R. J., Beadle-Brown, J. & Beecham, J. (2007). *Deinstitutionalisation and Community Living—Outcomes and Costs: A Report of a European Study: Vol. 2 Main Report*. Tizard Centre, University of Kent.

Netten, A., Beadle-Brown, J., Trukeschitz, B., Towers, A. M., Welch, E., Forder, J. E., Smith, J. E. & Alden, E. (2010). *Measuring the Outcomes of Care Hhomes.* Canterbury: Personal Social Services Research Unit. Retrieved 16 February 2017 from http://www.pssru.ac.uk/pdf/dp2696_2.pdf

Seifert, M. (1998). Wohnen—so normal wie möglich. In H. Jakobs, A. König & G. Theunissen (Eds.). *Lebensräume - Lebensperspektiven. Ausgewählte Beiträge zur Situation Erwachsener mit geistiger Behinderung* (150–190). Butzbach-Griedel: Afra Verlag.

Šiška, J. & Beadle-Brown J. (2011). Developments in deinstitutionalization and community living in the Czech Republic. *Journal of Policy and Practice in Intellectual Disabilities*, 8(2), 125–133.

Söderström, S. & Tøssebro, J. (2011). *Innfridde mål eller brudte visjoner* [Fulfilled Ideals or Broken Promises]. Trondheim: NTNU Social Research.

Stancliffe, R. & Lakin, K. C. (2005). *Costs and Outcomes of Community Services for People with Intellectual Disabilities*. Baltimore: Brookes.

Tøssebro, J. (1996). En bedre hverdag? [Improved Everyday Life?]. Oslo: Kommune forlaget.

Tøssebro, J., Bonfils, I., Teittinen, A., Tideman, M., Traustadóttir, R. & Vesala, H. (2012). Normalization fifty years beyond: Current trends in the Nordic countries. *Journal of Policy and Practice in Intellectual Disabilities*, 9, 134–146.

Townsley, R., Ward, L., Abbot, D. & Williams, V. (2010). *The Implementation of Policies Supporting Independent Living for Disabled People in Europe: Synthesis Report.* Leeds: University of Leeds, Centre for Disability Studies, Academic Network of European Disability Experts.

UK Commission (1957). Royal Commission on the law relating to mental illness and mental deficiency. *Report (Chair: Rt. Hon Lord Percy of Newcastle) Command Paper Cmd 169.* London: House of Commons.

UK Department of Health (1989). *Caring for People: Community Care in the Next Decade and Beyond* (Cm 849). London: HMSO.

UK Department of Health (1998). *Modernising Social Services: Promoting Independence, Improving Protection, Raising Standards* (Cm 4169). London: HMSO.

UK Department of Health (2001). *Valuing people: A new Strategy for Learning Disability for the 21st Century* (Cm 5086). London: HMSO.

UK Department of Health (2006). *Our Health, Our Care, Our Say: A New Direction for Community Services.* London Retrieved 21 February 2017 from https://www.gov.uk/government/uploads/system/uploads/attachment_data/file/272238/6737.pdf

UK Department of Health (2007). *Services for People with Learning Disabilities and Challenging Behaviour or Mental Health Needs: Report of a Project Group (Chairman: Prof J. L. Mansell). Revised Edition.* London: Department of Health.

UK Department of Health (2009). *Valuing People Now: A New Three-year Strategy for People with Learning Disabilities. 'Making it happen for everyone'.* London: Department of Health.

UK Department of Health and Social Security (1971). *Better Services for the Mentally Handicapped* (Cmnd 4683). London: HMSO.

UK Department of Health and Social Security (1975). *Better Services for the Mentally Ill* (Cmnd 6233). London: HMSO.

United Nations (1993). *The Standard Rules on the Equalization of Opportunities for Persons with Disabilities.* Adopted by the United Nations General Assembly, forty-eighth session, resolution 48/96, annex, of 20 December 1993. Retrieved 9 April 2016 from: http://www.un.org/esa/socdev/enable/dissre01.htm#concepts

United Nations (2006). *The United Nations Convention on the Rights of Persons with Disabilities.* Retrieved 7 April 2016 from: https://www.un.org/development/desa/disabilities/convention-on-the-rights-of-persons-with-disabilities.html

6 How to enhance Active Citizenship for persons with disabilities in Europe through labour market participation

European and national perspectives

Roy Sainsbury, Edmund Coleman-Fountain and Bruno Trezzini

Article 27 of the UN Convention on the Rights of Persons with Disabilities obliges signatories to seek to secure employment equality for persons with disabilities. This aim is supported by the European Disability Strategy 2010–2020 which calls for the European Union (EU) and member states to promote the active inclusion and full participation of persons with disabilities in the open labour market (European Commission, 2010b). While the challenge of lower employment rates in high-income countries for persons with disabilities is well reported (Greve, 2009; Haveman & Wolfe, 2000; Palmer, 2011), the task of understanding the mechanisms through which signatories seek to comply with the Convention is just beginning (Priestley & Lawson, 2015). This is the focus of this chapter, which presents a typology of policy responses to the employment gap in Europe and reflections on potential routes to securing employment equality for persons with disabilities.

To contextualise the discussion, the first part of the chapter begins by exploring employment as an area of policy intervention. It highlights the role employment plays as a symbol of the disability movement's commitment to equality, independence and inclusion (Beresford & Holden, 2000: 983). This is followed by a review of statistical data on employment rates across Europe. The next section sets out the policies used to secure labour market participation organised using DISCIT's disability policy system typology of *social regulations*, *social services* and *income maintenance* (see Chapter 2). Findings are then presented from interviews carried out with disability experts in the nine DISCIT countries on ways to increase the labour market participation of persons with disabilities. The chapter concludes by drawing on the statistical data, review of policies and expert interviews to suggest that future policy development should focus as much on employers and the demand for labour as on improving the employability of persons with disabilities.

Employment rights in Europe

Within social policy, the employment of disabled people has become an issue in light of economic concerns, including perceptions of a 'crisis' in disability benefits and income replacement schemes (Lindsay & Houston, 2013; Traustadóttir,

2008). More important for the DISCIT study has been the way employment has become a priority due to the efforts of the disabled people's movement. Challenges to definitions of disability as an individual tragedy incorporate a critique of economic and social processes that exclude persons with disabilities from society (Barnes & Oliver, 2012: 7). Tied to commitments to independence, this critique of the structural basis of disabled persons' exclusion has placed employment on the policy agenda as a matter of equality. As Beresford and Holden (2000: 984) explain:

> Its conception of independence rests not on people doing without any help or support, but on them having adequate and appropriate individual support as well as appropriate social conditions to live their life on equal terms with non-disabled people. The movements are thus much more likely to identify employment as a right rather than an obligation—a right which many of their members are still denied.

The UNCRPD can be seen as one important outcome of a growing recognition of persons with disabilities as rights-bearing subjects, matched by the gradual development of a rights-based approach to EU policy (European Commission, 2003; Traustadóttir, 2008). It is within this context that the DISCIT study focused on employment as an area of enquiry. Our aims were, first, to consider how Europe and European member states have so far aimed to secure the right to employment of persons with disabilities and second, to ask what 'new' thinking there might be with regard to disability employment policy.

Statistical data on labour market participation

The focus on employment as an equality issue has largely been driven by concerns with the employment gap. Drawing on data presented by the European Commission (2000), for example, Traustadóttir (2008: 78) argues that persons with disabilities 'are considered to be one of the most disadvantaged groups in Europe when it comes to labour force participation'. At the time the employment rate for persons with disabilities in Europe averaged 40 per cent (25 per cent for people categorized as severely disabled), in comparison with an employment rate of 70 per cent for non-disabled people. This situation had not improved by 2011 when Eurostat (2014e) stated that fewer than 1 in 2 disabled adults were in employment in the EU-28 (i.e. the countries that have been members of the EU since 2013).

Analysing available statistical data on labour market participation as indicators of the effectiveness of social inclusion policies (Atkinson et al., 2002), this section elaborates on the effectiveness of current disability policy systems as a whole. The analysis raises broad questions about how systems have so far aimed to enhance labour market participation and about enduring barriers experienced by persons with disabilities. To enhance comparability, data is collated from Eurostat which presents results of the 2011 EU Labour Force Survey ad-hoc module on employment and disability (see Eurostat 2016; Eurostat Database, 2016. No figures for Norway or Serbia were available.). No figures for Norway or Serbia were available.). Eurostat applies two primary disability definitions, namely disability as 'difficulties in carrying out basic activities (such as, hearing, seeing, walking, communicating)' and disability in employment as 'limitation in work caused by health problems/difficulties in basic activities' (Eurostat, 2015: 9).

Here, if not specified otherwise, data based on the second definition is used because it relates more closely to employment. It should be noted, however, that the gaps between disabled and non-disabled respondents tend to be larger for this definition than for the other.

Access to education and training

Participation in education and training are cornerstones of a person's future employment success and career advancement. Early school leaving in particular has been found to be related to unemployment, social exclusion and poverty. This is of particular significance to disabled children and young people who face a number of barriers to a full and comprehensive education. These include structural and relational barriers that prevent disabled young people from entering upper secondary or further education, and a failure to equip disabled children with the skills required to progress beyond compulsory education (Ebersold et al., 2011). As education is an important predictor of labour market outcomes, we present statistics on educational access and attainment at both the EU-28 aggregate and the individual country level, using general targets as a benchmark.

In its Training and Education 2020 strategic framework, the EU established a goal for the *rate of early leavers from education and training* aged 18 to 24. The target was set at below 10 per cent (Eurostat, 2014a; European Union, 2009). While by 2011 this goal was close to being achieved at the EU-28 level for persons without disabilities, nearly one disabled person out of three was still leaving school or training early. Of the DISCIT countries, only Sweden reached the 10 per cent target for this group, with Switzerland achieving a rate of 15 per cent. All other DISCIT countries had rates higher than the EU-28 average, with Germany at 42 per cent furthest from the target. Another target defined by the EU was that at least 40 per cent of people aged 30 to 34 should have completed some form of higher education by 2020. Looking at *tertiary educational attainment* for persons with disabilities, by 2011 Europe as a whole was halfway towards achieving that, with Italy and Czech Republic at 11 per cent showing the lowest rates of achievement among the DISCIT countries. Sweden (34 per cent) and Switzerland (33 per cent) were the closest to the 40 per cent target. Ireland and the UK had particularly large gaps between the attainment rates of disabled and non-disabled persons.

Finally, the EU also suggested a target of at least 15 per cent of adults who should participate in lifelong learning. Four of the DISCIT countries had not reached 10 per cent in 2011 (Germany, Italy, Czech Republic and Ireland) but Sweden and Switzerland had far exceeded the 15 per cent target (at 32 per cent and 26 per cent respectively).

Labour force participation: Rates of employment, unemployment and inactivity

The data suggests that persons with disabilities are less likely to be in employment and that this has proved to be so for some time. While the figures from the 2002 and 2011 EU Labour Force Surveys cannot be directly compared, there are some observations to be made about distributional patterns and relative magnitudes. In 2002 the weighted average rate of employment across the EU-25 countries (i.e. the countries that were members between 2004 and 2006) was nearly 50 per cent for disabled persons compared with an average rate of 68 per cent for persons without disabilities. Of the DISCIT countries, Italy showed the lowest rate of employment for persons with and without disabilities (38 per cent and 58 per cent respectively).

Eurostat data also reveals that a large proportion of the working-age population with limitations was inactive, meaning they were not in work and not actively seeking work. While the EU-25 average was 45 per cent, the country values ranged from 22 per cent in Sweden to 59 per cent in Italy. The inactivity status of working-age persons with disabilities may often be due to their having become discouraged from enrolling in or having dropped out of the unemployment rolls because they could not find paid work (Dupré & Karjalainen, 2003). However, inactivity may also be an intentional choice, reflecting a person's reduced ability to perform regular work in the mainstream labour market (due to the severity of impairment or the unavailability of partial disability benefits) or may be a result of a lack of suitable work opportunities such as part-time employment. The unemployment rate for disabled persons across all EU-25 countries reached 10 per cent (ranging from 5 per cent in Sweden to 17 per cent in Germany) as compared to 8 per cent for persons without a disability (varying from 4 per cent in Ireland to 9 per cent in Italy).

Almost a decade later and using the definition of disability as a 'basic activity difficulty', the employment rate in 2011 for disabled persons at EU level was, at 47 per cent, nearly 20 per cent lower than that for non-disabled persons. Defining disability as a limitation in work due to a *longstanding health problem and/or a basic activity difficulty* (LHPAD), the employment rate for disabled persons was almost 30 per cent less than that for those who did not declare such a limitation. Using the latter definition, countries such as Switzerland and Sweden had higher employment rates for disabled persons than others (for example, Ireland, Czech Republic, Germany, UK or Italy). Different countries had below-average employment gaps (for example, Sweden, Switzerland, Italy) or above-average (Ireland, UK, Germany). Data also indicate that more than half of the working-age population with limitations in work caused by a LHPAD were inactive. Sweden and Switzerland had lower inactivity rates than the EU average, while Ireland had the highest.

Reasons for inactivity and barriers to participation

The gap in employment rates can be explained in several ways. Eurostat data indicate that for those of working age with a disability who were inactive in 2011, the most cited reason for inactivity was *illness or disability*. This was particularly true for respondents from Ireland and the UK but in Czech Republic respondents stated retirement as the single most important reason. In contrast, for those without a disability, being in education or training was a more significant reason. Retirement was used as an explanation more often by working-age disabled persons than non-disabled persons. Furthermore, a majority of persons with a disability who were out of work also left their last job for health or disability reasons. For example, at the EU-28 level over 30 per cent of disabled persons aged 15 to 64 left a job due to illness or disability, especially among those aged between 35 and 44 (Eurostat, 2014d).

Reporting on barriers to employment for job seekers, Eurostat (2014b) shows that, at the EU-28 level, more than 1 in 3 people with a limitation in work due to a LHPAD felt that other personal or environmental factors limited their ability to work. In contrast, just 9 per cent of people without a LHPAD reported additional barriers. Of specific personal or environmental factors cited, lack of suitable jobs, poor transport, inflexible employers, family and other caring responsibilities, and lack of qualifications or experience were most common. Family and caring was a major factor for women in particular, reported by 27 per cent of women compared with 6 per cent of men (Eurostat, 2014b).

Working patterns

Of disabled persons in work in 2011, Eurostat (2014c) reports differences in working patterns. These include a marginally higher rate of home working. Over 15 per cent of disabled people in employment worked from home most or some of the time, compared with 13 per cent of non-disabled persons. Persons with disabilities were also more likely to report part-time working. Taking the EU-28 as a whole, 26 per cent of persons with disabilities in work were working part-time compared with nearly 18 per cent of working people without a disability. In other research, part-time work has also been shown to be associated with 'slight' disability in women (Salladarré & Hlaimi, 2014).

Eurostat (2014c) reported no statistically significant differences in the proportions of people with and without disability in supervisory roles, although in some countries (e.g. Czech Republic and Switzerland) persons with disabilities were less likely to be employed at a supervisory level. It is possible that part-time employment compounds this problem by making career progression more difficult. Finally, Eurostat (2015: 104) finds that contrary to expectations there was no significant difference in the prevalence of temporary employment in 2011 between persons with disabilities and those without.

The on-going challenge of the disability employment gap

Statistical data on disability and employment are beset by a range of problems, including difficulties defining disability and of measuring the prevalence of disability (Traustadóttir, 2008). Nevertheless, Eurostat analysis provides sufficient evidence to demonstrate clearly the labour market disadvantage of persons with disabilities. The employment gap is not only large but seemingly difficult to reduce. As the OECD (2010: 50) argues (referring to a 10 to 15 year period from the mid-1990s to the end of the first decade of this century), 'despite increased efforts to develop and expand employment integration measures, employment levels of people with disability have not improved.' In the next section we examine how the DISCIT countries have responded to the challenge of the disability employment gap.

Disability policies in Europe and the DISCIT countries

Aspiring to improve employment outcomes is central to current European policy agendas. EU 2020 sets a general target of increasing the employment rate of working-age adults and requires member states to address the problem of poverty among people with disabilities (European Commission, 2010a). The European Disability Strategy 2010–2020 sets a priority of increasing the numbers of disabled persons working in the open labour market (European Commission, 2010b). An employment rate of 75 per cent endorsed by EU leaders matches the target for persons aged 20 to 64 generally. This reflects the UN CRPD commitment to ensuring that disabled persons are able to work in the open labour market on an equal basis with others. Labour market integration is also supported by disabled people's organisations. The European Disability Forum (2015) calls on the EU to robustly support measures to improve the employment of persons with disabilities in the open labour market. In the context of these European-level policies this section presents an overview of policies in the DISCIT countries designed to increase the labour market participation of persons with disabilities, drawing mainly on the review of policies in DISCIT countries provided by the country research teams (rather than other published sources). Findings are organised using the DISCIT policy subsystems typology, namely: social regulations, social services and social benefits, rather than trying to cluster and map individual countries onto welfare state or disability typologies. The variation within and between the DISCIT countries did not allow the latter approach.

Social regulation subsystem

The subsystem of regulations covers laws and policies intended to change employer behaviour. One principal mechanism is anti-discrimination legislation, which defines discriminatory behaviour and appropriate responses. This is one area where the EU can claim some influence, and where disability activists have been able to effect change. For instance, Traustadóttir (2008: 91) notes that regulations have been one way in which principles of 'non-discrimination, universal design, human rights, and a rights-based approach to disability provisions' has been extended. At EU level, these principles are embedded in the 2000 Employment Equality Directive. This, Waddington and Lawson (2009: 10) note, is a significant piece of policy as it

> [...] addresses areas which had not previously been regulated in most Member States, such as the concept of reasonable accommodation, and requires reflection on the nature of disability based discrimination and the characteristics which an individual must possess before being able to claim protection from such discrimination.

Member states have subsequently sought to introduce or clarify anti-discrimination legislation in their own countries. In DISCIT, such regulations are now in place in Czech Republic (2009), Germany (2002 and 2006), Ireland (1998 and 2000), Norway (2008), Serbia (2006), Sweden (1999 and 2009), Switzerland (2004), and the United Kingdom (1995 and 2010). Most, though not all, were adopted after 2000 and incorporate notions of reasonable adjustment. In some cases, countries have a separate disability policy; in others, clauses on disability and reasonable adjustment are part of a general anti-discrimination law. As evidence of the influence of the EU on regulatory approaches, the European Commission retains powers to launch proceedings against member states that it considers to have failed to fulfil their obligations under the Employment Equality Directive, as happened with Italy in 2011 (Chopin & Germaine-Sahl, 2013: 10).

However, across DISCIT countries, there is no one single approach to regulation. For instance, in some countries anti-discrimination law is the sole means of regulating employer behaviour. In Germany, Italy, Czech Republic, Ireland and Serbia, employment quotas are also used, often alongside anti-discrimination laws. Most have been in place for many years, although Serbia's quota system was introduced in 2009. Quotas require employers to create positions for disabled persons as a proportion of employed staff. In Italy, Serbia and Czech Republic, reduced taxes and fees, and contributions to wages and the cost of workplace adaptations encourage compliance. Instead of offering direct employment, employers may also choose to make payments that support the employment of disabled persons elsewhere or use the services of external organisations with a larger proportion of disabled employees, as in Czech Republic. Levy money can be used to support employment services or to fund the costs of adjustments elsewhere. For instance, German integration offices are responsible for the management of levy funds that are made available to support employment services and activities. Quota legislation was repealed in the UK in favour of more individualised solutions (Thornton & Lunt, 1995). Wage subsidies also form a part of the social regulation subsystem and were used in a number of DISCIT countries (Norway, Sweden and Czech Republic).

It is typical for such regulations to apply differently depending on whether an employer is in the public or private sector. For instance, the German Disability Equality Act (BGG) has been criticised for applying notions of reasonable accommodation to public institutions only (BRK-Allianz, 2013: 18), while the Swiss Federal Act on the Elimination of Discrimination against People with Disabilities has no bearing on private sector practices. Ireland has a public sector employment duty set at 3 per cent but no target for private sector workplaces. Regulations may also be applied differently depending on company size; small organisations are exempt from equality rules in some countries.

Social services subsystem

Social services redistribute resources for accessing work, such as through education and training, job placements, assistive technologies, adaptations and assistance. As part of our review of policies, we found that there was far greater variability within the DISCIT countries in their services subsystems than in the range of regulatory mechanisms that were used. Variation was apparent in the types of services made available, in the distribution of services and money spent on them, on the ways people were referred to or made eligible for services, and in their integration into other mechanisms. This mirrored Traustadóttir's (2008: 91) claim that redistributive mechanisms, which cover services and income maintenance (Hvinden & Halvorsen, 2003), are typically more diversified compared to regulatory policies. Indeed, while there was an indication of similarities (for instance among the Scandinavian countries or between Ireland and the UK) in the service systems developed, there was also a sense that countries were trying different things. Here we set out some of the examples of policies being used.

Most DISCIT countries provide education and training. Germany has vocational training and retraining centres that provide education to disabled young people and adults. A similar system is in place in Switzerland. In Czech Republic, training is offered as rehabilitation, although this may not be linked to job integration, while the Serbian Anti-Discrimination Act (2009) introduced a right to professional rehabilitation. Rehabilitation is often provided to those who have fallen out of the job market due to illness or disability, and thus can be integrated as part of medical assistance. In Italy, employment services can negotiate training as part of a job placement. Norway offers training depending on individual capacity and background. Public sector traineeships are available to disabled persons with a higher education while vocational training provides a route to general labour market qualifications. In Ireland, internships are offered to people on benefits via a 'JobBridge' scheme, although this was initially not open to people in receipt of the main disability benefit. In the UK, training is available through the government 'Work Programme'. In Sweden, 'Special Introductory Support Measures' (SIUS) are available to people assessed as having a reduced work capacity. These can be used to meet training needs with the aim of securing regular employment.

Job placements, work experience schemes, internships and work trials are orchestrated by employment services in most countries. These are intended to enhance experience and skills, and may be offered for a time-limited period as part of training. In addition, government initiatives such as the German Job4000 scheme bolster existing provisions by funding additional apprenticeships and services. Access to such schemes may depend on an assessed level of impairment or need. Payment for placements may come directly from the employer or through the programme. Other services provide individualised support. The Swedish SIUS funds a personal advisor for a short time. Some countries provide money to fund technologies or adaptations. In Norway, disabled people have a right to assistive technology that will help them in work. The UK provides grants through the 'Access to Work' scheme to fund adaptations to workplaces and personal assistance, and to cover other costs such as travel. Money and support are sometimes also available to promote entrepreneurship, including in Czech Republic, Sweden and Switzerland. In cases where an employer employs someone on a longer-term basis, such as in Czech Republic, Norway and Sweden, wages can also be subsidised.

Finally, several countries maintain sheltered work facilities, including Germany, Norway, Sweden, Serbia, Switzerland and Czech Republic, although the UK had closed down or sold off its sheltered workshops by 2012. In Italy cooperatives provide work for disabled and other persons. Sheltered work is provided for people deemed to have a much reduced work capacity and in particular supports persons with intellectual and psychosocial impairments. Although it is usually intended to lead to work in the open labour market, the number of people moving out of sheltered work can be low. For instance, in Germany disabled people can spend much of their working lives in a sheltered workshop (Waldschmidt & Lingnau, 2007). In some cases payment may be given, although this is often low, while in others persons may receive incapacity benefit.

Income maintenance subsystem

The income maintenance subsystem redistributes money in the form of benefits, allowances and pensions. These typically replace work income where a person is deemed to have a fully or partially reduced work capacity. For example, full and partial disability pensions are offered in Switzerland, Germany, Serbia, Czech Republic and Norway. In Germany and Switzerland, a disability pension is granted after job integration has proved unsuccessful. In Sweden, a pension is granted if work ability is deemed to have been reduced permanently. A disability pension can have conditions. In Czech Republic, those on the highest disability pension have less access to job-seeker services. In Switzerland a person may return to work but might lose some or all of their pension.

In Sweden a form of benefit may be paid short of a pension for people assessed as 'unemployable'. In other countries benefits may be paid that enable a person to continue seeking work and accessing job services. This is the case with the UK 'Employment and Support Allowance' as well as the Irish 'Disability Allowance'. Such benefits stop when a person enters work, although in Ireland a small amount of 'rehabilitative' work, from which income does not exceed a certain amount, may be done. Increasingly, in both countries, access to benefits is based on a prior assessment of work capacity. In the UK, access to benefits is often now conditional and may require engagement with government employment services, for instance the 'Work Programme'. Low wages in the UK can be subsidised through the benefit system with higher levels of payment available to persons with disabilities.

Conditionality is also part of the Norwegian and Swedish systems. In Sweden, a person on sickness benefits will be routinely re-assessed. In Norway, a recently introduced 'work assessment benefit' is granted to people who are out of work but also in a work assessment or rehabilitation programme. Maximum stay on the benefit is four years and usually precedes the permanent incapacity benefit or disability pension. This benefit is meant to support a 'work first' policy. Often the general social benefits system, paid to people who are at risk of poverty (including notably people with psychosocial impairments who may face difficulty being recognised as disabled for the purpose of a benefits claim), supports a similar work-first view.

Promoting the labour market participation of persons with disabilities

One of the main aims of the DISCIT project has been to promote the Active Citizenship of persons with disabilities across Europe through participation in the labour market on an equal basis with non-disabled people. As mentioned earlier, the review of legislation and policies in the DISCIT countries and scrutiny of labour market statistics show that despite efforts of governments and European organisations over the course of several decades the challenge of closing the disability employment gap appears to be as difficult to resolve as ever.

In this section we draw on interviews with 84 expert informants in the nine DISCIT countries to explore a range of ideas designed to promote employment opportunities for persons with disabilities. Discussions about possible solutions and policy responses were preceded by an analysis of the problems that persons with disabilities faced in each country. Respondents not only offered some new ideas but argued for the maintenance and continuation of some current activities they saw as effective, and often also for their intensification and expansion. There was not always consensus among experts about what measures, or further measures, might be appropriate to adopt in each country. Differences were based sometimes on points of principle and sometimes on arguments about effectiveness.

Quota systems

Quota systems require employers to employ a specified percentage of disabled people in their workforces. They are in place in five of the nine DISCIT countries. Where they have been in place in the past but are no longer in use (the UK for example) the reason for discontinuing them has largely been their ineffectiveness. However, they were still seen as potentially useful by some experts despite the problems in enforcing them.

Creating jobs specifically for persons with disabilities

Creating jobs specifically for persons with disabilities represents a different focus to requiring disabled people to compete in the open market with non-disabled people. Examples include 'niche' jobs and 'job carving'. So-called 'niche' jobs are created purposively to be offered directly or through competition only to persons with disabilities. The tasks and duties required by the job are designed so that they are suited to a person with a particular type or types of impairment. 'Job carving' is similar but distinctive in that the idea here is to examine a single job or several jobs and select (or 'carve out') a set of tasks that would be suited to a person with disabilities, thereby 'carving' a new (though not additional) job.

On-the-job support

Although not a new idea, there was much support among the expert informants for the provision of *job coaches*, that is, trained staff who attend the workplace with disabled people and assist them in a variety of ways in order to become competent and confident enough to eventually carry out the functions of their job without assistance. Job coaches were seen as particularly helpful in assisting people with intellectual and psychosocial impairments enter the labour market.

Informed and inclusive workplaces

Some experts thought that opportunities available to employers and employees were not widely known and that programmes of education and knowledge building were necessary. *Disability awareness* training programmes were seen as appropriate mechanisms for promoting tolerance and understanding in the workplace, but needed to be used more.

Sheltered employment

Sheltered employment was a divisive topic among experts. Some opposed sheltered employment on principle because it did not promote employment in the open labour market while others were critical because it was seen as ineffective and wasteful of resources. However, an alternative perspective was offered by some who viewed sheltered employment more positively as a way of providing employment opportunities that otherwise would not be available to persons with disabilities. There was acknowledgment that problems did exist with sheltered employment but that it would be more constructive to address the problems rather than remove one mechanism for providing employment opportunities for disabled people.

Social enterprises

Social enterprises are companies and firms whose prime focus is to conduct business that benefits a local community or particular sector of the population. Social enterprises that employ persons with disabilities were seen as a model with the potential for helping larger numbers than at present. They offered a different (non-competitive) approach rather than trying to help people into the mainstream labour market and by definition the jobs within them were designed specifically for disabled people.

'Therapeutic' employment and rehabilitation–work transitions

The rationale behind 'therapeutic' employment is to integrate participation in work with health support. For instance, in relation to mental health, some proposed a model of employment in which therapy was received in the workplace, rather than outside it. It is contrasted with an approach that prioritises helping people to get well (or well enough) before employment help is offered. Persons with disabilities therefore receive support *in parallel* rather than *sequentially*. Such employment has a clear transitionary focus.

Expert informants also talked about the need for improved transitions out of rehabilitation and into work. Others felt that not enough was done to ensure that people in rehabilitation were able to move into work, as pathways from rehabilitation to work were not clear to many persons with disabilities. Greater interaction between employers and public sector actors and civil society within the health and social care spheres would allow for greater opportunities for the integration of work and health care.

Social security benefits

Problems with benefit systems were numerous and well understood by the expert informants, but ideas for how they could be improved were fewer in number. There were suggestions for improving the financial incentive to work and for ensuring that people on disability pensions had full access to employment services and were not, as they are at present in some countries, excluded from them.

Personal budgets

The principle of personal budgets has been adopted in some countries already to allow people to purchase health and/or care services. This principle could be extended to disabled job seekers so that they could buy any form of assistance desired (such as training, transport, clothing and equipment).

Improving attitudes towards disability

Improving attitudes is a change targeted specifically at the *multi-stakeholder system,* as it demonstrates the key role employers play in securing Active Citizenship for persons with disabilities. While improving the functioning of existing policies may represent a short- to medium-term goal, there was also the longer-term goal of enhancing the perception of disabled persons as employees. Such solutions, however, sit outside the disability policy system. Instead, they are an issue of education, and a cultural issue that can only be addressed by starting a dialogue around disability and employment. They also represent a way in which other stakeholders, including disabled persons' organisations and other representative organisations, may play a part in improving the circumstances of disabled persons.

Creating sustainable jobs and enhancing pay conditions

The working lives of disabled persons should be made more sustainable, by (for example) improving in-work support mechanisms and improving levels of pay. The first of these could be addressed through the *social services subsystem* in particular, by providing information and technologies that would enhance people's ability to work. *Social regulations* that allow for flexible working were also seen as an important means of allowing persons with disabilities to stay in work. Experts felt that work was still needed to be done in order to improve the pay conditions of disabled persons. There were concerns about the *disability pay gap*, meaning the gap in wages between non-disabled and disabled persons.

Building on existing provision by increasing resource allocations and scaling up existing solutions

A final perspective offered in the expert informant interviews was that there were already a number of promising ideas for enhancing the actual employment of persons with disabilities (as opposed to improving their employability), such as creating specific employment opportunities through niche jobs or job carving or via wage subsidies to employers. The issue was one of *scale*; there were simply not enough employers embracing these approaches to make a large impact on the employment rates of disabled people.

There were also many examples across the DISCIT countries of skills training and education programmes; work experience programmes; internship schemes; assistance with health, housing, debt and family issues; personal development courses; confidence building; CV preparation; job searching; interview training and other measures designed to increase the employability of persons with disabilities and move them towards a state of *job readiness*. It was thought that if resources could be increased for these existing provisions more persons with disabilities would be able to compete for employment in the open labour market and that in consequence employment rates for them would almost certainly improve.

Improving coordination between systems of social regulation, social services and social benefits

The current set of mechanisms used for integrating disabled persons into the open labour market are understood within the DISCIT study as falling within subsystems of social regulations, social services, and social benefits. Expert informants suggested that there were ways in which improvements could be made within each of these three systems by enforcing and monitoring existing legislation and policies, ensuring compliance and closing loopholes.

Many experts felt that work could be done to ensure a better coordination between services and benefits and to guarantee that entry into the *income maintenance subsystem* did not prevent persons from accessing provisions within the *social services subsystem*. It was also felt that there could be improvement in the *social regulation subsystem*, for example in monitoring quotas which too often do not support disabled people into work, where employers can circumvent rules or are not sufficiently regulated. Furthermore, while the benefits of anti-discrimination legislation for enhancing the employment of disabled people have been noted elsewhere (European Parliament, 2015), they have also been described as only weakly regulating employer behaviour, in particular in recruitment.

Policy ideas within the DISCIT disability policy framework

Earlier we linked current provisions in the nine DISCIT countries to the elements of the disability policy system—the social regulations subsystem, the social services subsystem and the income maintenance system. From this review of the ideas from the expert stakeholders we can see that many of these ideas also align with these three elements.

First, ideas to promote the employability of disabled people, to provide them with on-the-job support, to offer opportunities in sheltered employment environments and the provision of personal budgets are all associated with the social services subsystem. The social regulation subsystem has been identified as part of the solution to low employment rates in two different ways. First, the use of social regulations as *obligations and requirements* placed on employers still has support among some expert informants, as evidenced by the continued use and renewed interest in quota systems. The second way in which social regulation can be utilised is in creating *incentives* for employers to employ more disabled people. The suggestion that social enterprises might play a greater role in providing employment opportunities is based on them being granted favourable tax and other regulatory conditions through the social regulation system. Finally, suggestions for changes to social security benefits by definition fall within the income maintenance system.

Another set of suggestions seems to fall outside the disability policy framework however; these are aimed at educating employers, employees and the public about disability in order to reduce and, it is hoped, to eliminate the sorts of attitudes and prejudices that act as barriers to recruitment, sustained jobs and fulfilling employment. While it is possible to see roles here for governments, employers and civil society, it is less clear that the mechanisms required for changing attitudes necessarily lie within the disability policy system. Other forms of action—through education and publicity both within the workplace and externally—are arguably more appropriate.

Conclusion

The policy aim of improving employment rates of persons with disabilities is universal across Europe including the DISCIT countries, in which a wide variety of policy tools are currently being used or being introduced. These include regulatory, social service and income maintenance measures designed to promote employment, mediate barriers, and influence the behaviours of disabled persons and employers. As shown elsewhere, these policies work together to enhance people's prospects, although results vary for different people (see the accompanying Volume 2). However, as shown earlier, the disability employment gap is not only high but it has remained high for at least the last 10 to 15 years, despite the policy developments that have taken place in many countries.

One potential reason for this is that the tools available are not yet wholly effective in dismantling barriers. The policy experts interviewed suggest that outcomes can be improved by existing policy measures being properly resourced and enforced, a view shared by the European Disability Forum (2015) which calls on the EU to oversee the effective implementation of anti-discrimination and reasonable adjustment measures. Others see the existence of discriminatory attitudes as requiring more than regulation. Rather, greater integration of disabled people in mainstream schools and a programme of education are felt to be needed to challenge negative perceptions of disabled people's abilities.

It may also be that existing measures are only marginally effective given the current state of the labour market. Many, though not all, European countries have experienced the effects of a prolonged economic downturn from around 2008 onwards. The extent to which countries are emerging from recession is varied, and there may be an expectation that growing economies will eventually generate jobs for disabled people, but that remains uncertain. It has not always been the case that disabled people benefit from general improvements in countries' economies. The negative impacts of recession identified in the expert interviews included a general decline in employment opportunities, a rise in unemployment, a loss of low skilled jobs particularly those suited to some groups of disabled people (though this trend has been apparent in European economies since before the economic crisis), and the shrinking of the public sector in many countries where employers have historically been more inclusive of disabled people than the private sector. The overall effect has been to make the labour market increasingly competitive and hostile towards disabled people and in particular to restrict opportunities for younger disabled people to enter work.

The DISCIT study makes use of the concept of Active Citizenship to operationalise the phrase 'full and effective' participation in society and the economy. In particular, it focuses on the rights of disabled persons to make choices in key areas, including paid work, and to be protected from uncertainty and risks in those areas. Drawing on data from expert informants highlights the need for more critical thinking about work and also the need to consider how labour markets are structured, and how that is reflected in the demand for labour generally and for persons with disabilities in particular. A great deal of thought, effort and resources currently go into improving the skills and employability of disabled persons, and efforts are made to minimise exclusion and discrimination through anti-discrimination laws, notions of reasonable adjustment and quota systems, even if they are felt to have only limited impact. This emphasis on employability and removing barriers is based on a desire to respond to two 'problems'. The first reflects what Traustadóttir (2008: 90) sees as an on-going perception of persons with disabilities as individually lacking. The other reflects a more recent focus on rights and equality, and a perception of injustice as being a product of the behaviours of employers. However, labour market structure, labour market demand and the nature of jobs also exclude and deny choice for persons with disabilities. The need is for long-term thinking about work and the kinds of work people can and hope to do.

Rethinking work from a disability perspective may contribute as much, and possibly more, to enhancing Active Citizenship for persons with disabilities through open labour market participation than programmes designed to integrate disabled people into an exclusionary mainstream. How people engage with the labour market and the extent to which they are able to do so is clearly partly a matter of personal choice and preference. The assumption that being an 'active citizen' necessarily includes having paid work in the open labour market is challenged by the accounts of some of the people interviewed in the DISCIT project. Voluntary and caring roles or participation in other activities may also give people a sense of being Active Citizens in ways that make participation in the labour market less important to them or even irrelevant.

The three components of the DISCIT project—the review of policy, life-course histories of persons with disabilities and interviews with disability experts—have given us a better understanding of the complex interplay of personal and structural factors that shape the employment experiences of persons with disabilities across Europe. That some people manage to create long and rewarding careers demonstrates what is possible. Nonetheless, the statistical evidence across countries and across decades shows that still far too few persons with disabilities enjoy the benefits of employment. While it is important that practices aimed at increasing the employability of people are maintained and improved, the DISCIT project has shown that only by refocusing our attention on employers and the demand for labour can we expect to make the necessary progress towards closing the employment gap and achieving equality in the labour market for persons with disabilities.

References

Atkinson, A. B., Cantillon, B., Marlier, E. & Nolan, B. (2002). *Social Indicators: The EU and Social Inclusion*. Oxford: Oxford University Press.

Barnes, C. & Oliver, M. (2012). *The New Politics of Disablement*. Basingstoke: Palgrave Macmillan.

Beresford, P. & Holden, C. (2000). We have choices: Globalisation and welfare user movements. *Disability and Society*, 15(7), 973–989.

BRK-Allianz (2013). *For Independent Living, Equal Rights, Accessibility and Inclusion!* Retrieved from: http://tbinternet.ohchr.org/Treaties/CRPD/Shared%20Documents/DEU/INT_CRPD_NGO_DEU_16323_O.pdf

Chopin, I. & Germaine-Sahl, C. (2013). *Developing Anti-discrimination Law in Europe: The 28 EU Member States, the Former Yugoslav Republic of Macedonia, Iceland, Liechtenstein, Norway and Turkey Compared*. Luxembourg: Publications Office of the European Union.

Dupré, D. & Karjalainen, A. (2003). Employment of disabled people in Europe in 2002. *Statistics in Focus: Population and Social Conditions. Theme*, 3(26), 1–7.

Ebersold, S., Schmitt, M. J. & Priestley, M. (2011). *Inclusive Education for Young Disabled People in Europe:* Trends, *Issues and Challenges*. Retrieved 15 April 2016 from: http://www.disability-europe.net/content/aned/media/ANED%202010%20Task%205%20Education%20final%20report%20-%20FINAL%20(2)_0.pdf

European Commission (2000). *Benchmarking Employment Policies for People with Disabilities*. Brussels: European Commission.

European Commission (2003). *Equal Opportunities for People with Disabilities: A European Action Plan*, Vol. 30 (10). Brussels: European Commission.

European Commission (2010a). *Europe 2020: A strategy for Smart, Sustainable And Inclusive Growth*. Brussels: European Commission.

European Commission (2010b). *European Disability Strategy 2010–2020: A Renewed Commitment to a Barrier-Free Europe*. Brussels: European Commission.

European Disability Forum (2015). *Alternative Report to the UN Committee on The Rights of Persons With Disabilities*. Brussels: European Disability Forum.

European Parliament (2015). *Reasonable Accommodation and Sheltered Workshops for People with Disabilities: Costs and Returns of Investments*. Brussels: European Parliament.

European Union (2009). Council conclusions of 12 May 2009 on a strategic framework for European cooperation in education and training ('ET 2020'), Official Journal of the European Union, C 119/2, 28.5.2009. Retrieved 20 February 2017 from http://eur-lex.europa.eu/legal-content/EN/TXT/PDF/?uri=CELEX:52009XG0528(01)&from=EN

Eurostat (2014a). *Disability Statistics: Access to Education and Training*. Retrieved 15 April 2016 from: http://ec.europa.eu/eurostat/statistics-explained/index.php/Disability_statistics_-_access_to_education_and_training

Eurostat (2014b). *Disability Statistics: Barriers to Employment*. Retrieved 15 April 2016 from: http://ec.europa.eu/eurostat/statistics-explained/index.php/Disability_statistics_-_barriers_to_employment

Eurostat (2014c). *Disability Statistics: Employment Patterns*. Retrieved 15 April 2016 from: http://ec.europa.eu/eurostat/statistics-explained/index.php/Disability_statistics_-_employment_patterns

Eurostat (2014d). *Disability Statistics: Labour Market Access*. Retrieved 15 April 2016 from: http://ec.europa.eu/eurostat/statistics-explained/index.php/Disability_statistics_-_labour_market_access

Eurostat (2014e). *Situation of People with Disabilities in the EU*. Retrieved 15 April 2016 from: http://ec.europa.eu/eurostat/documents/2995521/6181592/3-02122014-BP-EN.pdf/aefdf716-f420-448f-8cba-893e90e6b460

Eurostat (2015). *Employment of Disabled People: Statistical Analysis of the 2011 Labour Force Survey ad hoc Module*. Luxembourg: Publications Office of the European Union.

Eurostat (2016). Statistics explained. Disability statistics. Retrieved 20 February 2017 from http://ec.europa.eu/eurostat/statistics-explained/index.php/Disability_statistics

Eurostat Database (2016). Disability. Retrieved 20 February 2017 from http://ec.europa.eu/eurostat/web/health/disability/data/database

Greve, B. (2009). *The Labour Market Situation of Disabled People in European* Countries *and Implementation of Employment Policies: A Summary of Evidence from Country Reports and Research Studies*. ANED. Retrieved from: http://www.disability-europe.net/content/aned/media/ANED%20Task%206%20final%20report%20-%20final%20version%2017-04-09.pdf

Haveman, R. & Wolfe, B. (2000). The economics of disability and disability policy. In A. J. Culyer & J. P. Newhouse (Eds.), *Handbook of Health Economics* (995–1051). Amsterdam: Elsevier.

Hvinden, B. & Halvorsen, R. (2003). Which way for European disability policy? *Scandinavian Journal of Disability Research*, 5(3), 296–312.

Lindsay, C. & Houston, D. (2013). Fit for work? Representations and explanations of the disability benefits 'crisis' in the UK and beyond. In C. Lindsay & D. Houston (Eds.), *Disability Benefits, Welfare Reform and Employment Policy* (1–14). Basingstoke: Palgrave Macmillan.

OECD (2010). *Sickness, Disability and Work: Breaking the Barriers, A Synthesis of Findings across OECD Countries*. Paris: OECD.

Palmer, M. (2011). Disability and poverty: A conceptual review. *Journal of Disability Policy Studies*, 21(4), 210–218.

Priestley, M. & Lawson, A. (2015). Mapping disability policies in Europe: Introducing the disability online tool of the commission (DOTCOM). *ALTER—European Journal of Disability Research*, 9(1), 75–78.

Salladarré, F. & Hlaimi, S. (2014). Women and part-time work in Europe. *International Labour Review / International Labour Office*, 153(2), 293–310.

Thornton, P. & Lunt, N. (1995). *Employment for Disabled People: Social Obligation or Individual Responsibility*. York: University of York, Social Policy Research Unit.

Traustadóttir, R. (2008). Work, disability, and social inclusion. In M. DeVault (Ed.), *People at Work: Life, Power, and Social Inclusion in the New Economy* (74–93). New York: New York University Press.

Waddington, L. & Lawson, A. (2009). *Disability and Non-discrimination Law in the European Union: An Analysis of Disability Discrimination Law within and beyond the Employment Field*. Luxembourg: Publications Office of the European Union.

Waldschmidt, A. & Lingnau, K. (2007). *Report on the Employment of Disabled People in European Countries—Country: Germany*. Academic Network of European Disability experts. Retrieved 20 February 2017 from: http://www.disability-europe.net/downloads/338-de-employment-report

7 To what extent is the assistance and support provided by social services capable of enhancing Active Citizenship for persons with psychosocial disabilities? A comparative perspective

Rafael Lindqvist, Marie Sépulchre and Victoria Schuller

Introduction

Over the past few years mental health has increasingly been recognised as a major issue for European countries (EC, 2005; WHO, 2005). It is estimated that 38.2 per cent of the EU population is affected by a mental disorder each year (Wittchen et al., 2011) and figures indicate that suicide is one of the top ten leading causes of premature death in Europe (Knapp et al., 2007: 1). Mental disorders also have a huge total societal cost estimated at €798 billion in 2010 (Gustavsson et al., 2011: 720). Furthermore, Wittchen et al. (2011) found that less than one-third of people with a mental disorder receives any treatment, which points to a considerable level of unmet needs. Research has shown that a mental disorder is likely to appear in childhood or youth, and that psychosocial disabilities are usually long-term conditions (OECD, 2012: 175–198). Individuals can recover but are likely to continue experiencing psychosocial disabilities throughout their life course. Mental ill health is strongly stigmatised in society and persons experiencing psychosocial disabilities have been deprived of their fundamental rights and locked up in segregated institutions. The UN Convention on the Rights of Persons with Disabilities (CRPD) reaffirms their fundamental human rights and the fact that persons with mental impairments, including persons with psychosocial disabilities (Minkowitz, 2007), have the right to participate in society on the same basis as others. This chapter draws on this perspective and uses the concept of Active Citizenship to explore the possibilities for citizens with psychosocial disabilities to participate in society. Furthermore, we use the term 'psychosocial disabilities' to signify that mental ill health results from a complex interplay of individual, social and structural factors.

This chapter focuses on the structural level and discusses how European disability and mental health policy systems—consisting of social services, benefits and regulations—influence the possibility for persons with psychosocial disabilities to be active citizens. The main focus is on services but the interdependencies between services, cash benefits and, to some extent, social regulation are taken into account. We look at both the European and national levels and cover nine different countries: the Czech Republic, Germany, Ireland, Italy, Norway, Serbia, Sweden, Switzerland and the United Kingdom. The aim of the chapter is not to give a detailed account of the disability and mental health policy systems of each country but to investigate how these systems relate to Active Citizenship. Drawing on interviews with experts in the disability and mental health field, the chapter also sheds light on the main challenges that countries face in relation to psychosocial disabilities.

The first part of the chapter outlines the general context of mental health in Europe and provides an overview of the process of de-institutionalisation, decentralisation, the austerity measures and the international legislation and strategies concerning mental health. The conceptual framework is presented in the following section and the main concepts are: psychosocial disabilities, Active Citizenship, disability and the mental health policy system, and welfare regimes. Next, we present our data and the methodology used to collect expert interviews in the nine countries. The chapter's fourth part outlines the disability and mental health policy systems of the various countries, categorised into four welfare regimes. This part also presents the findings of the expert interviews. Finally, the chapter closes with a comparative section about the disability and mental health policy systems in the four welfare regimes and discusses how these can affect Active Citizenship for persons with psychosocial disabilities.

Contextual framework

De-institutionalisation and decentralisation

During the second half of the 20th century, major changes occurred in the way the state provides for persons with psychosocial impairments in Western societies. Until the 1960s, people with mental health problems usually lived in segregated residential institutions (Scull, 1979; Wright & Digby, 1996) but such services were widely criticised because of their poor conditions, residents' lack of autonomy and segregation from the wider community and reported human rights abuses (Goffman, 1961; Sayce, 2000). Furthermore, factors including the huge cost of residential institutions, the evolution in treatments and the claims of mental health service users' organisations resulted in a movement away from institutional living towards 'life in the community'. This de-institutionalisation process happened differently across Europe; while psychiatric hospitals were eliminated in some countries, institutional care continued to exist alongside community living arrangements in other countries. Italy was a pioneer in this process and began to close down all psychiatric hospitals in the 1970s (Leff & Warner, 2006: 64). Sweden followed this example a decade later (Markström et al., 2004). In contrast, large psychiatric institutions still prevail in other countries such as Germany, Switzerland and the post-communist countries (WHO, 2011a).

Another important change that happened in parallel to de-institutionalisation was the process of decentralisation through which national governments transferred the responsibility for organising welfare from central government to local authorities. In several countries, this process was accompanied by the privatisation of care. These changes spawned new challenges such as the coordination and collaboration between different administrative levels and between public, private and third-sector actors. This brought potential difficulties in terms of multiple assessments, coping with different eligibility criteria and dealing with staff with diverging levels of knowledge about disability. If the various welfare providers do not cooperate, the clients do indeed risk being endlessly circulated between agencies (Hasenfeld, 2009; Lindqvist & Grape, 1999). One response to such developments in community mental health services has been to emphasise the role of joined-up health and social services, and more generally one-stop-shop arrangements for benefits and services (see e.g. the arrangement provided by the Social Services Act of 2009 in Norway). Such arrangements were designed to improve the user's ability to influence and control the social services he or she receives.

The European legal framework and action plans

Apart from national and local policies developed by individual countries to respond to the challenges related to mental health, strategies and action plans have been developed at an international and European level. In 2005, the WHO (2005) European Ministerial Conference on Mental Health identified the main issues concerning mental health and suggested viable solutions. A few months later, the EU (2005) published a Green paper entitled 'Improving the mental health of the population: Towards a strategy on mental health for the European Union'. Further, in 2008 the EU ratified the CRPD, which also covers persons with psychosocial disabilities (Minkowitz, 2007: 407). The CRPD has important consequences for persons with psychosocial disabilities; it does not only reassert their most fundamental Human Rights, but also prohibits the deprivation of liberty on the basis of a disability—Article 14 protects persons against non-consensual psychiatric interventions (Minkowitz, 2007)—and recognises that persons with disabilities should enjoy legal capacity on an equal basis with others in all aspects of life and should be given the support they may require to enjoy this right (Art 12; see also Weller, 2014). Further important documents are the 'European pact for mental health and well-being' (EU, 2008) and the 'European mental health action plan 2013–2020' (WHO, 2015), which outline priority areas and objectives to strengthen mental health and well-being. Finally, the importance of mental health is highlighted in the EU 2020 flagship initiatives relative to mental health in the workplace (EC, 2010). These different documents form a legal and strategic framework to promote mental health in general and protect the rights of persons with psychosocial disabilities in Europe.

Economic crisis and austerity measures

Another development influencing welfare provisions for persons with psychosocial disabilities concerns the economic crisis of 2008 and the austerity measures taken by most European governments (see Chapter 2). The WHO Regional Office for Europe (WHO, 2011b) investigated the effects of the economic crisis on mental health and concluded that there were several factors influencing mental health such as poverty, unemployment, poor working conditions, substandard housing and poor education. Although the WHO (2015) recommended developing schemes that secure the resources of individuals in order to prevent mental ill health, European countries have adopted austerity measures when it comes to funding their welfare systems. However, the situation varies across Europe. Concerning the countries covered by this chapter, the UK made the biggest cuts in its welfare budget; the Czech Republic, Germany, Italy, Serbia, Sweden and Switzerland had relatively stable levels of spending on disability benefits; and Ireland and Norway had a substantial growth in their levels of spending over the period 2003–2013 (see Chapter 2). The socio-economic crisis and austerity measures are important contextual factors that influence the ability of persons with psychosocial disabilities to participate in Active Citizenship because they affect their job opportunities, their financial security and the provision of mental health treatments.

Conceptual framework

A psychosocial approach to mental health

This chapter draws on a psychosocial approach to mental distress. This was developed as a reaction to the biomedical approach that conceives mental distress as a biological defect and an illness that needs to be treated by medication. The major critique of the medical model was that it denied the impact of the social context on mental distress (Ramon & Williams, 2005: 14). In contrast, psychosocial approaches consider that mental distress implies a combination of individual psychological and socio-structural elements (Williams & Ramon, 2005: 1). The term ‘psychosocial disabilities’ used in this chapter refers to disabilities that are caused by psychological and social factors. This definition does not deny the existence of medical diagnoses but holds that a biomedical understanding of mental distress is insufficient for understanding the complexity at stake. Furthermore, the concept of psychosocial disabilities covers both persons with and without a medical diagnosis because it focuses on the lived experiences of the individuals and not on a medical assessment. Finally, the psychosocial approach recognises the importance of viewing psychosocial disabilities in a life-course perspective and takes the view that mental distress occurs differently over the life span (WHO, 2015: 4).

Active Citizenship

Following the theoretical framework elaborated for DISCIT, we consider that the core of Active Citizenship consists of three main dimensions: influence, autonomy and security (see Chapter 1 in this volume). This framework fits the psychosocial approach to mental health because it goes beyond the medical aspects and holds that a person with psychosocial disabilities is not only a patient but a citizen who has rights and should be given the possibility to enjoy these rights and participate in society on an equal basis with others (see CRPD, Art. 19).

Disability and mental health policy systems

In this volume, the term 'disability policy systems' refers to the policies, benefits and regulations directed to persons with disabilities (see Chapter 2 in this volume). However, since mental health is sometimes included in general disability policies and sometimes treated separately, in this chapter we use the term 'disability and mental health policy systems' to cover the range of policies, benefits and regulations affecting persons with psychosocial disabilities. In order to compare different welfare systems in relation to the individual citizens, their families and the labour market, many studies start from Esping-Andersen's typology (1990), distinguishing between liberal, conservative and social-democratic welfare regimes. Following this typology, which has been further elaborated to include post-communist welfare regimes (see Cook, 2010; Cerami & Vanhuyesse, 2009), we tentatively group the nine European countries included in the study into four different welfare regimes: liberal (the UK and Ireland); continental conservative (Germany, Italy and Switzerland); social democratic (Norway and Sweden); and post-communist (the Czech Republic and Serbia).

Data and methodology

International reports and expert interviews

Disability and mental health policy systems are complex because they apply to a heterogeneous group of people and because they are organised at different levels and delivered by various actors. Furthermore, there is a dearth of data about these systems and the available datasets are often not comparable (see for instance WHO, 2011a and Chapter 4 in this volume). As a consequence, it is very complicated to sketch a picture and compare disability and mental health systems across countries. This chapter draws on various sources of secondary data and on original interviews. The secondary data consists of the following international and national reports: WHO, 2011a; EC, 2013; OECD, 2014; FRA, 2014; MDRI-S, 2016; SSA, 2014. The second dataset consists of the summaries of 84 'expert interviews'; that is interviews with experts in the field of mental health and disability.

Disability and mental health policy systems in nine European countries

The different European strategies and plans for mental health mentioned earlier indicate that the issue of mental health is placed high on the European agenda. However, countries organise their welfare provisions in various ways and these have different impacts on Active Citizenship. This section offers a comparative perspective on the disability and mental health policy systems in nine European countries categorised in four welfare regimes. The scope of this chapter does not permit a discussion of all the aspects of the policy systems. Therefore, apart from considering whether the country in question has a national mental health policy, we have decided to base the comparison on three aspects that are related to the three dimensions of Active Citizenship: the number of beds in psychiatric hospitals (autonomy), the organisation of welfare services (security) and the right to vote (influence).

The continental conservative regimes

In the continental conservative group of countries we tentatively count Germany, Switzerland and Italy. Their common features identified by Esping-Andersen (1990) are that their welfare systems tend to preserve status differentials between social and occupational groups and have a strong emphasis on traditional family values. Table 7.1 summarises different features of their disability and mental health policy systems.

Concerning the strategies to tackle mental health we can observe that Italy and Switzerland have elaborated a national plan for mental health but that such a strategy on the national level does not exist in Germany. Furthermore, mental health

Table 7.1 Characteristics of the continental conservative welfare regimes

	Germany, DE	*Switzerland, CH*	*Italy, IT*
National mental health plan	No	Yes	Yes
Number of beds in mental hospitals	High	High	Low
Right to vote	Can be restricted for persons who by a court order are in a psychiatric hospital	Can be restricted for persons subject to tutorship due to mental illness or 'weakness of the mind'	No limitations on the right to vote
Organisation of disability and mental health policy systems	Decentralised to Federal States; Private practitioners play important role	Decentralised to cantons; Private practitioners play important role	Decentralised to (local) public and NGO providers and social cooperatives
Role of the state and public actors: Social services Social benefits	Public-private mix Sickness funds: tripartite model of state and social partners; Social assistance for poor households	Public-private mix Mandated social insurance provided by cantonal, industrial or federal funds; Social assistance for poor households	Public (local) + NGOs + social cooperatives financed by public and private sources Selective social security benefits + social assistance

Sources: Alzheimer Europe, 2010; FRA, 2014; SSA, 2014; WHO, 2011a.

treatments are organised differently in the three countries; in Italy where mental hospitals closed down from the late 1970s onwards, inpatient care is provided by general hospital psychiatric units with a maximum of 15 beds (EC, 2013). In contrast, mental health care in Germany and Switzerland can be provided in psychiatric hospitals (EC, 2013). However, a shift from psychiatric hospitals to community- based inpatient facilities has taken place over the last 25 years in Germany; psychiatric wards in general hospitals now form the main part of community-based inpatient care (EC, 2013). In addition, outpatient clinics, general practitioners and office-based psychiatrists play an important role in community-based psychiatric care. The Swiss mental health plan promotes a shift of services and resources from psychiatric hospitals to community mental health facilities (WHO, 2011a). However, inpatient care is common in Switzerland as well as a large number of psychiatrists in private practice (OECD, 2014: 125–148). Despite the fact that Italy was a pioneer in Europe in terms of de-institutionalisation in mental health care, the development of new district-based community services (rehabilitation and day care services) has been slow and differences between regions in Italy are significant (Goodwin, 1997: 17–18). Hence, although a limited number of community mental health services, including residential facilities for long-term psychiatric care and day hospital/centres, exist (EC, 2013), the care of persons with psychosocial disabilities is mostly put on the shoulders of the families (De Girolamo et al., 2007).

The three countries are similar as regards the subsidiary role of public authorities and the decentralised organisation of welfare services. In Germany, federal authorities are only involved if the private and voluntary organisations fail to provide services (Schulz, 2012: 111). The Swiss approach to dealing with mental ill-health presents a combination of public, private subsidised and fully private systems; cantons plan and provide mental health services resulting in significant variation between cantons (OECD, 2014). In Italy, non-government organisations (NGOs) and social cooperatives play a significant role in providing services and support for persons with psychosocial disabilities. The three countries in the continental conservative welfare regime have developed different programmes for income protection and social security. The German social insurance system has been described as 'quasi-universal', providing better benefits to core industrial workers and public servants (Palier, 2010: 605). The system is administered by separate sickness funds organised within federations at the national or state level with representatives from employers and the insured (SSA, 2014: 118). Social benefits for persons with psychosocial disabilities can be provided by either the health insurance system or the social assistance system in terms of integration support granted if other means of support are not sufficient (SSA, 2014: 119–120). Switzerland has fairly generous social insurance benefits within a framework of public and private insurance-based regulations. Health insurance (compulsory for every person in Switzerland) usually pays for medical examinations and treatments, nursing costs and medical prevention. Income protection can be provided in terms of daily sick cash benefits or a disability pension administered by a network of cantonal, industrial and federal compensation funds (SSA, 2014: 301). Since 2012, 'rehabilitation before a pension' is the new motto of the Swiss Invalidity Insurance (AHV/AI Information Centre, 2017). Means-tested social assistance exists in cases where the person is not eligible for a disability pension. In Italy, which has the least generous social benefits system, many poor households, including persons with psychosocial disabilities, fail to fulfil the narrow eligibility criteria stipulated by the social security programmes (EC, 2013; Ferrera, 2010: 622).

Concerning the right to vote, there are no restrictions on persons with mental health issues voting in Italy (FRA, 2014) but a person's right to vote may be restricted in Germany and Switzerland. In Germany, the right to vote can be restricted by court order for persons who are in psychiatric hospitals because they have committed a crime, or persons who have a custodian who takes care of their affairs (FRA, 2014). Similarly, the right to vote of persons with mental illness can be restricted in Switzerland if they are subject to tutorship (Alzheimer Europe, 2010).

Challenges facing the conservative continental model

The expert interviews in Italy, Germany and Switzerland indicate that the three countries are preoccupied by the high number of persons living with psychosocial problems and by the fact that they often live in poverty. The increase of psychosocial disabilities is, according to German experts, mainly due to stress-related conditions, high pressure at work, increased temporary work contracts, increased competition and decreased job security. Swiss experts made similar observations and were worried that, although people with psychosocial difficulties are the biggest group of invalidity pension recipients, they are not in the focus of Swiss disability policy (see also OECD, 2014). In Italy, our informants also commented on an increase in psychosocial disabilities and were especially worried about the mental health of younger and older people.

According to the experts in Switzerland and Germany, the fact that persons with psychosocial disabilities are not a main target group for the social security systems entails a risk of poverty. Swiss experts therefore emphasised the importance of supporting people, and young people in particular, so that they can retain their job and/or can return to work. Another Swiss expert underlined the need for employers and psychiatrists to collaborate on these issues. Italian experts contended that families suffered from the lack of public support for persons with psychosocial disabilities. They also explained that, although Italy has ambitious plans and strategies, these are not implemented because of a lack of resources. Finally, the experts of the three countries found that people with psychosocial disabilities face more difficulties than persons with other types of disabilities and believed that this was mostly due to the stigmatisation of mental ill health.

The liberal welfare regimes

Key characteristics of the liberal welfare regimes are, according to Esping-Andersen (1990: 27), means-tested assistance, modest social insurance plans and benefits for the poor. Selectivity and low benefits are a consequence of a vision that work is always preferable to welfare benefits. In this model, welfare policies target the most vulnerable groups and are seen as a last resort that should be used by as few as possible. Hence, family, charity organisations, NGOs and private providers and insurance often play an important role in terms of income maintenance and social services. Table 7.2 summarises different features of the British and Irish disability and mental health policy systems.

Ireland and the UK share similar characteristics when it comes to the centralised organisation of mental health care and both countries have national strategies promoting a shift towards community mental health services. Hospital care still prevails when it comes to care of persons with psychosocial disabilities in Ireland, but a number of large mental hospitals have been closed down in recent years according to the Irish mental health plan. It follows that short-term inpatient acute care is increasingly provided in psychiatric units in general hospitals (EC, 2013). In the UK, the number of psychiatric beds supplied by the National Health Service has dropped by almost a half since 1989 and psychiatric wards in general hospitals and psychiatric hospitals (some privately run) form the main core of inpatient provision (EC, 2013). Moreover, the British mental health plan intends to develop a collaborative programme of action that ensures local planning and priority-setting, providing for mental health needs across a full range of services.

Mental health systems in Ireland and the UK consist of a combination of public and private systems and NGO providers. Community mental health services are delivered by multidisciplinary teams including day centres, day hospitals and high-, medium- and low-care hostel provision (EC, 2013). Services in the

Table 7.2 Characteristics of the liberal welfare regimes

	Ireland, IE	*United Kingdom, UK*
National mental health plan	Yes	Yes
Beds in mental hospitals	Medium	Low to medium
Right to vote	Certain limitations exist for persons with mental disorders	No limitations
Organisation of disability and mental health policy systems	Centralised, organised within health care system; Divide between health care and social services	Centralised responsibility for services, but local planning and priority-setting
Role of the state and public actors:	Public-private mix;	Public-private mix, emphasis on care in the community;
Social services	NGOs play significant role	Private providers play important role
Social benefits	Strong component of income- and needs-test	Universal with flat-rate benefits; Strong component of income- and needs-test

Sources: Alzheimer Europe, 2010; FRA, 2014; SSA, 2014; WHO, 2011a.

UK, though, when compared to Ireland are more oriented towards care in the community and primary mental healthcare services.

Income protection in the form of cash benefits in the case of sickness and disability in Ireland and the UK is characterised by a low level of compensation, limited duration and by means-testing and the patient's own contribution (SSA, 2014). The Irish Disability Allowance, which is means-tested and can be claimed by persons with psychosocial disabilities, is paid to people who are substantially restricted in their capacity to take on suitable work because of a specified disability, including mental illness. The level of benefit depends on the individual's financial resources (SSA, 2014: 143). The UK national social security system provides cash benefits in the case of reduced capacity to work due to sickness under strict assessment procedures of the capacity to work. Means-tested social assistance can be provided if the person is not eligible for social security. Persons with mental disorders can claim generic benefits in terms of unemployment benefits, means-tested income support and long-term sickness benefit based on the assessment of the claimant's ability to carry out a range of activities (SSA, 2014: 312–318). In terms of social benefits Ireland is more of a clear-cut liberal welfare regime than the UK. The right to vote for persons with mental health problems differs between Ireland and the UK; while Ireland still has formal restrictions (though rarely practised) the UK does not have any such restrictions.

Challenges for the countries of the liberal welfare regime

According to the expert interviews, the Irish disability policy and mental health system has yet to accomplish the shift of services from hospital care to services in the community. In the UK, compared to Ireland, this process has proceeded further. However, although many large residential institutions have been closed down, experts pointed to a trend of 're-institutionalisation' because treatment units look increasingly like institutions. Given the sharp divide between health care and social services, an Irish expert said there are not enough connections between medical and vocational rehabilitation. In contrast to Ireland, there is a strong emphasis in the UK on care in the community. Hence, the UK experts found that health service reforms made services more fragmented and the collaboration between different services for disabled people difficult.

Experts in both countries talked about challenges in terms of labour market participation for persons with psychosocial disabilities and contended that mental ill-health is probably the issue employers are most frightened about. They also pointed to the fact that negative attitudes to mental health problems are important barriers that prevent access to the labour market. British experts talked about the effects of the financial crisis 2007–2008; when tax revenue fell, there were cuts in public services and the difficulties in funding mental health services increased. They pointed to the detrimental consequences of the financial crisis for persons with mental health conditions because employers are less flexible and less prepared to make accommodations.

The social democratic regimes

Social democratic regimes have been characterised by the importance attached to an active state, a large public sector and universal social benefits and services (Esping-Andersen, 1990; Kautto, 2010: 586–600; Kvist et al., 2012: 201–206). In this regime, the right to work is encouraged by active labour market policies and conceived as equally important as the right to income protection in the case of sickness, disability and old age. This model is based on a complex relationship between the state and local municipalities, in which the state decides on policy formulation and semi-autonomous local municipalities take on implementation. Few measures specifically target persons with psychosocial disabilities. Instead, the main rule is mainstreaming welfare provisions on the basis of an assessment of the need for social support or assistance. However, eligibility criteria for services and benefits have become stricter during the last decade. The main characteristics of the disability and mental health policy system in Norway and Sweden are summarised in Table 7.3.

Both Norway and Sweden have a national plan for mental health. The Norwegian Action Plan was established for the time period 1997–2009 and was revised in 2011 (WHO, 2011a). Its goal was to expand mental health services in regional and local areas, improve coordination within and between the different

Table 7.3 Characteristics of the social democratic welfare regimes

	Norway, NO	*Sweden, SE*
National mental health plan	Yes	Yes
Beds in mental hospitals	High	Non-existent
Right to vote	Voting on Election Day may be denied if the voter manifestly suffers from a seriously weakened mental state or a reduced level of consciousness	No limitations
Organisation of disability and mental health policy systems	Combined hospital care and decentralised community care; Coordinated organisation of benefits and services	Basically decentralised, lack of inpatient care facilities; Poor coordination of benefits and services
Role of the state and public actors:		
Social services	State and local municipalities have strong role	State, county and local municipalities have strong role; Publicly financed private providers play an increasing role;
Social benefits	Universal social insurance; Means-tested social assistance	Universal social insurance; Means-tested social assistance

Sources: Alzheimer Europe, 2010; FRA, 2014; SSA, 2014; WHO, 2011a.

levels of administration and strengthen user influence. The inter-organisational coordination was especially addressed by the Coordination Reform, which established a joint administration for work and welfare in 2012. Concerning psychiatric care, it is noteworthy that there is still a high number of psychiatric hospitals in Norway. In contrast, Sweden closed down most of its psychiatric hospitals in the late 1970s (with the exception of forensic facilities) and enhanced the municipalities' responsibility to organise community mental health services following the psychiatry reform of 1995 (Markström, Sandlund & Lindqvist, 2004). The Swedish national mental health plan, which was revised in 2010, encourages municipalities to expand their community mental health services and increase the cooperation between health and social services. As in Norway, available community mental health services in Sweden tend to vary due to the highly decentralised system (Markström & Lindqvist, 2015). In cases where persons with psychosocial disabilities are not eligible for generic social security benefits they have access to means-tested social assistance and financial support, special residence or housing support services or a personal agent who helps them to get in touch with the relevant welfare agencies.

Norway and Sweden provide rather generous income-related sick cash benefits and disability pensions, albeit under an increasingly strict assessment of the capacity to work and medical conditions. In Norway, a training programme exists for persons of working age who have significantly reduced work capacity, and in Sweden return-to-work policies now require that the claimant takes part in activation measures to increase motivation and employability. In both countries, means-tested social assistance rests with the municipalities, which have considerable scope for discretion to set conditions on financial support (e.g. they can decide that the person must accept offers of treatment, rehabilitation training or referral to the employment service).

Norway and Sweden differ when it comes to the right to vote; whereas the right to vote can be limited for persons with mental illness in Norway (Alzheimer Europe, 2010), no such limitations on the right to vote based on psychosocial disabilities exist in Sweden (FRA, 2014).

Challenges faced by the social democratic welfare regime

Swedish experts pointed out that the welfare system was fragmented and implied barriers for people with disabilities who run the risk of being endlessly circulated among welfare agencies. Swedish experts also emphasised the need for flexible community mental health service arrangements allowing for increased user influence on the treatments and services offered. In both Sweden and Norway, the experts found that there were problems recruiting qualified staff to mental health services posts. Experts also emphasised the need for personalised services in mainstream education, vocational rehabilitation and employment. Norwegian experts suggested that employers and government agencies should be creative and develop new policies and approaches to combat the unemployment of persons with disabilities. In both countries experts commented that there is a need to change attitudes and to increase the awareness and acceptance of persons with psychosocial disabilities. Experts pointed to the stigma attached to mental health problems (both social stigma and self-stigma), which is very negative for persons with psychosocial disabilities.

The post-communist regimes

After the fall of the communist regimes, many countries in Eastern Europe began to reform their health systems in line with Western European principles (Cook 2010: 671–686). State monopolies in welfare provision ended and means-tested benefits replaced universal subsidies and family benefits. The post-communist regime is characterised by both path dependency and path-departure, i.e., by egalitarian legacies of communism, globalising influences, interventions of international financial institutions and the potential influence of a European Social Model (Cook, 2010: 672, 686). Table 7.4 summarises the characteristics of the disability and mental health policy systems in the Czech Republic and Serbia.

Both the Czech Republic and Serbia have a national mental health plan which aims to integrate mental health services into primary care and to shift mental health care from psychiatric hospitals to community mental health facilities (WHO, 2011a). In the Czech Republic, although the mental health care organised by the state is mostly provided in psychiatric hospitals, the number of beds

Table 7.4 Characteristics of the post-communist welfare regimes

	Czech Republic, CZ	*Serbia, SR*
National mental health plan	Yes	Yes
Beds in mental hospitals	High	Medium
Right to vote	Court decisions may restrict the right to vote for persons with mental disorders	Court decisions may restrict the right to vote for persons with psychosocial disabilities
Organisation of disability and mental health policy systems	Basically hospital-based; Slow shift to community-based services	Basically hospital-based; Plans for shift to community-based care exist
Role of the state and public actors:	Strong, but poor coordination between central and local levels;	Strong, but poor coordination between central and local levels;
Social services	Increasing role for NGOs and private providers	Increasing role for NGOs and private providers
Social benefits	Public sickness insurance + flat-rate + earnings-related disability pension; Own insurance contribution required; Means-tested social assistance	Public sickness insurance; Strict criteria for disability pension; Own insurance contribution required; Means-tested social assistance.

Sources: Alzheimer Europe, 2010; FRA, 2014; SSA, 2014; WHO, 2011a.

in mental hospitals has decreased in recent years (Höschl et al., 2012: 280). In addition, NGOs provide community mental health services but these are usually situated in larger cities (EC, 2013) and are largely insufficient, which means that many patients have to rely on psychiatric hospitals. In Serbia, outpatient services exist in municipal health centres (Lecic Tosevski & Pejuskovic, 2005). As in the Czech Republic, NGOs have an important role within the mental health system through various psychosocial programmes.

Concerning social benefits, in the Czech Republic, people with psychosocial disabilities may claim sick cash benefits or a disability pension (which is the most widely used benefit) if their capacity to work is reduced to a certain level and if they have made sufficient contributions to the social insurance system (WHO, 2011a: 74–77). Entitlement is not linked to requirements of activation (or work-for-welfare). Means-tested basic income protection and a housing allowance exist for people who have urgent needs (SSA, 2014). Corresponding arrangements exist in Serbia for persons considered 'incapable of all work' (WHO, 2011a: 260–264). However, in Serbia the 2011 Law on Social Welfare significantly improved benefit levels and coverage, particularly for beneficiaries living in multi-member households and for households where members are unable to work. In contrast to the Czech Republic, welfare policies in Serbia expect recipients to become more active in addressing their problems (Petrovic, 2011). According to the WHO (2011a), the Czech Republic seems to rely more on care in mental hospitals than does Serbia.

In both countries there are limitations on the right for persons with psychosocial disabilities to vote in public elections (FRA, 2014; MDRI-S, 2014).

Challenges faced by the post-communist model

Czech experts voiced concern about the fact that psychiatric care was predominantly provided in terms of inpatient facilities. There are only limited community mental health services and few connections between the mental health care sector and social services at all administrative levels. Many patients remain in inpatient facilities because there are no community alternatives. As a consequence, the workload of hospital social workers is extremely heavy because they are expected to follow up on patients. According to Czech experts, developing community mental health services is a challenge because of the resistance from stakeholders who want to preserve hospital care and inpatient facilities. Similarly, the experts in Serbia pointed to the continuing lack of an integrated approach of the mental health care and social services systems to provide services to persons with psychosocial disabilities. They also draw attention to the lack of implementation mechanisms, the lack of funds for developing social and community health services and the lack of professionals. Experts in both countries also pointed to the lack of coordination and integration between the mental health system and the labour and welfare departments. Such coordination was increasingly urgent as decision-making and the provision of services are placed on the local level.

In terms of social security and income protection, Czech experts recalled that the socialist system was quite generous; however, when new market-oriented policies were launched, persons with disabilities found themselves in a vulnerable position both in terms of income protection and social services. Social benefits in Serbia are strictly income-tested and not sufficient in order to live an independent life. A challenge facing persons with psychosocial disabilities in the Czech Republic and in Serbia is that this group often do not meet the eligibility criteria because of a too short or irregular work history and too few years of making insurance contributions.

Discussion

The previous sections sought to sketch a picture of various aspects of the disability and mental health policy systems in Germany, Italy, Switzerland, Ireland, the UK, Norway, Sweden, the Czech Republic and Serbia. Although they were presented in four different regimes, the differences between the regimes are not clear-cut (see Table 7.5). In this section we discuss the results of the analysis of the disability and mental health policy systems in relation to Active Citizenship

Table 7.5 Comparison between welfare regimes

	Continental conservative	*Liberal*	*Social democratic*	*Post-communist*
Beds in mental hospitals	DE: medium IT: none CH: high	IE: medium UK: medium to low	NO: high SE: none (except for forensic care)	CZ: high SR: medium
National mental health plan	DE: no IT: yes CH: yes	IE: yes UK: yes	NO: yes SE: yes	CZ: yes SR: yes
Right to vote	DE: limited IT: full CH: limited	IE: limited UK: full	NO: limited SE: full	CZ: limited SR: limited
Organisation of disability and mental health policy systems	Strong component of mental hospital care; Private or public community care	Lingering hospital based care (IE)—developments towards community care and services	Basically integrated in primary care and community service-oriented	Mental hospital-based
Role of the state and public actors in terms of social services and benefits	Modest, fragmentary—oriented towards preserving status differentials	Modest, selective	Strong, universal, fragmentary	Weak; Increasing role for NGOs

in order to provide some insights into the ways in which these systems enable or hamper the right of persons with psychosocial disabilities to participate fully in society.

With regard to the dimension of autonomy, which we connected to the level of the de-institutionalisation of mental health services, it appears that persons with psychosocial disabilities still receive care in psychiatric hospitals in all countries except for Italy and Sweden. However, all countries seemed to strive to reduce this segregated form of care in line with the CRPD and the European strategies for mental health promoted by the EU and WHO. Concerning the dimension of security, the analysis indicates that income protection and measures to avoid poverty are crucial. Social benefits that provide adequate compensation for loss of income and additional costs due to disability can increase social security and have the potential to help individuals avoid or manage major life risks. Narrow eligibility criteria, the requirement of long work histories and insurance contribution periods make this difficult. In sum, the dimension of security seemed to be problematic in all nine European countries. Moreover, the provision of social benefits for persons with psychosocial disabilities was insufficient in all countries. Even in the social democratic welfare regimes, which are characterised by a universal welfare system, persons with psychosocial disabilities risk not receiving mental health care and falling into poverty. The organisation of adequate disability and mental health policy systems forms, thus, an important challenge in all nine countries covered by this chapter. On the basis of our data, we can argue that the major difficulties are the coordination of the different levels and actors involved in these services, the lack of funding, the disparities within countries and the negative attitudes towards psychosocial disabilities. Where public support is insufficient, NGOs and families provide services and these are particularly active in Italy, the Czech Republic, Serbia, the UK and Ireland. In Switzerland and Germany, private insurance schemes seem to play an important role. The level of social services and benefits seems to be higher in Norway and Sweden but the data on which this chapter draws clearly indicates that persons with psychosocial disabilities have difficulties accessing adequate services. Finally, there are differences between countries when it comes to the dimension of influence, which was discussed as based on the right to vote. There are restrictions on the right to vote on the basis of mental illness in all countries except for Sweden, Italy and the UK. Hence, it seems that the countries that reduced or closed down all psychiatric hospitals also removed their restrictions on the right to vote.

Conclusions

This chapter sought to shed light on the main challenges that countries face in regard to psychosocial disabilities. In conclusion, we want do draw attention to three aspects. First, the lack of data about disability and mental health systems makes it very difficult to compare the situation of persons with psychosocial disabilities across Europe, let alone examine the extent and impact of the processes of de-institutionalisation and decentralisation, international strategies and legal frameworks, welfare retrenchment and austerity measures. This means that countries need to gather more evidence and comparable data so that they can improve their disability and mental health policy systems. Second, although data is scarce some trends can be identified on the basis of previous research and the data analysed in this chapter. In particular, it is clear that persons with psychosocial disabilities live in precarious conditions in all European countries. The levels of welfare benefits and the degree of institutionalisation vary but all nine countries need to invest resources and commit to creating disability and mental health policy systems that enable Active Citizenship for persons with disabilities. Third, the conceptual framework of the psychosocial approach to mental health and Active Citizenship proved to be a valuable conceptual tool with which to discuss the situation of persons with disabilities. Active Citizenship highlights three complementary aspects of participation in society—autonomy, security and influence—which are otherwise overlooked by approaches that focus on health or welfare. Finally, the psychosocial approach to mental health calls attention to the structural factors that discriminate against persons with psychosocial disabilities, including age, gender, financial situation, work opportunities, place of residence and stigma. These cannot be overlooked if countries want to create conditions that will enable persons with disabilities to enjoy full participation in society and Active Citizenship.

References

AHV/AI Information Centre (2017). *Social Security in Switzerland*. Retrieved on 16 February 2017 from: https://www.ahv-iv.ch/p/890.e

Alzheimer Europe (2010). Legal capacity and proxy decision making. Retrieved on 16 February 2017 from: http://www.alzheimer-europe.org/Alzheimer-Europe/Our-work/Completed-projects/2010-Legislation-relating-to-legal-capacity-and-proxy-decision-making

Cerami, A and Vanhuyesse, P. (Eds.) (2009). *Post-Communist Welfare Pathways: Theorizing Social Policy Transformations in Central and Eastern Europe*. Basingstoke: Palgrave Macmillan.

Cook, L.J. (2010). Eastern Europe and Russia. In J. Castles, S. Leibfried, J. Lewis, & C. Pierson (Eds.). *The Oxford Handbook of The Welfare State* (671-686). Oxford: Oxford University Press.

De Girolamo, G., Bassi, M., Neri, G., Ruggieri, M., Santone, G. & Picardi A. (2007). The current state of mental health care in Italy: Problems, perspectives, and lessons to learn. *European Archives of Psychiatry and Clinical Neuroscience* 257:83-91.

Esping-Andersen, G. (1990). *The Three Worlds of Welfare Capitalism*. Cambridge: Polity Press.

European Commission (EC) (2005). *Green Paper. Improving the mental health of the population: Towards a strategy on mental health for the European Union*. Brussels: European Commission, Health and Consumer Protection Directorate-General.

European Commission (2010). *Europe 2020: For a Healthier EU*. Brussels: European Commission. Retrieved on 16 February 2017 from: https://ec.europa.eu/health/europe_2020_en

European Commission (2013). *Mental Health Systems in the European Union Member States: Status of Mental Health in Populations and Benefits to be Expected from*

Investments into Mental Health. European profile of prevention and promotion of mental health (EuroPoPP-MH). Brussels: European Commission.

European Union (2008). *European Pact for Health and Well-being. EU High-Level Conference. Together for Mental Health and Well-being.* Brussels 12-13 June. Retrieved on 16 February 2017 from: http://ec.europa.eu/health/ph_determinants/life_style/mental/docs/pact_en.pdf

Ferrera, M. (2010). The Southern European Countries. In J. Castles, S. Leibfried, J. Lewis, & C. Pierson (Eds.). *The Oxford Handbook of The Welfare State* (616–629). Oxford: Oxford University Press.

FRA (European Union Agency for Fundamental Rights) (2014). *Can Persons deprived of Legal Capacity Vote? Indicators on the right to Political Participation of Persons with Disabilities.* Vienna: FRA.

Goffman, E. (1961). *Asylums: Essays on the Social Situation of Mental Patients and Other Inmates.* New York: Penguin Books.

Goodwin, S. (1997). *Comparative Mental Health Policy: From Institutional to Community Care.* London: Sage.

Gustavsson, A., Svensson, M., Jacobi, F., Allgulander, C., Alonso, J., Beghi, E., … Olesen, J. (2011). Cost of disorders of the brain in Europe 2010. *European Neuropsycho pharmacology*, 21(10), 718–779. (http://doi.org/10.1016/j.euroneuro.2011.08.008)

Hasenfeld, Y. (Ed.) (2009). *Human Services as Complex Organizations.* London: Sage.

Höschl, P., Winkler P. & Pěč, O. (2012). The state of psychiatry in the Czech Republic. *International Review of Psychiatry*, 24(4), 278–285.

Kautto, M. (2010) The Nordic Countries. In J. Castles, S. Leibfried, J. Lewis, & C. Pierson (Eds.). *The Oxford Handbook of The Welfare State* (686–600). Oxford: Oxford University Press.

Knapp, M., McDaid, D., Mossialos, E. & Thornicroft, G. (2007). *Mental Health Policy and Practice across Europe: The Future Direction of Mental Health Care.* Berkshire: Open University Press.

Kvist, J., Fritzel, J., Hvinden B. & Kangas, O. (Eds.) (2012). *Changing Social Equality: The Nordic Welfare Model in the 21st Century* (201–206). Bristol: The Policy Press.

Lecic Tosevski, D. & Pejuskovic, B. (2005). Mental health care in Belgrade: Challenges and solutions. *European Psychiatry*, 20(Suppl. 2), 266–269.

Leff, J. & Warner, R. (2006). *Social Inclusion of People with Mental illness.* Cambridge: Cambridge University Press.

Lindqvist, R. & Grape, O. (1999). Vocational rehabilitation of the socially disadvantaged long-term sick: Inter-organizational co-operation between welfare state agencies. *Scandinavian Journal of Public Health*, 1: 5–10.

Markström, U. & Lindqvist, R. (2015). Establishment of community mental health systems in a postdeinstitutional era: A study of organizational structures and service provision in Sweden. *Journal of Social Work in Disability & Rehabilitation*, 14(2), 124–144.

Markström, U., Sandlund, M. & Lindqvist, R. (2004). Who is responsible for supporting 'long-term mentally ill' persons? Reforming mental health practices in Sweden. *Canadian Journal of Community Mental Health*, 23(2), 51–63.

MDRI-S (Mental Disability Rights Initiative) (2016). *Serbian Country Report on Legal Capacity.* Person Country Report. Belgrade: Mental Disability Rights Initiative of Serbia. project.

Minkowitz, T. (2007). The United Nations Convention on the Rights of Persons with Disabilities and the Right to be Free from Nonconsensual Psychiatric Interventions. *Syracuse Journal of International Law and Commerce*, 34(d), 405–428.

OECD (2012). *Sick on the Job? Myths and Realities about Mental Health and Work.* Paris: OECD. DOI:http://dx.doi.org/10.1787/9789264124523-en

OECD (2014). *Mental Health and Work: Switzerland.* Paris: OECD Publishing. DOI:http://dx.doi.org/10.1787/9789264204973-en

Palier, B. (2010). Continental Western Europe. In J. Castles, S. Leibfried, J. Lewis & C. Pierson (Eds.). *The Oxford Handbook of The Welfare State* (601–615). Oxford: Oxford University Press.

Petrovic, M. (2011). *Social Assistance and Activation in Serbia: In Search of Inclusive Policy Options.* Belgrade: Center for Liberal-Democratic Studies (CLDS). Retrieved on 28 March 2016 from: http://www.clds.rs/newsite/Social%20Assistance-%20web.pdf

Ramon, S. & Williams, J. E. (2005). Towards a conceptual framework: The meanings attached to the psychosocial, the promise and the problems. In J. E. Williams & S. Ramon (Eds.). *Mental Health at the Crossroads: The Promise of the Psychosocial Approach* (13–24). Aldershot: Ashgate.

Sayce, L. (2000). *From Psychiatric Patient to Citizen. Overcoming Discrimination and Social Exclusion.* Basingstoke: Palgrave Macmillan.

Schulz, M. (2012). Mental health services in Germany. In N. Brimblecombe & P. Nolan (Eds.). *Mental Health Services in Europe: Provision and Practice* (97–120). London: Radcliffe.

Scull, A. T. (1979). *Museums of Madness: The Social Organization of Insanity in 19th Century England.* New York: St. Martin's Press.

SSA (Social Security Administration) (2014). *Social Security Programs Throughout the World: Europe.* Washington, DC: Social Security Administration. SSA publication No. 13-11801.

Weller, P. (2014). Reconsidering legal capacity: Radical critiques, governmentality and dividing practice. *Griffith Law Review,* 23(3), 498–518. DOI:http://doi.org/10.1080/10383441.2014.993499

Williams, J. E., & Ramon, S. (2005). *Mental Health at the Crossroads: The Promise of the Psychosocial Approach* (1–10). Aldershot: Ashgate.

Wittchen, H., Jacobi, F., Rehm, J., Gustavsson, A., Svensson, M., Jönsson, B. & Steinhausen, H. (2011). The size and burden of mental disorders and other disorders of the brain in Europe 2010. *European Neuropsychopharmacology,* 21(9), 655–679.

World Health Organization (WHO) (2005). *Mental Health—Facing the Challenges, Building Solutions:Report from the WHO European Ministerial Conference.* Geneva: WHO. Retrieved from http://public.eblib.com/EBLPublic/PublicView.do?ptiID=284778

World Health Organization (2011a). *Mental Health Atlas 2011.* Geneva: WHO.

World Health Organization (2011b). *Impact of Economic Crises on Mental Health.* Copenhagen: WHO Regional Office for Europe.

World Health Organization (2015). *The European Mental Health Action Plan 2013–2020.* Copenhagen: WHO Regional Office for Europe.

Wright, D. & Digby, A. (1996). *From Idiocy to Mental Deficiency: Historical Perspectives on People with Learning Disabilities.* London: Routledge.

8 Enabling people with disabilities through effective accessible technology policies

Jennifer Kline and Delia Ferri

Introduction

In the most recent disability scholarship (Macdonald & Clayton, 2013), the advantages and the challenges that technology poses to persons with disabilities have become a hot topic of debate. Even though a certain degree of scepticism towards technology remains (Sheldon, 2003), several scholars acknowledge that advances in technology have enabled more persons with disabilities than ever before to actively participate in society (Halvorsen, 2010; Blanck, 2014). In particular, accessible technology can serve as an equalising force in education, employment, transportation and social life (Ripat & Woodgate, 2011). Under International Organization for Standardization (ISO) guidelines, accessible technology encompasses both assistive technology and universally designed products (ISO/IEC, 2001). Assistive technology refers to any product intended to support the tasks and activities that people do during the course of everyday life by enabling the technology's user to perform tasks that would otherwise be difficult or impossible (ISO, 2011: 2.3; Ferri, 2015a, 2015b). Researchers have considered assistive technology as a facilitator of independent living, and a tool to enable people with disabilities to realise their full potential and participate in society (Borg et al., 2012; Berry & Ignash, 2003; Alper & Raharinirina, 2006). Universally designed technologies are digital goods and services that are readily usable by the widest possible population without any modification. They are produced in line with the principle of universal access, taking into account human differences and allowing all individuals to interact with the environment and society to the best of their ability (Gassmann & Reepmeyer, 2008; Ferri et al., 2015).

The entry into force of the UN Convention on the Rights of Persons with Disabilities—UN CtRPD (UN, 2006)—has greatly boosted the move towards more comprehensive research on the role that accessible technology can play in eliminating societal barriers. The UN CtRPD places a great emphasis on both assistive devices and universally designed technology, and bestows upon Parties to the Convention a range of duties related to the provision of accessible technology and the promotion of universally designed goods.

All DISCIT countries except Ireland (i.e. Czech Republic, Germany, Italy, Norway, Sweden, Serbia, Switzerland and the UK) have ratified the Convention, and the European Union (EU) is also a party to the UN CtRPD (Council of the

European Union, 2010). This means that all the DISCIT countries and the EU must undergo a review of legislation and policies to ensure conformity with the UN CtRPD and pass new legislative instruments to implement the provisions of the Convention. In practical terms and with reference to accessible technology, both EU and national legislation must promote accessible technology, its availability on the market and its affordability, within the scope of the promotion and protection of the rights of people with disabilities.

Against this background, this chapter aims to contribute to the current debate and to assess both EU and national legislation on accessible technology in light of the UN CtRPD. It also aims to verify whether international, EU and national laws, and their intersection, sufficiently enhance the rights of people with disabilities by providing them with clear rights and scope for choice with regard to accessible technology. Although it does not endeavour to carry out a comparative legal analysis, this chapter attempts to detect current trends and patterns in regulating accessible technology, by taking into account the conceptual framework of Active Citizenship (see Chapter 1).

This chapter is divided into three main parts that focus respectively on the UN CtRPD, EU law and national law on accessible legislation. The next section discusses how accessible technology features in the UN CtRPD. We then examine to what extent EU disability law and policy promote accessible technology. Finally, we turn to examining national laws. It is important to note that none of the countries reviewed has uniform legislation on accessible technology. The patchwork of legislation is due both to the variety of technological tools encompassed by the definition of accessible technology, and to the contexts in which technology is used. For assistive devices, a unique system for the provision of assistive technology to persons with disabilities does not seem to exist in any of the countries considered. Rather, legislation differentiates the provision of technology into three main contexts: the health/social integration context, the educational context and the employment context. Thus, we refer to the health/social integration context and to the provision of assistive technology through the health and/or welfare systems. Secondly, we refer to where the educational system provides assistive technologies to pupils with disabilities. We finally look at the employment context and focus on whether and to what extent the employer provides assistive technology, which may be in part subsidised or reimbursed by the State. The concluding section discusses the relationship between the UN CtRPD, EU law and national law, and examines to what extent the UN CtRPD and EU have played a proactive role in promoting the availability and affordability of accessible technology in the DISCIT countries.

Accessible technology in the UN CtRPD: An overview

For a long time, the dominant view was that persons with disabilities faced significant barriers in many areas of life directly as a result of their impairments, rather than as a result of discrimination or inadequate respect for their human rights. The UN CtRPD embodies the first official recognition, at international level, of disability as a human rights issue, and takes as its point of departure the fact that disability stems primarily from the failure of the social environment to meet the needs and aspirations of people with disabilities (Kayess & French, 2008).

The UN CRPD consists of a Preamble and fifty Articles. It includes an introductory set of articles outlining its purpose and key definitions (Arts. 1–2), and general provisions to be applied throughout the treaty text (Arts. 3–9). Articles 10 through 30 enumerate specific rights that cover the whole range of life activities of persons with disabilities such as access to employment, education, housing and family. Its scope is broad and covers civil and political rights as well as economic, cultural and social rights (Quinn, 2009; Lord, 2010).

In putting a great emphasis on accessibility, the UN CtRPD also explicates the role that accessible technology might play in the promotion and protection of the rights of people with disabilities. The Convention mentions technology in various articles generally in relation to accessing other rights and makes clear that technology is (often) an indispensable condition for the exercise of human rights in the disability context.

First, Article 2 adopts a wide definition of 'communication', encompassing among other things display of text and accessible multimedia as well as written, audio, plain-language, 'human-reader and augmentative and alternative modes, means and formats of communication, including accessible information and communication technology'. Further, Article 4(1)(g) obliges Parties to 'undertake or promote research and development of, and to promote the availability and use of new technologies, including information and communications technologies, mobility aids, devices and assistive technologies, suitable for persons with disabilities, giving priority to technologies at an affordable cost'. Article 4(1)(h) requires Parties to provide 'accessible information to persons with disabilities about mobility aids, devices and assistive technologies, including new technologies'. Article 9 imposes a range of duties on Parties to the Convention, making it clear that accessibility covers more than technical design specifications for products, information and signage or the built environment. It also establishes that technologies must be accessible, and explicitly requires that information and communication technologies are made accessible to people with disabilities at a minimum cost. Article 20, on personal mobility, imposes on Parties to the Convention the obligations to facilitate access 'to quality mobility aids, devices, assistive technologies and forms of live assistance and intermediaries, including by making them available at affordable cost'. It also imposes on Parties the duty to encourage 'entities that produce mobility aids, devices and assistive technologies to take into account all aspects of mobility for persons with disabilities'. Article 21, which focuses on the freedom of expression and opinion, and access to information, explicitly states that Parties to the Convention must provide information in accessible formats and technologies 'appropriate to different kinds of disabilities in a timely manner and without additional costs'. Article 26 obliges Parties to organise, strengthen and extend comprehensive habilitation and rehabilitation services and programmes. The latter provision clarifies the importance of technology to enhance rehabilitation and make it possible. The role of technology is evoked also in Article 29, in order to make political participation of people with disabilities possible and feasible. Article 32, on international cooperation, requires State parties *inter alia* to facilitate access to and sharing of accessible and assistive technologies.

Notably, the Convention includes the obligation to spread 'universal design' (Article 4(1)(f)). In fact, according to the Committee on the Rights of Persons with Disabilities (CtRPD) 'the strict application of universal design to all new goods, products, facilities, technologies and services should ensure full, equal and unrestricted access for all potential consumers, including persons with disabilities, in a way that takes full account of their inherent dignity and diversity'. However, the Convention explicitly provides that the enhancing of universal design shall not exclude assistive devices for particular groups of persons with disabilities where this is needed.

The UN CtRPD does not include any explicit reference to technology when it defines the concept of reasonable accommodation. Art. 2 UN CtRPD uses the words 'necessary and appropriate modification and adjustments' with no further specification. The Convention itself gives no more specific guidance than is contained in its definition in Article 2. However, the Committee has specified that reasonable accommodation is an individualised adjustment, which might fall outside the scope of any accessibility standard (UN CtRPD, 2014). This clearly encompasses assistive technologies, such as screen readers, page-turners, voice recognition software, screen magnification software, switches, keyboards and wrist supports.

Overall, it is apparent that the Convention does not use the term 'accessible technology'. However, the concepts of technology and accessibility are inextricably linked. On the one hand, technology itself must be accessible. The General Comment No. 2 on Accessibility, released by the Committee on the Rights of Persons with Disabilities, clarifies that 'new technologies can be used to promote the full and equal participation of persons with disabilities in society, but only if they are designed and produced in a way that ensures their accessibility' (UN CtRPD, 2014). In addition, the Convention makes it crucial that technology must be available at affordable prices. In this respect, the General Comment highlights that the Convention requires Parties' accessible technologies (namely ICT) to 'become accessible at minimum cost'. On the other hand, technology is a tool to ensure accessibility, to increase autonomy and participation, and is at least to a certain extent essential for people with disabilities to enjoy their rights, such as the right to education, freedom of expression or the right to move.

The UN CtRPD embraces the idea that technology is a means to achieve autonomy, inclusion in society, and a tool that allows people with disabilities to exert an influence on societal structures. In line with this conceptualisation, the UN CtRPD obliges Parties to the Convention to adopt laws and policies that enhance the production of accessible technologies and promote their availability among persons with disabilities.

Accessible technology in EU law and policy

EU disability law and accessible technology in a nutshell

During the last few decades, the EU has developed a significant body of disability laws and policies (Waddington, 1999). Until the 1980s, EU action focused on stimulating a policy debate, rather than on laying down concrete actions (Perjul, 2011). However, a major quantitative and qualitative change in EU disability policy occurred with the entry into force of the Amsterdam Treaty in 1997, which conferred on the EU the competence to combat disability discrimination. The Amsterdam Treaty also included a Declaration stating that EU institutions must take account of the needs of persons with disabilities in drawing up measures under former Article 95 EC, now Art. 114 of the Treaty on the Functioning of the European Union (TFEU) (2012). Further to these constitutional changes, the 'Employment Equality Directive' (Council of the European Union, 2000) marked the first legislative intervention to address discrimination on the grounds of disability. The Charter of Fundamental Rights of the European Union (2012), proclaimed in 2000, shed a new light on the rights of persons with disabilities. Besides the prohibition of discrimination, Article 26 of the Charter recognises the right of persons with disabilities to benefit from measures aimed to ensure their independence, integration and participation in the life of the community.

The ratification of the UN CtRPD by the former European Community (now, of course, the EU) contributed to increasing the EU commitment towards people with disabilities. The UN CtRPD currently enjoys a quasi-constitutional status in the EU legal system, beneath the Treaties but above secondary law (Ferri, 2010). As a consequence, EU secondary law must be interpreted in the light of the Convention (see Court of Justice of the European Union, 2013, 2014).

Since the 2000s, disability-related provisions have been introduced in various areas of EU legislation, such as transport, lifts, public procurement, and electronic communications networks and services. Accessible technology as such is not an essential element of this EU legislation or of disability-related provisions. This trend has not been changed after the ratification of the UN CtRPD. However, we can find implicit or explicit references to accessible technology in several pieces of legislation. For example, Directive 2000/9/EC on cableway installations to carry persons sets standards to ensure that children and persons with reduced mobility can use the installation safely (European Parliament and Council, 2000). Similarly, in the legislation on lifts, transport, and radio equipment and telecommunications, accessibility provisions are included (Arsenjeva, 2014). Legislation on the provision of services also includes sparse accessibility provisions. For example the Cross Border Healthcare Directive, Directive 2011/24/EU, which promotes the rights of patients to access healthcare in other EU Member States, requires Member States to establish national contact points for cross-border healthcare which must, among other things, provide 'information on the accessibility of hospitals for persons with disabilities' (European Parliament and Council, 2011). Further, all the information provided by these contact points must be 'made available by electronic means and in formats accessible to people with disabilities, as appropriate'. The latter point certainly includes the use of accessible technology. In general, these provisions, most of which predate the ratification of the UN CtRPD, aim to ensure access for persons with disabilities, on an equal basis with others, to certain services. These provisions attempt to ensure both that technology is not a barrier in itself and that, when needed, additional technological aid is provided to make the service fully accessible.

To date, the above-mentioned Employment Equality Directive probably remains the most important act that protects and promotes the rights of people with disabilities. This Directive provides minimum standards that Member States must ensure are met in their national laws. These take the form of requiring Member States to prohibit discrimination on the grounds of disability in the spheres of employment, occupation and vocational training. The Directive does not mention accessible technology explicitly. However, on closer inspection, technology implicitly features in the broader provision on reasonable accommodation included in the text. Article 5 of the Directive recognises that, in order to ensure equality of opportunity for disabled people, it is necessary to address both work practices and barriers within the physical environment that tend to exclude persons with disabilities. It obliges the employers to 'take appropriate measures, where needed in a particular case, to enable a person with a disability to have access to, participate in, or advance in employment, or to provide training for such a person'. As noted by Waddington and Lawson (2009), this provision does not elaborate on the meaning of 'reasonable accommodation'. Additional guidance can be derived from some of the recitals in the Directive's non-binding preamble. Recital 20 affirms that appropriate accommodations can consist, for example, in adapting premises and equipment. These adaptations and technical solutions include assistive technology, which is mostly required for employees with physical and sensory disabilities such as wheelchair-users or persons with visual impairments (Ferri & Lawson, 2016). Reasonable accommodation is concerned with the removal of the disadvantage to which a disabled person would otherwise be subjected by an employer's standard working practices. In this context, technology is a means to ensure equality, and the enjoyment of the right to work.

In 2008, the Commission proposed a new Directive extending the scope of the provisions against discrimination on the grounds of religion and religious belief, disability, age and sexual orientation beyond the area of employment and into the fields of social protection, including social security and healthcare, social advantages, education and access to and supply of goods and other services which are available to the public, including housing (European Commission, 2008). The proposed Directive should complement the Employment Equality Directive, and purports to implement the principle of equal treatment even in sectors other than employment. The proposed Directive shows an ambitious approach with regard to the prohibition of disability discrimination, and includes a number of additional provisions to strengthen disability discrimination law. The original text of the proposal included reference to the UN CtRPD, and a specific provision on 'Equal treatment of persons with disabilities'. This provision, without mentioning technology, deals with effective access for disabled people to social protection, social advantages, health care, education and access to and supply of goods and services that are available to the public, including housing. Individual measures of reasonable accommodation are also mentioned. In this provision, the requirement to make reasonable accommodation does not only imply making physical changes to the service itself, but may entail an alternative means (including technological ones) of providing a service. If adopted, the Directive will contribute to both making technology more accessible and to increasing the use of accessible technology in the provision of services. However, to date, the proposal is buried in the Council and there is not any evidence that this proposal will be approved soon.

Although it does not explicitly mention accessible technology, EU State aid law is also relevant. EU State aid law concerns subsidies and other forms of public intervention. In general, these subsides are prohibited (Art. 107 TFEU). However, the Treaty itself and other legislation specify a number of cases in which national support measures are permissible. Among these, the General Block Exemption Regulation or GBER (European Commission Regulation 651/2014) includes a provision to encourage subsidies that protect the rights of persons with disabilities. In particular, Article 34 GBER allows Member States to provide aid for compensating the additional costs of employing workers with disabilities, including costs of adapting premises and of adapting or acquiring and/or validating specific equipment and software, that is, assistive devices or—more broadly—accessible technology (Ferri, 2015b). By allowing state subsidies to cover the cost of specific technological adaptations, the GBER constitutes an essential element in the effort to ensure that the right to work is enjoyed by people with disabilities on an equal basis with others, and contributes to making them active citizens. The GBER has been clearly influenced by the UN CtRPD, which is also quoted in the preamble of this regulation.

Finally, in December 2015 the Commission released the proposal for a new 'European Accessibility Act', that is, a directive aimed to ensure the cross-border provision of accessible services across the EU, thus increasing accessibility for people with disabilities (European Commission, 2015a). The proposed act, clearly inspired by the UN CtRPD, aims to harmonise the different accessibility requirements across the EU Member States. However, being an internal market piece of legislation, explicitly directed to eliminate barriers to the circulation of services across the EU, it covers a closed list of products and services for which 'accessibility features are most needed, in areas where there is most legislative divergence and greatest market fragmentation, or where there is a very strong likelihood that these will occur, with consequential risks to the working of the single market' (European Commission, 2015b). The list of products and services covered by the proposed directive include: ticketing machines, check-in machines, automatic teller machines (ATMs), general purpose computer hardware and operating systems, consumer terminal equipment, banking services, passenger transport services (air, bus, rail and boat), telephony services and audio-visual media services. The proposed directive defines accessible products and services as those that are 'perceptible, operable and understandable for persons with functional limitations including persons with disabilities, on an equal basis with others' (Art. 2). Although this directive may (if and when approved) potentially improve access to commercial services for people with disabilities, it does not per se fulfil the obligations purported by the UN CtRPD. The scope of the directive is in fact limited, and many people with disabilities will still be limited in their access to accessible products and services (European Disability Forum, 2016). In addition, the Directive does not address the obligation to ensure adequate access to assistive technology enshrined in the UN CtRPD. It is still very early to predict any outcome, as the text will have to be approved by both the Council and the European Parliament (which are also likely to amend the original text).

The role of accessible technology in EU disability policy

EU legislation does not exist in a vacuum, but alongside a myriad of policy documents that have contributed to the creation of a comprehensive approach towards disability. In 1996, the former European Community launched the European Community Disability Strategy (European Commission, 1996), which advocated the identification and removal of barriers preventing individuals with disabilities from achieving equality of opportunity and full participation in all aspects of social life. The 1996 Strategy was then followed by the EU Disability Action Plan (DAP) for the years 2004–2010 (European Commission, 2003), which was in turn followed by the European Disability Strategy (EDS) 2010–2020 (European Commission, 2010a).

The EDS 2010–2020 proposes comprehensive policy action, and complements the legal framework in force. It has also been conceived of as a roadmap for the implementation of the UN CtRPD. Although it is 'soft-law', meaning law that is not a legally binding document, the Strategy is a driver for new legislative intervention in the field of disability, and aims to empower people with disabilities and to make them able to fully enjoy their rights.

The EDS 2010–2020 is articulated in eight interconnected key areas of action, which were selected to take into account also the obligations the EU has undertaken internationally by concluding the UN CtRPD: accessibility, participation, equality, employment, education and training, social protection, health and external action. For each of these areas, the Strategy identifies key actions. While accessible technology is not identified as such as an area of policy intervention, the Strategy proposes the use of legislative instruments and standardisation to optimise accessibility of the built environment, transport and ICT, in line with the Digital Agenda and Innovation Union flagship initiatives adopted within the frame of the EU2020 Strategy (European Commission, 2010b). The EDS promotes the use of public procurement as a means of ensuring accessible goods and services. In addition, there is an explicit commitment to promote an EU-wide market of assistive devices, and to improve the availability and choice of assistive technology. The Strategy also includes the EU commitment to 'make workplaces more accessible'.

The Commission recently launched a mid-term consultation for the review of the European Disability Strategy, which closed on 18 March 2016. The idea behind the consultation was to gather opinions on the achievements of the Strategy and to identify areas that need prioritisation for future action. The consultation document did not include any specific question on accessible technology as such (European Commission, 2015c). However, significantly, it mentioned the lack of access to ICT among possible problems to be tackled, and the 'accessibility of goods and services including public services and assistive devices' among the areas that required action. At this stage, it is not at all clear which revisions of the Strategy will be put in place, and whether more emphasis will be placed on accessible technology. However, the consultation might represent the first big test of how the EU is advancing disability policy, and accessible technology in particular, further to the EU ratification of the UN CtRPD.

Accessible technology in National Law

This section will look primarily at the laws that govern public provision of assistive technology. Assistive technology provision allows people with disabilities to access employment, housing and education as well as simply lead active lives. When looking at how laws impact on accessible technology it is important to look at assistive technology provision in addition to accessibility laws since access to assistive devices is often needed by people with disabilities to fully access Active Citizenship. As important as EU law and policy is in both directing and influencing the availability and access to accessible technology at the national level, it is important to recognise that, in most cases, public provision of assistive technology largely falls outside the scope of EU law. This is because in many EU countries assistive technology is still provided through the health system or through social services, which remain largely in the hands of Member States, with the EU having only a supporting competence exercised mainly through the mere coordination of social security systems (see Chapter 12).

In looking at accessible technology we have focused mainly on assistive devices, and the way in which they are provided. Considering the conceptual framework of Active Citizenship and the obligations set forth in the UN CtRPD, this section first examines whether national law provides for a right to assistive technology. It then goes on to analyse whether people with disabilities have choices of different technologies, and can acquire ownership of the technology.

Is there a right to assistive technology?

We first looked at whether a right to assistive technology for people with disabilities is granted. A fundamental right to technology translates into reliable and consistent access to assistive technology, which is a precondition to accessing aspects of Active Citizenship such as social inclusion, education and employment, in compliance with the UN CtRPD.

In the DISCIT countries, access to assistive technology through the health or social security systems is rarely provided through the recognition of a right. In fact, access to assistive technology is often provided based on the meeting of certain predetermined qualifications beyond medical need for assistive technology or disability. Examples of such conditions include residency, nationality and income-based restrictions. For example, access to free or heavily subsidised assistive devices accessed through the Health Service Executive (HSE) in Ireland generally requires meeting strict income guidelines. Norway requires residency for two years prior to access to assistive technology. Only Norway declares a specific right to assistive technology under their social security legislation, meaning that the government cannot ration or limit the access of eligible beneficiaries to assistive technology (Norway, 1997a). Serbia also recognises a right to certain types of accessible technology through their right to health (Tatic, 2007). Rights of access to other accessible technology are prescribed through a different provision that—in practice—is often not fully realised by people with disabilities. Italy grants a right to the assistive technologies provided by the National Health Service, but only the technologies listed in the *Nomenclatore Tariffario* (Italian Ministry of Health, 1999), which was finally updated and amended in June 2016. This list would cover much of the accessible technology related to independent living.

With regards to the employment context, all the EU Member States and Norway include, in their legal frameworks, a provision on reasonable accommodation for people with disabilities. Within the EU countries, reasonable accommodation was, in the majority of cases, introduced to implement Art. 5 of the Employment Equality Directive. Sometimes, following the wording of Recital 20, national laws provide examples of accommodations or include non-exhaustive lists of adjustments (Ferri & Lawson, 2016). In Ireland, for example, reasonable accommodation requires 'adaptation of premises and equipment, patterns of working time, distribution of tasks or provision of training or integration resources' (Employment Equality Act Section 16(4), 2004). In all the DISCIT countries, however, it appears that accommodations include assistive devices or other adaptations of the workplace linked to a specific type of disability.

Is there a choice of assistive technology?

By mapping that question onto assistive technology policy, we looked specifically at how laws and policies facilitate choice of devices and allow for ownership of publicly provided assistive technology. Thus, in order to evaluate how laws respect the autonomy of people with disabilities, we look at whether people with disabilities are able to own and freely use and modify their devices, and who under law chooses the assistive device that is given to the person with a disability.

With regard to choice, systems vary greatly in the level of choice afforded to persons with disabilities attempting to access assistive technology. For example, the Czech Republic created a system that allows eligible persons with a disability to freely choose the accessible technology they wish to use. The Czech Republic has a Special Aid Allowance that is available to persons with 'serious disability of the supporting or musculoskeletal system, serious hearing disability, or a serious visual disability' who require a special aid (Czech Republic, 2011). A decree lists the types of aids covered under the scheme but does not name specific brands or devices (Czech Republic, 2011). There is then a tiered system of compensation based partially on the income of the family and on the price of the aid (Czech Republic, 2011). According to the legislation, this system would give persons with a qualifying disability in the Czech Republic full choice and freedom to explore the products available to them and choose what would work best.

Other countries like Germany and Italy restrict the choices of persons with disabilities through the use of lists of eligible products. In Germany, there is a Directory of Appliances which is not a formal law or regulation but strongly influences what is provided through the Statutory Health Insurance scheme (Germany, 2008, S 139). As mentioned above, Italy has a similar list of devices and products in the *Nomenclatore Tariffario* and those are the devices and products covered by the National Health Service.

Sweden has a very localised system governing the provision of assistive technology, where the councils and municipalities have the responsibility for providing assistive technology to people with disabilities. Within their responsibilities of provision the councils and municipalities choose what to provide and what the associated costs and fees are (Kylberg, 2015). Thus, even before the person with the disability gets to the local municipality, choices have already been made about what is available to them, what will be funded and what is considered necessary. There is no provision in the law that mandates the inclusion of persons with disabilities at this higher level of decision-making. This is similarly true for the lists of *Nomenclatore Tariffario* in Italy and the Assistive Devices Directory in Germany.

In the employment context, there is not any explicit provision concerning a duty to enquire of or consult with the worker with disabilities with regard to the choice of technology as reasonable accommodation. It is not clear whether the worker has a real choice and/or whether employer and workers choose together (Ferri & Lawson, 2016). Employers are not prevented from seeking the views of, and might choose to consult with, the person with a disability with regard to the accessible technology or the assistive device that best meets their needs. In Norway (McClimans, 2011) and the UK, employers are, however, expected to do so. In the UK, best practice establishes that the first step in making reasonable adjustments is consultation with the disabled worker about what the worker wants by way of adjustment. The Code states, ‘It is a good starting point for an employer to conduct a proper assessment, in consultation with the disabled person concerned, of what reasonable adjustments may be required. It is advisable to agree any proposed adjustments with the disabled worker in question before they are made’ (UK Equality and Human Rights Commission, 2010). In Norway, the employee has a corresponding duty to collaborate and suggest solutions. In Ireland there is a precedent establishing a duty to consult. In *A Health and Fitness Club v. A Worker,* the Labour Court held that the burden was on the employer to ensure that an employee is fully capable of performing the duties for which they are employed by making ‘adequate enquiries so as to establish fully the factual position in relation to the employee’s capacity’.

Ownership of the technology

Ownership of the provided technology varies greatly not only between countries, but also between the points of access within the country (home/health/social integration, employment and education). A person with a disability may own the technology if they access it through the health system but not through the education system. Lack of ownership of the technology can result in several problems. If a person does not own the technology they may not be able to modify it to better fit their specific needs. Lack of ownership can also result in the person with a disability having a lack of consistent access to the technology they are most familiar with and able to use. In Germany the person with the disability owns the assistive technology, regardless of the point of access (Cullen et al., 2012). In Norway the opposite is the case: here the National Labour and Welfare Administration (NAV) lend out the assistive technology and it is the property of the assistive technology centre (Nordic Centre for Rehabilitation Technology 2007). In the UK, it depends on who provided the technology as well as the context in which it was provided: if the person received the technology through the National Health Service they are sometimes the owner; if it is provided through the local authority then the local authority is the owner; and if it is provided to assist in employment then the employee with the disability is the owner (Cullen et al., 2012). Italy also has a fractured system where the person with a disability does not own the assistive technology if it is provided through the employment and education systems but does own it if it is provided through the National Health Service (Cullen et al., 2012). This is similar to Ireland where the person with a disability does own the device if it is provided through the health service, through an NGO or for private employment, but not usually if it is provided through the education context. In that instance, it is the school that owns the technology (Department of Education and Skills (Ireland), 2013).

Concluding remarks

It has been widely acknowledged that technology cannot eliminate every potential barrier, but can be a means for a person with a disability to retain choice and autonomy in his or her life (see Chapter 8 in accompanying volume 2). Accessible technology impacts quite visibly and directly on the enjoyment of the rights of people with disabilities. As recognized by the UN CtRPD, accessible technology is in fact essential to independent living, to free, movement and to community inclusion.

To date the EU has enacted various provisions aimed at ensuring the availability of accessible technology in various contexts. The action of the EU is, however, insufficient to meet the objectives set forth in the UN CtRPD and comply with the obligations that the Convention places on parties. The EU is currently reforming its own policy, and has recently presented a long-awaited proposal for a new European Accessibility Act. However, it is not yet clear whether these reforms will boost the availability of accessible technology within the EU market.

At the national level, aside from some general provisions on accessibility, legislation has mainly focused on the provision of assistive technology to people with disabilities in certain contexts. On the basis of the data available, this legislation seems not to be influenced by the UN CtRPD. It appears that none of the DISCIT countries has undertaken any palpable reform of these systems to meet UN CtRPD obligations. EU law has had little or no influence on these systems. By contrast, the only area in which EU law has clearly shaped national legislation is in that of reasonable accommodation in the employment context. A certain affordability of the technology is ensured given that national laws allow for people with disabilities to obtain assistive devices free of charge or at a low price. However, people with disabilities have very little (sometimes no) choice with regard to the type of technology they can acquire, and often they do not own the technology itself. The fast changing nature of technology and the greater use of universal design are often not adequately accounted for in the existing legal schemes that govern assistive technology provision. Schemes that rely on lists of subsidised assistive technology may not be amended often enough to incorporate the latest advances in assistive technology. The rise of universally designed ICT that people with disabilities are using as a replacement for assistive devices is often ignored. For example, iPhones are often accessible to people with visual impairments who then can download different applications that carry out a variety of operations such as give directions, read menus, read currency, detect clothes colour as well as talking camera aids. However, most national laws would not cover or subsidise the purchase of an iPad or iPhone even though a person with a visual impairment could use such a device to access applications that would replace a host of physical assistive technology aids. For example, it seems that Norwegian assistive technology laws specifically prohibit the government provision of devices that are commonly used in the house such as appliances and electronics (Norway, 1997b: §2).

Overall, there is the need for both the EU and individual nation states, within their respective fields of competence, to bring laws and policy on accessible technology into closer alignment with the UN CtRPD.

References

Alper, S. & Raharinirina, S. (2006). Assistive technology for Individuals with Disabilities: A review and synthesis of the literature. *Journal of Special Education Technology*, 21(2), 47–66.

Arsenjeva, J. (2014). Annotated review of European Union law and policy with reference to disability, prepared under the direction of Prof. Lisa Waddington on behalf of the Academic Network of European Disability experts (ANED). Retrieved 10 April 2016 from: http://www.disability-europe.net/theme/eu-law-and-policy

Berry, B. E. & Ignash, S. (2003). Assistive technology: Providing independence for individuals with disabilities. *Rehabilitation Nursing*, 28(1), 6–14.

Blanck, P. (2014). The struggle for web e-quality by persons with cognitive disabilities. *Behavioral Sciences and The Law*, 32(1), 4–32.

Borg, J., Larsson, S., Östergren, P-O., Rahman, A. S. M. A, Bari, N., Khan, A. H. M. N. (2012). Assistive technology use and human rights enjoyment: a cross-sectional study in Bangladesh. *BMC International Health & Human Rights*, 12(18), 1–11.

Charter of Fundamental Rights of the European Union, [2012] OJ C 326/391.

Collection of Laws c. 388/2011, (2011). Sbírkazákonu c. 388/2011. Retrieved 10 April 2016 from: http://www.mpsv.cz/files/clanky/11911/vyhlaska_388.pdf

Council of the European Union (2000). Directive 2000/78/EC of 27 November 2000 establishing a general framework for equal treatment in employment and occupation. OJ L 303/16.

Council of the European Union (2010). Decision of 26 November 2009 concerning the conclusion, by the European Community, of the United Nations Convention on the Rights of Persons with Disabilities 2010/48/EC. OJ L 23/35.

Court of Justice of the European Union (2013). *Ring and Werge*, Joined Cases C-335/11 and C-337/11. ECLI:EU:C:2013:222.

Court of Justice of the European Union (2014). *Z. v A Government Department and the Board of Management of a Community School* Case C-363/12. ECLI:EU:C:2014:159.

Cullen, K., McAnaney, D., Dolphin, C., Delaney, S. & Stapleton, P. (2012). Research on the provision of Assistive Technology in Ireland and other countries to support independent living across the cycles. Work Research Centre, Dublin. Retrieved 10 April 2016 from: http://nda.ie/File-upload/Research-on-the-provision-of-Assistive-Technology1.pdf

Czech Republic (2011). Providing benefits for people with disabilities and Amendments of Related Acts, (2011). (*o provedení některých ustanovení zákona o poskytování dávek osobám se zdravotním postižením, Sbírka zákonů*). č. 388/2011.

Department of Education and Skills (Ireland) (2013). Circular to the Management Authorities of Primary Schools, Special Schools, Secondary, Community and Comprehensive Schools and the Chief Executive Officers of Vocational Education Committees (2013). Circular No 0010/2013. Retrieved 10 April 2016 from: https://www.education.ie/en/Circulars-and-Forms/Active-Circulars/cl0010_2013.pdf

European Commission (1996). Communication of the Commission of 30 July 1996 on equality of opportunity for people with disabilities: A New European Community disability strategy. COM(96) 406 final.

European Commission (2003). Communication from the Commission to the Council, the European Parliament, the European Economic and Social Committee and the Committee of the Regions: Equal opportunities for people with disabilities—A European action plan. COM/2003/0650 final.

European Commission (2008). Proposal for a Council Directive on implementing the principle of equal treatment between persons irrespective of religion or belief, disability, age or sexual orientation. COM (2008) 426 final.

European Commission (2010a). Communication from the Commission to the Council, the European Parliament, the European Economic and Social Committee and the Committee of the Regions: European disability strategy 2010–2020—A renewed commitment to a barrier-free Europe. COM(2010) 636 final.

European Commission (2010b). EUROPE 2020: A strategy for smart, sustainable and inclusive growth. COM/2010/2020 final.

European Commission (2014). Regulation (EU) NO 651/2014 declaring certain categories of aid compatible with the internal market in application of Articles 107 and 108 of the Treaty. OJ L 187/1.

European Commission (2015a). Proposal for a Directive of the European Parliament and of the Council on the approximation of the laws, regulations and administrative provisions of the Member States as regards accessibility requirements for products and services. COM(2015) 615 final.

European Commission (2015b). Commission staff working document—Executive Summary of the Impact Assessment accompanying the document 'Proposal for a Directive of the European Parliament and of the Council on the approximation of the laws, regulations and administrative provisions of the Member States as regards the accessibility requirements for products and services'. SWD/2015/0265 final—2015/0278 (COD).

European Commission (2015c). Public consultation on the review of the European disability strategy 2010–2020: Consultation document. Retrieved 10 April 2016 from http://ec.europa.eu/social/main.jsp?catId=699&langId=en&consultId=19&visib=0&furtherConsult=yes.

European Commission, Employment, Social Affairs and Inclusion (2016). Moving and working in Europe. Your rights by country: Czech Republic—Persons with disabilities. Retrieved 10 April 2016 from: http://ec.europa.eu/social/main.jsp?catId=1106&langId=en&intPageId=2495

European Disability Forum (2016). EDF initial position on the proposal for a European Accessibility Act. Retrieved 10 April 2016 from: http://cms.horus.be/files/99909/MediaArchive/EDF%20Initial%20response%20European%20Accessibility%20Act%20Feb%202016%20-%20final.pdf

European Parliament and Council (2000). Directive 2000/9/EC of the European Parliament and of the Council of 20 March 2000 relating to cableway installations designed to carry persons. OJ L 106/21.

European Parliament and Council (2011). Directive 2011/24/EU of the European Parliament and of the Council of 9 March 2011 on the application of patients' rights in cross-border healthcare. OJ L 88/45.

European Union (2012). Consolidated version of the Treaty on the Functioning of the European Union (TFEU). OJ C 326/01.

Ferri D. (2010). The conclusion of the UN Convention on the Rights of Persons with Disabilities by the EC/EU: A constitutional perspective. *European Yearbook of Disability Law*, 2, 47–71.

Ferri D. (2015a). Does accessible technology need an 'entrepreneurial state'? The creation of an EU market of universally designed and assistive technology through state aid. *International Review of Law, Computers, and Technology*, 29, 137–161.

Ferri D. (2015b). 'Subsidising accessibility': Using EU state aid law and policy to foster development and production of accessible technology. *ESTAL—European State Aid Law Quarterly*, 14, 51–67.

Ferri, D., Giannoumis, A. G. & O'Sullivan, C. E. (2015). Fostering accessible technology and sculpting an inclusive market through regulation. *International Review of Law, Computers and Technology*, 29(2–3), 81–87.

Ferri, D. & Lawson, A. (2016). *Reasonable Accommodation for Disabled People in Employment* Contexts. *A legal analysis of EU member States, Iceland, Liechtenstein and Norway*. European Commission European Network of legal experts in gender equality and non-discrimination. Retrieved 10 April 2016 from: http://www.equalitylaw.eu/downloads/3724-reasonable-accommodation-for-disabled-people-in-employment-contexts

Gassmann, O. & Reepmeyer, G. (2008). Universal design: Innovations for all ages. In F. Kohlbacher & C. Herstatt (Eds.) *The Silver Market Phenomenon: Business Opportunities in an Era of Demographic Change* (125–140). Berlin: Springer-Verlag.

Germany, Federal Republic of (2008). Social code book five: Statutory health insurance—Aid list, quality assurance tools. (*Sozialgesetzbuch (SGB) Fünftes Buch (V) Gesetzliche Krankenversicherung (2008). Hilfsmittelverzeichnis, Qualitätssicherung bei Hilfsmitteln* §139).

Startseite, *Krankenversicherung*, *Hilfsmittel*, *Hilfsmittelverzeichnis*, Retrieved 10 April 2016 from: https://www.gkv-spitzenverband.de/krankenversicherung/hilfsmittel/hilfsmittelverzeichnis/hilfsmittelverzeichnis.jsp

Halvorsen, R. (2010). Digital freedom for persons with disabilities: Are policies to enhance e-accessibility and e-inclusion becoming more similar in the Nordic countries and the US? *European Yearbook of Disability Law*, 2, 77–102.

International Organization for Standardization (ISO) (2011). *Assistive Products for Persons with Disability: Classification and Terminology* (ISO 9999:2011). Geneva, Switzerland: ISO.

International Organization for Standardization and International Electrotechnical Commission (ISO/IEC) (2001). *Guidelines for Standards Developers to Address the Needs of Older Persons and Persons with Disabilities* (ISO/IEC Guide 71:2001). Geneva, Switzerland: ISO.

Ireland (2004). *Equality Act 24/2004*, Irish Statute Book.

Italian Ministry of Health (1999). Regulation on prosthetics assistance granted by the National Health Service: Types of supply and tariffs. (*Regolamento recante norme per le prestazioni di assistenza protesica erogabili nell'ambito del Servizio sanitario nazionale: modalita' di erogazione e tariffe*). Decree 27 August 1999 No. 332.

Kayess, R. & French, P. (2008). Out of darkness into light? Introducing the Convention on the Rights of Persons with Disabilities. *Human Rights Law Review*, 8, 1–34.

Kylberg, M. (2015). A European perspective on the service delivery systems for assistive technology: Differences and similarities between Latvia and Sweden. *Journal of Cross-Cultural Gerontology*, 30, 51–55.

Lord, J. E. (2010). The UN disability convention: Creating opportunities for participation. *Business Law Today*, 19(5), 22–27. Retrieved 10 April 2016 from: http://www.jstor.org/stable/23297735

McClimans, E. L. (2011). Report on measures to combat discrimination. Directives 2000/43/EC and 200/78/EC. *Country Report 2011 Norway*. Retrieved 10 April 2016 from: http://www.refworld.org/pdfid/525534ee0.pdf

Macdonald, S. & Clayton, J. (2013). Back to the future, disability and the digital divide. *Disability and Society*, 28(5), 702–718.

Nordic Centre for Rehabilitation Technology (2007). *Provision of Assistive Technology in the Nordic Countries* (2nd ed, 53). Retrieved 10 April 2016 from: http://www.hinnovic.org/wp-content/uploads/2008/11/pdf_provisionassistivetechnology.pdf

Norway (1997a). *National Insurance Act*. No 19 of 1997. *Lov (Nr 19 av 1997) om folketrygd (Folketrygdloven)*.

Norway (1997b). Regulations on benefits for utilities, etc. to improve the functioning of the labour marker and in daily life and to the modification of machinery in the workplace,. (*Forskrift om stønad til hjelpemidler mv til bedring av funksjonsevnen i arbeidslivet og i dagliglivet og til ombygging av maskiner på arbeidsplassen*). F15.04. 1997 No. 318.

Perjul, V. (2011). Impairment, discrimination, and the legal construction of disability in the European Union and the United States. *Cornell International Law Journal*, 44, 279–348.

Quinn, G. (2009). The United Nations Convention on the Rights of Persons with Disabilities: Toward a new international politics of disability. Jacobus tenBroek Disability Law Symposium 15 *Tex. J. on C.L. & C.R.* 33 (2009–2010).

Ripat, J. & Woodgate, R. (2011). The intersection of culture, disability and assistive technology. *Disability and Rehabilitation: Assistive Technology*, 6(2), 87–96.

Sheldon, A. (2003). Changing technology. In J. Swain, S. French, S, Barnes & C. Thomas (Eds.). *Disabling Barriers—Enabling Environments*. London: Sage.

Tatic, D. (2007). Report on situation of persons with disabilities in Serbia: Analysis of legislation and practice, European Disability Forum. Retrieved 10 April 2016 from: http://www.cilsrbija.org/ebib/200707251930150.Izvestaj%20-%20engleski.pdf

UK Equality and Human Rights Commission (2010). *Employment Statutory Code of Practice*. §6.32, p 86

United Nations (2006). Convention on the rights of persons with disabilities. Retrieved from: http://www.un.org/disabilities/convention/conventionfull.shtml

United Nations, Committee on the Rights of Persons with Disabilities (UN CtRPD) (2014). General Comment N. 2 on Accessibility. Retrieved from: http://www.ohchr.org/EN/HRBodies/CRPD/Pages/GC.aspx

Waddington L. (1999). The European Community's response to disability. In M. Jones & A. Basser Marks (Eds.), *Disability, Divers-Ability and Legal Change* (139–151). The Hague: Martinus Nijoff.

Waddington, L. & Lawson, A. (2009). *Disability and Non-discrimination Law in the European Union: An analysis of Disability Discrimination Law* Within and *Beyond the Employment Field*. European Commission Directorate-General for Employment, Social Affairs and Equality, Unit G.2.

9 Towards positive wealth accumulation strategies for persons with disabilities

Linking social protection with social inclusion

Sinéad Keogh, Gerard Quinn, Eilionóir Flynn and Jennifer Kline

Introduction

Article 28 of the UN Convention on the Rights of Persons with Disabilities (2006) ensures a right of

> access by persons with disabilities, in particular women and girls with disabilities and older persons with disabilities, to social protection programmes and poverty reduction programmes
>
> (Art. 28, b)

The twin animating philosophies of the convention—restoring power to people over their own lives and creating pathways for social inclusion—means that the task of designing effective social protection systems is not business as usual. As is well known, the UN Convention blends together civil and political rights with economic, social and cultural rights. Disability policy in the future cannot be all about civil rights such as non-discrimination and it cannot be all about social protection without folding in the goals of civil rights: enhancing autonomy and influence.

There is therefore a need to go beyond the traditional focus of social protection, which is primarily designed to place a material floor underneath the individual. The system harbours well-known poverty traps that must be alleviated. And the relative inattention of traditional social protection systems to individual choice and control leads to a search for new ways of complementing social protection systems so as to ensure more personal choice as well as a more direct pathway to social inclusion. One way of enhancing choice is to devolve or personalise existing social care budgets to the person with a disability. That is beginning to happen in most EU countries—Ireland being the latest example with the 2016 Programme for Partnership Government including a dedicated Taskforce on personalised budgets for persons with disabilities (Ireland, 2016: 71). But perhaps the best way to ensure choice and control is to allow, enable and facilitate the growth of personal assets out of which individuals can express their own preferences and effectuate them without risk to their underlying social entitlements.

The recent focus in some (non-EU) countries on wealth or asset building for those unlikely to build wealth through their labour (at least given the structure of existing labour markets) offers one way of complementing our social protection systems into the future—a phenomenon that deserves to be explored in a European context. That is the core focus of this chapter.

The operative assumption for decades has been that persons with disabilities—especially intellectual disabilities—are and will remain poor and dependent on social protection. Lately, some (non-EU) States have attempted to turn that assumption on its head with affirmative wealth accumulation strategies in favour of persons with disabilities (or at least certain categories of persons with disabilities). To some extent the pressure exerted by austerity measures have forced a re-examination of existing systems. But austerity is not the main reason why a new approach is needed. Correctly viewed, wealth- or asset-building measures are not a replacement for social protection income or programmes but a necessary complement to enable persons with disabilities to emerge from the margins and needless dependency.

This chapter will explore three specific topics. First, it will briefly recount the well-known phenomenon of poverty traps within existing social protection systems. This will be brief because the traps are well known. Second, it will examine the philosophical and political premises of innovative asset-building mechanisms and programmes in the United States, Canada and Australia and their operation. These are countries where the poverty traps have been, if anything, even more pronounced. The third part of this chapter draws on some of the lessons learned from comparative analysis and the case for considering wealth accumulation strategies in favour of persons with disabilities in Europe.

Social protection, means-tested benefits and poverty traps

The redistributive system: Meeting needs and enhancing income

Wealth—and by direct implication personal autonomy and power—is largely generated through direct market participation. In the absence of this, the loss is either allowed to lie where it falls or some redistributive mechanism is put in place to ameliorate its consequences. The great twentieth century response has been the growth of the welfare state and associated systems of social protection.

Social protection, narrowly defined as the transfer of cash through social insurance and social assistance, is concerned with preventing, managing, and overcoming situations that adversely affect people's well-being (United Nations, 2014). In other words, social protection constitutes a safety net or a guarantee of minimum resources to citizens who lack sufficient income from other sources (usually employment). Traditionally, social protection systems have two objectives, though Cantillon et al. (2013) note that more recently these objectives have been complemented with a third, the cultivation of social inclusion. It is this goal that wealth- or asset-accumulation strategies aim, in part at least, to enhance.

The first objective of social protection is the maintenance of living standards in the event of social risks such as unemployment, social exclusion, sickness, disability or old age. Second, social protection strives to combat poverty by guaranteeing a minimum income that is sufficient to live on. Third, social protection seeks to cultivate social inclusion, defined by the World Bank (2013) as the process of improving the ability, opportunity and dignity of people—disadvantaged on the basis of their identity—to take part in society, as a means of preventing or rectifying damage. The addition of social inclusion as an explicit or intentional goal is only very recent.

As is well known, especially across the first two objectives of social protection systems, there are fundamental tensions, particularly with respect to programmes for persons with disabilities. These tensions create many unintended poverty traps. For example, to make oneself eligible for certain direct or cash benefits one might need to keep one's assets under a certain monetary threshold that can be set quite low. Usually the impact is huge in the sense that the very people who need assets to get a life are stripped of them to remain entitled to a wide variety of programmes. Having that extra asset base could make all the difference, enabling a person not merely to survive but to thrive as an active citizen.

To recall briefly, there are several mechanisms through which redistributive policy is effectuated. Universal benefits that are not related to income or employment status might be allocated to all individuals within a certain category of deemed entitlement. Social insurance benefits are benefits that arise from a person's contribution paid into to a social insurance scheme (usually from employment). This of course assumes that the person is employed and employable. It also assumes that the labour market is inclusive and operates rationally and without discrimination (a very big assumption for persons with disabilities). Fiscal policy, and specifically the allocation of tax credits, is another way in which the State can alleviate costs. For example, Canada has non-refundable disability tax credits that reduce taxes for all qualified persons.

Finally, income-related or means-tested benefits (which overlap but are not the same thing) are benefits whereby eligibility is dependent upon the current or recent resources of the beneficiary. Income-tested or income-related benefits are generally taken to be those where the level of benefit to which an applicant is entitled is based on an assessment of his or her earnings or other income and where capital or other property and assets may or may not be taken into account. It assumes some level of economic activity or some level of income or capital from other sources. It aims to complement this income where deemed insufficient. Means-tested benefits are generally afforded those who are without or largely without an income or some other capital. They are usually withdrawn from the individual or household when a certain income threshold is surpassed (Eardley et al., 1996). One of the main problems with means-tested benefits is that persons lose their entitlements (or they are tapered away) when assets (e.g., savings, inheritance, the notional value of capital assets) exceed a certain amount, which is usually set at a fairly low threshold. This means that, to remain eligible, persons must either deliberately impoverish themselves or they are forced into the cruel dilemma of either lying about their assets or revealing them and losing their entitlements.

Means-tested benefits, sometimes referred to as targeted benefits, are those where both income and assets are taken into account. In Ireland, for example, if a person receiving disability-related benefits earns more than €120 per week, their disability allowance will be reduced. Furthermore, capital in the form of savings, investments, shares or property exceeding the value of €50,000 will negatively affect a person's disability allowance as well as ancillary supports such as free medical care in the form of the medical card. That capital allowance looks large. But, if the person wishes to receive housing supports (e.g., in the shape of rent support in the private rental sector) then the person is only allowed approximately €5,000 in assets. The net effect is that if they wish to benefit from housing benefits they will have to reduce their overall capital base—notwithstanding that a higher threshold was allowable for disability benefits—thus impoverishing themselves in the process.

In France, to qualify for Adult Disability Allowance, any income received must not be in excess of €711.95 per month, though this ceiling is higher if the person is married, cohabiting or has children. The Norwegian disability benefit system, replacing the disability pension in January 2015, makes it easier for those who are able to work to do so while receiving disability benefits by ensuring that a person's income and disability benefit combined will always be higher than disability benefit alone (Stove et al., 2015). The United Kingdom replaced the Disability Living Allowance (DLA) with a Personal Independence Payment (PIP) benefit system with the passing of the Welfare Reform Act in 2012. The PIP has two components, daily living and mobility needs, and each component can be paid at standard or enhanced rates. The Personal Independence Payment is based upon the effects of a disability on a person rather than the condition itself. It is dependent on an assessment of a person's disability; however, it is not means-tested and is therefore not affected by income or assets.

Recipients of disability allowances are usually subject to means-testing, the requirement being that they are totally unable to earn income, or have a severely reduced earning capacity. For example, in Bulgaria, Greece and Croatia, to qualify for disability allowance, recipients must have at least a 50 per cent reduction in working capacity but in Hungary individuals must have a permanent severe disability to be eligible for the disability benefit. Eligibility in Ireland is not restricted by level of impairment, though individuals must be incapable of work for a minimum of 12 months or permanently incapable of work. In Poland individuals must have at least a moderate level of impairment to qualify for disability allowance while severity of disability also determines eligibility for the Estonian disability allowance.

Finally, a number of European countries provide disabled people with extra tax deductions or credits, though these benefits are sometimes only available to taxpayers with a disability. However, in Norway, for example, such a benefit can also be claimed if the taxpayer has a dependent disabled child. Disability pension is usually determined by employment history and contributions to the social security scheme, but is sometimes determined by the number of years of residency in the country in question.

Across the EU Member States, there is also a range of benefits related to specific extra needs (or costs) that arise because of disability. Such benefits can cover the added costs of owning, modifying and running a private vehicle; they can subsidise driving lessons, provide free access or reduced fares to public transport or provide alternatives to public transport such as specialised transport. A number of countries, including Austria, Czech Republic, Hungary, Latvia, France, Norway and Poland, provide flat-rate payments for care or personal assistance while others such as Finland, Lithuania, Malta and Slovakia, subsidise the purchase of technical aids or assistive equipment for people with a disability. Eligibility for the benefits described above is determined by a complex set of criteria relating to employment history and insurance status, income level, residence, impairment level and age.

The poverty traps in the system

Several distinct poverty traps typically arise with respect to both income-related benefits as well as means-tested benefits.

First, and with respect to income-related benefits, the current systems in Member States generally reduce benefits as a person's earnings increase (or if their asset base is considered too large). If the person returns to employment he or she loses whatever benefits they were entitled to (or these are drastically reduced). In the policy environment created within many European countries, people with a significant functional limitation and a relatively low capacity to earn wages potentially face the following choice: they can work, receive wages, perhaps obtain some in-kind supports, and live in or near poverty. Alternatively, they can severely limit their work, navigate the support system, and receive income and in-kind benefits that also leave them in or near poverty.

Second, poor coordination between different elements of support systems can force persons with disabilities to effectively impoverish themselves. This does not happen with respect to benefits-in-kind, which are made available universally to meet the acknowledged higher costs of disability. But where the relevant benefits are not universally available, they may indeed have different capital or asset thresholds beyond which benefits are lost. The example was already given in Ireland of a high capital threshold for disability benefits but a low capital threshold for housing rental supplement. The net result is that, even though the person has a high capital allowance for disability benefit, they are forced to reduce their asset base drastically if they wish to remain eligible for housing. One cause is the fact that the various benefits and allowances may be under the aegis of different government departments—with their budgets to watch and their own cultures and modus operandi. The affected persons can always opt to remain on disability allowance—but remain effectively homeless. This lack of intelligent inter-operability between the various allowances, benefits and such like creates huge cracks through which highly vulnerable persons may fall. Or rather the cracks create the vulnerability. This poverty trap, in particular, is what asset- or wealth-accumulation strategies seek to compensate for.

Yet another poverty trap arises as a result of the fact that social protection (and especially the funding of social protection) is largely a responsibility of the EU Member States. That being so, entitlements do not generally cross borders. For example, an individual with a budget for a personal assistant in Ireland will not be allowed to carry that budget with them when they travel, for example to Belgium to take up paid employment or simply to live. Their entitlements will depend on Belgian law. This is not, of course, a poverty trap in the strict sense in as much as the individual can opt to remain at home where the allowances are available. But it does expose the free movement of persons and workers as rather hollow unless and until the free exportability of social benefits is allowed.

In sum, the poverty traps in the system—especially with regard to means–tested benefits—are well known. The utopian solution is a more universalistic social protection system as well as one that allows for the free exportability of benefits. That is unlikely given the diversity of social protection systems in Europe and the hard reality that the EU lacks legal competence to require it. The results are needless impoverishment, a general lack of choice and control over how benefits are operationalised, and a focus on meeting material needs as distinct from affording citizens the means to be active and included in their community. There are ways of ameliorating all of the above. Indeed, we have to do so if we take the third general goal of social protection seriously—namely, social inclusion. Nonetheless it is worth examining a radical departure in thinking which focuses less on mitigating the loss of income or wealth and more on intentionally building an asset base to expand the individual's opportunities to gain and retain control as well as participate actively in society.

Breaking free from the traps? The value of wealth- or asset-accumulation strategies

The philosophy: Going beyond a floor and giving more choice and control

What if, for the sake of avoiding traps as well as enhancing choice and increasing the possibilities of Active Citizenship, our social protection systems were nudged to encompass not merely interventions that alleviated the impact of a lack of income or income-gaining ability but instead (or in addition) focused on building a person's asset base?

You don't have to subscribe to the philosophy of Frederick Hayek to understand that some degree of economic autonomy is vital to ensure autonomy in other aspects of one's life and to provide a secure base from which to interact and participate actively (Hayak, 1978). It is of course not the function of Government (at least not in most EU States) to directly enhance people's wealth or asset base. But where the above-mentioned poverty traps have a hugely disproportionate effect on certain categories of persons with disabilities (especially those with intellectual disabilities) then perhaps it is time to think again.

Intentional government programmes designed to grow a person's asset base help to avoid poverty traps—especially ones arising from low capital thresholds as well as from conflicts between thresholds and between different benefits and programmes. Such programmes also afford direct power and choice to the individual who, as a typical consumer, shops around for what meets his or her felt needs as distinct from those adjudged prudent by his or her social services. This ties into a larger trend that has to do with the individualisation of social benefits. The flip side has to do with the need for entirely different business models within traditional service providers. And such programmes also enable individuals to plan better for the future with an added capital margin. Again, what they can plan for is not just a life of social *security* but also a life of *social inclusion* and, importantly, *on their own terms.*

As far back as 1991 Sherraden (1991) offered a rationale as to why government policy should aim to broaden asset ownership. Assets not only provide an economic cushion and enable people to make investments in their futures, but they provide a psychological motivation to connect and participate. Galen's aphorism that 'work is nature's medicine' often proves true. However, assets and the promise of a better future for one's children are nature's motivator and, if managed properly, should be the ultimate employment incentive and the first step in changing the economic expectations of people with disabilities (World Institute on Disability, 2015).

Asset building refers to strategies that increase financial and tangible assets, such as savings, a home and businesses of all kinds. Therefore, through asset-building programmes, people with disabilities can own their own homes, fund retirement accounts, and continue or even start a business. These kinds of goals and outcomes are absent from the current discussion within disability civil society and the policy community in Europe.

When governments intentionally design asset-building programmes it is important to ensure that they interact fairly with existing social protection entitlements. To put this another way, the capital accrued should not generally be taken into account when determining social protection entitlements—or render the person ineligible. This is key to protecting any assets accumulated to enable persons with disabilities to build their lives rather than just survive. How is this done? The next sections address relevant asset-building innovations in the US, Canada and Australia.

Innovation in the United States of America: ABLE Act *2014*

In March 2014, the US Federal Congress enacted far-reaching legislation on asset accumulation: *Achieving a Better Life Experience Act (ABLE)* 2014. What led up to it was Individual Development Accounts (IDAs), which will be superseded by ABLE as the new programme is commenced.

IDAs were matched savings accounts designed to enable low-income families to save towards a targeted amount, usually used for building assets in the form of home ownership, post-secondary education or small business ownership. Account holders generally make monthly contributions to an account, usually over a one- to four-year period, and their savings are matched by funds drawn down from a variety of private and public sources, typically at a rate ranging from one dollar for each dollar saved to three dollars for each dollar saved. There is no national assessment of how many people with disabilities have participated in IDA programmes, though the World Institute on Disability (2004) speculated that as many as 53.2 per cent of IDA holders had a physical disability.

Since the 1990s IDAs have been placed on a statutory basis in *The Personal Responsibility and Work Opportunity Reconciliation Act* of 1996 and in the domestic laws of more than 40 US States. Once recruited, participants open IDA accounts with a partnering financial institution and begin making deposits. Match dollars for IDAs come from many different places, such as government agencies, private companies, churches or local charities. Any individual, organisation or business can contribute match dollars to IDAs.

In most cases, donors can get a tax deduction for contributions to IDAs. Each month, IDA participants receive a report telling them how much money is accumulating in their IDA, which is a sum of their individual savings, matched dollars and interest. Individual and matching deposits are never co-mingled; all matching dollars are kept in a separate, parallel account. When the IDA account holder has accumulated enough savings and matching funds to purchase the asset and has completed the required financial education course, payments from the IDA are made directly to the asset provider to complete the asset purchase. Withdrawals are usually restricted to the purchase of assets, such as buying a home, pursuing post-secondary education and training or starting small businesses. Other uses, especially the purchase of a car or computer for work-related purposes, are sometimes permitted. Account holders are usually required to attend financial education courses prior to an asset purchase.

Advocates of IDAs argue that those with assets are more economically secure, have more options in life and can pass on status and opportunities to future generations. They further argue that assets have potential social, psychological and civic effects that are independent of the effects of income (Boshara, 2005). Over the last decade, research and demonstration projects have been initiated to address these claims and their findings suggest that IDAs do lead the poor, including those with disabilities, to save or acquire assets (Schreiner, 2002, Mills et al., 2004). Junior Individual Savings Accounts in the United Kingdom and Canada's LearnSave project have both been directly inspired by the experience of IDAs in the US and informed by research on IDAs. It is considered by most in the US that the use of the IDAs by persons with disabilities will be replaced with ABLE accounts.

Signed into law in the United States of America by President Obama on 19 December 2014, the *Achieving a Better Life Experience (ABLE) Act* amends the Federal tax code to allow for Section 525A tax-exempt saving accounts for disability-related expenses. Importantly, this allows federal law to disregard ABLE account funds for means-tested federal programmes such as Supplemental Security Income (SSI) and Medicaid (the US national healthcare system). Such means-tested federal programmes usually cap the amount an individual can save at $2,000. The money that is saved in an ABLE account is not taxed and is also not counted as an asset when determining eligibility for federal means-tested benefits (United States, 2014). The passing of the *ABLE* Act through Congress was the culmination of a nine-year campaign to gain approval for tax-free savings accounts that would help individuals and families to finance various disability needs. The *ABLE* Act had 454 co-sponsors in the House and Senate (85 per cent of Congress), making it the most bipartisan, bicameral bill in the 113th Congress (National Down Syndrome Society, 2016).

It is important to note that the *ABLE* Act allows a State to establish an ABLE programme, but it does not obligate States to do so. Therefore, each of the fifty states must pass their own ABLE laws. To date, 33 States have enacted their own versions of the *ABLE* Act and are in the process of setting up State ABLE programmes.

There are a number of criteria that a person must meet in order to be eligible for an ABLE account. An eligible individual is someone who has become disabled before the age of 26. They must be in receipt of Social Security Disability Insurance (SSDI) or Supplemental Social Income (SSI). SSI is a means-tested cash support for disabled persons on low income. SSDI is an insurance-based programme that covers mainly workers who acquire disabilities whether on the job or otherwise. Medicaid is a means-tested health care assistance programme (funded by the federal government and state governments) for people on low income. Expenses (or allowable expenditures) that are covered under ABLE are those that are for the benefit of the person with the disability, including education, housing, transportation, employment training and support, assistive technology and personal support services, health, prevention and wellness, financial management and administration services, legal fees, expenses for oversight and monitoring, funeral and burial expenses and any other expenses approved under the regulations.

The following features characterise an ABLE account:

- Individuals with a disability, their families, their employers, and any other person wishing to contribute assets for the individual with a disability, may contribute up to $500,000 into an ABLE account for that individual until the individual reaches the age of 65. Direct tax breaks are given to incentivise investments.
- The owner of an ABLE account may save up to $100,000 in their account before their public benefits (SSI) are suspended.
- The person would retain eligibility for the SSI programme but would not receive any payments while their ABLE account has in excess of $100,000 in it.
- The ABLE account has no impact on Medicaid eligibility.
- Any excess contributions (and earnings attributable to them) would be subject to a six per cent excise tax. The earnings of the assets held in an ABLE account are not subject to federal income tax while they remain in the account.
- Withdrawals from an ABLE account that are not for qualified expenses are taxable in respect of the beneficiary. Specifically, if the annual withdrawal from an ABLE account exceeds the beneficiary's annual qualified disability expenses, a portion of the withdrawal is subject to income tax plus an additional 10 per cent excise tax. The taxable portion of the withdrawal represents the interest earned on assets in the ABLE account.

Importantly, prior to the passing of the *ABLE* Act, while persons with disabilities in the USA could save for future expenses in tax-advantaged ways, such savings were counted as assets and thus persons with disabilities risked the loss of other supports like SSI and Medicaid. As outlined previously, living with a disability can be expensive. Treatments, therapies, transportation and housing are just some of the items that can be more expensive living with a disability. Saving in an ABLE account allows the affected individuals and their families to save for these added expenses without losing other supports and benefits. The $2,000 asset limitation in the United States, above which all benefits like SSI and Medicaid would be cut off, created a disincentive for persons with disabilities to work. With this asset limitation removed, individuals can work as hard as they are able, become at least partially self-sufficient and continue to receive needed benefit.

Grandparents, parents, other family members and friends can now leave money through a will or gift money to individuals living with disabilities without concern that it would eliminate their entitlement to benefits like SSI. Before the passing of the *ABLE* Act, Special Needs Trusts, a complicated and expensive process that required a lawyer and cost as much as $10,000, were used by families to amass assets for their children. Individuals living with a disability can actively seek work, contribute to their own support and save for their own future without fear of losing necessary support and services. ABLE encourages individuals living with a disability to become active and productive and participate in the workforce and society, and thus benefits everyone.

On 19 June 2015 the US Department of Treasury, in conjunction with the Internal Revenue Service, released a Notice of Proposed Rule Making regarding the *ABLE* Act. The draft rules (subject to consultation and final adoption) will serve to assist states and programme administrators in understanding how to develop and maintain an ABLE programme. They give clarification to parts of the law.

The proposed regulations provide that the eligible individual is responsible for establishing his or her own account and that the designated beneficiary is the owner of the account. However, 'if an eligible individual is unable to establish an ABLE account on his or her own behalf, the ABLE account may be established by the eligible individual's agent under a power of attorney or, if none, by a parent or legal guardian of the eligible individual' (United States, 2015: 35613). Also, 'if the designated beneficiary is not able to exercise signature authority over his or her ABLE account or chooses to establish an ABLE account but not exercise signature authority, the designated beneficiary's agent under a power of attorney or, if none, a parent or legal guardian of the designated beneficiary' (National Disability Institute, 2015: 2) may be given signature authority.

Innovation in Canada: Registered disability savings plan

As a result of many years of advocacy by Planned Life Advocacy Network (PLAN), families and supporters, the Canadian federal government implemented the Registered Disability Savings Plan (RDSP) on 1 December 2008. A Registered

Disability Savings Plan is a long-term savings plan designed to enable individuals with disabilities and their families to save for their future financial security.

The first of its kind in the world, the programme consists of the Canada Disability Savings Grant, which matches personal contributions, and the Canada Disability Savings Bond, that provides funding to RDSPs of people on low and moderate incomes. A person who establishes an RDSP can make contributions to the plan up to a lifetime contribution limit of CAD $200,000 for the benefit of the person named the beneficiary. With written permission from the RDSP holder, anyone such as family, friends, charities or neighbours, may contribute to the RDSP.

The Canada Disability Savings Grant works as follows: for every deposit a person makes in an RDSP account, the federal government can (if the family income is below $87,123) match with up to $3 per $1. The Canada Disability Savings Bond is slightly different in that for people living on a low income (less than $25,356), the federal government will put $1,000 in the account each year for 20 years. People living on an income of between $25,356 and $43,561 still receive a partial bond. As there are no restrictions on how the money is spent, people with disabilities can choose what to do with the money when it comes out of the savings plan (Canada RDSP, 2015).

To open an RDSP, a person must have a long-term disability, be eligible for the Disability Tax Credit, be under of the age of 60 (if the person is 59, they must apply before the end of the calendar year in which they turned 59), be a Canadian resident with a valid Social Insurance Number and be looking for a long-term savings plan (Canada RDSP, 2015). The Disability Tax Credit supports persons with disabilities by reducing the amount of income tax they have to pay. It is non-refundable in that the person pays less tax initially and therefore they do not get any money back in the future. The aim of the Disability Tax Credit is to provide equity among tax payers by allow relief for the additional costs that persons with disabilities incur due to the nature of their disability (Canada RDSP, 2015).

Only one RDSP account may be set up per individual, and only that beneficiary is entitled to any payments. An RDSP arrangement must be between the issuer (bank) and either the beneficiary, a qualifying person in relation to the beneficiary or a legal parent who is not a qualifying person, but who is a holder of another RDSP of the beneficiary. A qualifying person can only establish and administer an RDSP on behalf of the beneficiary if the beneficiary lacks the mental capacity to do so. An adult with a disability and with mental capacity who wishes to benefit from an RDSP must establish the plan himself or herself. However, family members, friends or others could contribute to a plan established by the person with disabilities, with his or her permission.

A person receiving disability benefits can set up an RDSP without going through an asset test and without it affecting their disability benefits. Contributions are not tax-deductible, and earnings and growth accrue on a tax-deferred basis. The contributions grow tax-free until withdrawn, at which time a proportion of the plan (earnings and growth received) is taxable and will need to be declared as income in the hands of the beneficiary at that time. In most cases it does not affect eligibility for provincial disability benefits. Contributions can be made up to the end of the year in which the beneficiary turns 59 years old.

There are complex rules governing the withdrawal of funds from RDSPs because RDSPs were created to encourage long-term savings. In line with this, a Registered Disability Savings Plan encourages a person with a disability to seek gainful employment as those with an income of between CAD $25,356 and $43,561 still receive a partial bond. It is generally felt that this is one of the better solutions to the poverty traps faced by persons with disabilities as it permits them to accumulate wealth, retain some of their disability allowances and still work to earn their own income and secure their own independence.

Innovation in Australia: National Disability Insurance Scheme Act *2013*

Australia does not have a wealth- or asset-accumulation strategy as such. However, it is to the very forefront in the world in affording persons with disabilities direct control over their various social protection benefits and allowances. This trend—the personalisation of supports (whether insurance-based or means-tested)—strongly complements other more direct wealth-accumulation strategies. Optimally, asset accumulation strategies should be accompanied by the direct personalisation of social protection supports. Australia is now the exemplar in that regard.

The Australian *National Disability Insurance Scheme (NDIS)* Act 2013 is, as the title suggests, insurance-based and paid into by all the working-age and employed population. It provides individualised support for eligible people with disabilities, their families and carers. The NDIS provides funding for support, services and equipment that help persons with disabilities to achieve their goals, do things on their own and become independent, develop skills for day-to-day living, take part in the community and work and earn money. The NDIS helps to improve mobility and learning and aims to promote self-care and self-management while helping persons with disabilities to build capacity for social and economic participation. The scheme was launched in July 2013, following years of discussion about the need for a major reform of disability services in Australia. The NDIS is being introduced across Australia in stages with the first stage rolled out in South Australia, Tasmania, the Hunter Region in New South Wales and the Barwon area of Victoria in July 2013 (Australia, 2015).

In 2010 the Australian Government commissioned a pubic enquiry into a long-term disability care and support scheme. The enquiry was undertaken by the Productivity Commission and received over one thousand submissions indicating that the existing social protection system did not work. Published in August 2011 and paving the way for the NDIS, the Productivity Commission's report outlined how a disability and support scheme should be designed and funded and how those most in need should be identified; it listed the funding options of alternative schemes, including service delivery arrangements, and the costs, benefits and feasibility as well as how the scheme would interact with the health, aged care, informal care, income support and injury insurance systems. The report detailed the expected impacts on the workforce, recommended how any scheme should be introduced and governed and, finally, what protections and safeguards should be part of such a scheme. Following the publication of the report, the Council of Australian Governments agreed to the need for a reform of disability services through a national disability insurance scheme (NDIS). It was agreed that mid-2013 would be the benchmark date for implementation.

Conclusions

The innovations outlined above are startling. They break embedded assumptions that persons with disabilities (or at least certain cohorts) are fated to remain dependent and with no direct power over their entitlements and assets. Wealth-accumulation strategies complement the trend toward the personalisation of supports that gives people more choice and control. They enable persons with disabilities to grow their assets, which, in turn, expands their opportunities to participate in the community. From a conceptual point of view they are a tool to give meaning to the goal of social inclusion in our traditional social protection systems. They would seem to be not only compatible with the letter and spirit of the UN CRPD but arguably demanded by it.

However, there are big risks—risks worth pondering as we begin to think how this innovation could be replicated in EU Member States.

Perhaps the biggest risk is that asset- or wealth-accumulation strategies will be seen (if not immediately then maybe over the medium term) as a substitute for social protection programmes themselves. They most assuredly are not. Traditional social protection programmes are themselves becoming more personalised—a trend that is set to continue and increase in the future. A nice symmetry could therefore emerge between personalised social protection entitlements and personalised control over capital accumulated through asset accumulation strategies. This symmetry will not happen if one (asset accumulation) is seen as a substitute for the other (social protection). However, it has to be frankly admitted that the risk remains real.

A related and even deeper fear is that the reliance on market forces (at least in part) represented by asset accumulation strategies represents an unacceptable harnessing and intrusion of market thinking into the traditional social protection field. For example, some say it is no accident that these strategies have emerged in strong market-based economies (and societies). However, it is by now incontrovertible that innovation is required to breathe fresh life into the European social model to go beyond providing for material needs in order to give a voice and choice back to the individual and to achieve greater levels of social inclusion and active citizenship. It could be argued that wealth-accumulation strategies do not, directly or indirectly, surrender the future of our social protection systems to the market. Rather, they simply seek to complement social protection with capital that can be intelligently obtained from market forces. Seeking to achieve social ends through market forces is inherently dangerous. However, the difficulty of doing it should not stop innovation and the learning that can come from it.

Another risk is that the relevant capital thresholds (upon which entitlements are lost) will be set too low which means that wealth will not be allowed to grow to a meaningful point. These thresholds will vary from state to state and will depend, to a certain extent, on the degree to which there are other (i.e., more universalistic-based) entitlements in the system. The point is that the thresholds should be realistic. The big risk is that they won't be.

Of course, the higher the threshold the greater the hit that is taken by the treasury (in foregone tax income). It follows that another risk is that governments will only be persuaded to implement asset accumulation strategies if it can be shown that, somehow, the individual will cost the state less at some point in the future and therefore generate savings. Interestingly, wealth accumulation strategies in the US and Canada were not advocated for on the basis that they would save the state money in the long term. Whatever argumentative strategy is adopted to persuade states to move in this direction, this should not be one of them. It may well turn out to be true—or partly true, but this is a dangerous line of advocacy. A much better line of argument is that the outcomes for individuals in terms of active citizenship are measurably enhanced at a relatively low cost to the state.

A related risk is that the allowable expenditures (payable from the funds) will be set too narrowly thus constraining the range of choice normally afforded to ordinary consumers. For example, ABLE funds in the US may only be used to cover 'qualified disability expenses' whereas a person with a RSPD account in Canada can use their fund on any expense they wish. An incidental by-product of asset-accumulation strategies is that they can incentivise new business models among service providers. If the range of allowable expenditure is too constrained this systems change will not happen. It is therefore preferable to keep the range of expenditures relatively open.

All of these risks are real. Nevertheless, the authors believe that a substantial case exists to give active consideration to complementing our European social protection system with some form of wealth accumulation strategies. This essay is, it is to be hoped, a first step in that direction.

References

Australia, NDIS (2015). *National Disability Insurance Scheme*. Retrieved Retrieved 22 August 2015 from: http://www.ndis.gov.au/

Boshara, R. (2005). Individual Development Accounts: Policies to Build Savings and Assets for the Poor. *The Brookings Institution Policy Brief.* 32, 6. Washington, DC: Brookings Institution.

Cantillon, B., Van Mechelen, N., Pintelon, O. & Van Den Heede, A. (2013). Social redistribution, poverty and the adequacy of social protection in the EU. *GINI Discussion Paper 54*. GINI Research.

Eardley, T., Bradshaw, J., Ditch, J., Gough, I. & Whiteford, P. (1996). Social assistance in OECD counties. *Department of Social Security Research Report No. 46*. York: University of York.

Hayak, F. A. (1978). *The Constitution of Liberty*. Chicago: University of Chicago Press.

Ireland (2016). A programme for partnership government Retrieved 29 May 2016 from: http://www.merrionstreet.ie/MerrionStreet/en/ImageLibrary/Programme_for_Partnership_Government.pdf

Mills, G., Patterson, R., Orr, L. & Demarco, D. (2004). *Evaluation of the American Dream Demonstration*. New York: The Ford Foundation.

National Disability Institute (2015). *IRS Issues Proposed ABLE Act Regulations*. Washington DC: NDI. Retrieved from: https://www.aucd.org/docs/ABLE%20Reg%20Highlights%20Ltrhd(2).pdf

National Down Syndrome Society (2016). *Stephen Beck, Jr. Achieving a Better Life Experience (ABLE) Act in 50 States*. Retrieved 6 June 2016 from: http://dsagno.org/wp-content/uploads/2015/01/ABLE-Act-Update.pdf

RDSP (2015). *Registered Disability Savings Plan*. Retrieved 16 August 2015 from: http://www.rdsp.com/

Schreiner, M. (2002). *Saving Performance in the American Dream Demonstration: A National Demonstration of Individual Development Accounts*. Washington: Centre for Social Development, George Brown School of Social Work, Washington University.

Sherraden, M. (1991). *Assets and the Poor: A New American Welfare Policy*. New York: M. E. Sharpe.

Stove, B., Overgaard, H. M., Rodevand, S. & Sollie, M. (2015). The Norwegian Disability Pension System: Actuarial challenges arising from new regulations. *Working Paper*. Bergen, Norway: University of Bergen.

United Nations (2006). The United Nations Convention on the Rights of Persons with Disabilities. Retrieved 2 April 2014 from https://www.un.org/development/desa/disabilities/convention-on-the-rights-of-persons-with-disabilities.html

United Nations (2014). *Social Policy and Development, 2000–2009*. United Nations Research Institute for Social Development (UN RISD). Retrieved 5 July 2014 from: http://www.unrisd.org/research/spd

United States, Congress (2014). *ABLE Act of 2014*. Retrieved 2 September 2015 from: https://www.congress.gov/bill/113th-congress/house-bill/647

United States, IRS (2015). Guidance under Section 529A: Qualified ABLE Program. *Federal Register* Vol. 80, No. 119. Monday 22 June 2015. Retrieved 5 August 2015 from: https://www.gpo.gov/fdsys/pkg/FR-2015-06-22/pdf/2015-15280.pdf

World Bank (2013). *Inclusion Matters: The Foundation for Shared Prosperity*. Washington, DC: The World Bank.

World Institute On Disability (2004). *Integrating Universal Design Principles in Asset Building Programs*. Retrieved 11 August 2015 from: https://worldinstituteondisabilityblog.files.wordpress.com/2016/01/integrating-universal-design-principles-in-asset-building-programs.pdf

World Institute on Disability (2015). Equity. Asset Building Strategies for People with Disabilities. A Guide to Financial Empowerment. Retrieved on February 14th 2017 from: https://worldinstituteondisabilityblog.files.wordpress.com/2015/11/equity-asset-building-strategies-for-people-with-disabilities.pdf

10 Exercising influence at the European level

Political opportunity structures for disability rights advocacy and the impact of the UN CRPD

Andreas Sturm, Anne Waldschmidt, Anemari Karačić and Timo Dins

Historically, international disability rights movements have been crucial collective actors in promoting disabled persons' interests. These movements gained new momentum in the 1970s, when the first cross-disability coalitions were formed. Since then, both the integration of the European Union (EU) and globalisation have progressed, changing not just conditions of economics and politics on an international scale, but also having effects on civil society and non-governmental organisations (NGOs).

Against this background, the main objective of this chapter is to shed light on the current prospects of disability rights advocacy to enhance Active Citizenship through political influence at the European level in the age of the Convention on the Rights of Persons with Disabilities (CRPD). By describing existing opportunity structures for interest representation and drawing on original data we explore how European organisations of and for persons with disabilities make use of political opportunities provided by the EU and the Council of Europe. Based upon earlier research (Waldschmidt, 2009), we investigate the relations between European institutions and civil society organisations. Bearing in mind that not only most European countries, but also the EU, have ratified the Convention, we also explore the question of how the adoption of the CRPD has changed these relations.

After having presented our theoretical framework, we delineate the existing opportunity structures at the European level. We explain our approach for the empirical study, which started with investigating how European civil society organisations that are active in disability policies use coalition building at the European level. We present the results of a series of interviews with representatives of European disability organisations about the impact of the CRPD. Finally, we discuss the findings and draw conclusions about how European disability organisations are most likely to influence policy development at the European level.

What are political and legal opportunity structures?

Eisinger (1973) coined the term 'opportunity structure' in order to address the question of when social protest is most likely to occur. He argues that it emerges 'in systems characterized by a mix of open and closed factors', being 'vulnerable or responsive to political efforts combined with the persistence of inequities [...]' (Eisinger, 1973: 15). Similarly, Tarrow (1994: 85) understands opportunity structures as 'consistent—but not necessarily formal or permanent—dimensions of the political environment that provide incentives for people to undertake collective action [...]'. As our study is less concerned with the analysis of social protest, but focuses on classic interest representation conducted by formal organisations addressing official institutions, we find the concept of Princen and Kerremans (2008: 1130) useful. They define political opportunity structures as 'set[s] of characteristics of a given institution that determine [...] the relative ability of (outside) groups to influence decision-making within that institution'. In addition, we draw on the work of Marks and McAdam (1999: 99), who identify four major dimensions of these structures:

- Openness versus closure of an institutionalised political system
- Stability or instability of 'elite alignments'
- Presence or absence of 'elite allies'
- Capability and willingness of the state to use repressive measures.

In the following, we focus on the first dimension—openness versus closure of an institutionalised political system—as proposed by Marks and McAdam. 'Openness' and 'closure' are not univocally defined concepts; however, there is consensus that they denote the degree of 'receptivity' (della Porta, 1996: 65) or 'responsiveness' of a political system to political protests, claims and actions (Eisinger, 1973; Kitschelt, 1988: 62).

The EU Commission can strategically use funding to 'privilege a few large and well-connected' and 'resource rich NGOs' which often become 'administrative partners' (Maloney, 2008: 24). Some European NGOs receive up to 90 per cent of their total funding from the EU (Johansson & Lee, 2015: 71), which in turn enables the EU to threaten these organisations' existence by withdrawing financial resources. In this study, we consider the providing of financial resources as an indicator of an open political system and the withholding of resources as an indicator of closure.

Drawing on Princen and Kerremans (2008: 1131), we address the structural aspects of responsiveness by exploring 'the ease of access for political actors' on the basis of 'objective structural factors' as 'outside constraints'. In addition, Princen and Kerremans' (2008) concept of 'resource exchange' is also helpful for investigating European disability politics. This aspect refers to the fact that both the official institutions as well as the NGOs can benefit from mutual cooperation (Princen & Kerremans, 2008: 1134ff).

Last but not least, recent literature tends to widen the concept of political opportunity structures by specifying 'legal opportunity structures' as a distinct dimension of the structural conditions. With regard to the CRPD, Vanhala (2011) argues that legal dimensions need more consideration. Hilson (2002) contends that the lack of political opportunity structures 'may *influence* the adoption of litigation as a strategy in place of lobbying, and that the choice of protest as a strategy may be *influenced* by poor political and legal opportunities' Hilson, (2002: 239; emphasis in original). Justifiably, these approaches emphasise that legislation and jurisdiction need to be integrated in the picture of (political) opportunity structures. Yet, the political system is usually comprised of the legislative, executive and judiciary dimensions anyway. Therefore, this chapter refrains from specifically conceptualising the CRPD as a legal opportunity structure in itself, but understands it as potentially offering specific legal opportunities within given political systems.

Political opportunity structures at the European level: The European Union

Regarding the political system of the EU, it is worth noting that the Treaty of Lisbon, which entered into force in 2009, stipulates that EU 'institutions shall maintain an open, transparent and regular dialogue with representative associations and civil society' (European Union, 2007: Art. 8.B.2; 2012a: Art. 11.2; 2012b). Yet, in this regard the EU institutions differ from each other. Whereas the Council of the European Union offers only limited access for the civil society sector (Waddington et al., 2013: 339), the European Parliament and also the European Commission are said to provide relatively open political opportunity structures for lobbying activities (Kohler-Koch, 1997: 6). Even more, the latter is often portrayed as a door-opener for civil society organisations (Quittkat & Kohler-Koch, 2011). Further, both the European Economic and Social Committee (EESC) and the Committee of the Regions (CoR) are influential advisory bodies within the EU. While the EESC functions as a bridge between the EU system, workers' and employers' organisations and other interest groups, it has no official say in law-making. In contrast, the CoR has the right to 'intervene at several stages in the EU law-making process' (Committee of the Regions, n.d.), concerning EU legislation at regional and local levels. Lastly, the EU Agency for Fundamental Rights (FRA) endeavours to maintain a dialogue with NGOs through its Fundamental Rights Platform. In the following, we concentrate on the European Parliament, the European Commission and the Committee of the Regions as significant political institutions, then consider the EU's Monitoring Framework.

First, as one of the two EU institutions with legislative power (the other being the Council of the European Union), the European Parliament (EP) can look back on a long tradition of cooperation with civil society. As to participation opportunities for disability rights advocacy, the establishment of the Disability Intergroup in 1980 clearly marks a milestone. In spite of not being a part of the EP's official structure, as one of the oldest European Intergroups it enhances the dialogue between Members of the European Parliament (MEPs) from all political groupings and stakeholders from European organisations representing disabled persons.

Whereas the Disability Intergroup's composition of participant MEPs remains fixed during each parliamentary term, the civil society stakeholders attending the group vary with each of the meetings held per year (European Disability Forum, n.d.-a). The European Disability Forum provides secretarial services to the

Disability Intergroup, while its bureau, composed solely of MEPs, is responsible for its organisation and management, including the admission of the civil society organisations to its meetings (European Disability Forum, n.d.-b).

Another opportunity to gain access to the European Parliament is the European Transparency Register, which was established in 2011, with the goal of implementing the aforementioned provisions of the Lisbon Treaty. The inter-institutional 'Agreement [...] on the establishment of a transparency register for organisations and self-employed individuals engaged in EU policymaking and policy implementation' (European Union, 2011) sets out the rules; it stipulates, for instance, that registration is voluntary. The provision of 'badges affording long-term access to the European Parliament's buildings' (European Union, 2011: Part VII, Art. 22) is supposed to make registration attractive. Yet, this privilege may be somewhat out of date. As White (2013: 276) points out: 'Whilst direct observation of meetings takes place in the Parliament building, and whilst observation of such meetings helps to keep lobbyists au fait with developments, more significant contacts with MEPs and with their staff may take place elsewhere.'

Second, the European Commission is both the EU's executive body and the only institution within the EU that has the right of initiative to propose law. In media coverage and public debates the Commission is often criticised as being non-transparent and lacking political legitimacy (Moravcsik, 2004). In actual fact, it has a key role in EU policy processes. With its need for expert advice and socio-political legitimacy, the Commission has created a variety of advisory bodies that interact with the civil society sector.

The administrative 'core unit within the European Commission on disability issues' (Waddington et al., 2013: 233) is the Disability Unit, at present affiliated to the Commission's Directorate General for Employment, Social Affairs and Inclusion (European Commission, 2015). In its mission statement this Unit pledges 'to promote equal opportunities for people with disabilities at EU level' in the following ways:

- by facilitating the cooperation of the EU Member States in the development of their disability policies
- by endeavouring to ensure that the disability perspective is taken into account in the Commission's own internal affairs and in the formulation of relevant Community legislation, programmes and policies
- by contributing to the raising of awareness levels throughout the European Union by supporting non-governmental organisations and relevant activities. (European Commission, n.d.)

The Disability Unit cooperates with a variety of European organisations representing disabled persons and offers several participation opportunities to these organisations, for instance, by inviting them to annual conferences and events such as the European Day of Disabled People. It also presides over the Inter-Service Group on Disability, a platform that brings together policy-makers and EU officials from all Directorates General (DGs) to enhance disability mainstreaming at EU level (Waddington et al., 2013: 233). Additionally, the Unit collaborates with the Academic Network of European Disability Experts (ANED), which was set up in 2008 and funded by the EU Progress Programme 'to support [disability] policy development' (Human European Consultancy, n.d.).

Last but not least, the Commission and its Directorates General have established several advisory bodies or Expert Groups, which are also significant parts of the opportunity structures within the Commission. To start with, there are the European Expert Group on the Transition from Institutional to Community Based Care (hereinafter: EEG Community Based Care) and the EU Stakeholders for the Platform against Poverty (hereinafter: Stakeholders against Poverty). Both are coordinated by the DG Employment, Social Affairs and Inclusion. Further, the DG Health and Consumers leads the EU Health Policy Forum (EU HPF), and the DG Regional Policy manages the Commission Expert Group entitled Structured Dialogue with European Structural and Investment Funds' Partners Group of Experts (ESIF SD). Another relevant Expert Group is the Consultative Group of Stakeholders on Air Passenger Rights (APRCG), which is affiliated to the DG Mobility and Transport. This list of Expert Groups illustrates that disability politics at EU level is not confined to 'classic' policy areas such as employment and social security, but addresses a wide range of policy fields in which a variety of stakeholders exercise political influence.

As one of the most important Commission Expert Groups, the Disability Unit hosts the High Level Group on Disability (HLGD), which has the goal 'to promote—in collaboration with the Member States and with non-governmental organisations of and for people with disabilities—the exchange of useful information and experience especially concerning innovative policies and good practice' as set out in a Council Resolution on equal opportunities for persons with disabilities (Council of the European Union, 1997: Part III, Art. 2). The HLGD's main task is to generate common European guidelines for disability-related policy issues; for this purpose it maintains a regular dialogue between national as well as European policy-makers and organisations representing persons with disabilities.

Third, besides the European Parliament and the Commission there is the Committee of the Regions (CoR), which was founded in 1993 under the Maastricht Treaty (Kaniok & Daďová, 2013: 115). This advisory body is also a channel to influence EU disability policy, as it cooperates, often at the regional and local level, with both formal and informal interest groups (Kaniok & Daďová, 2013: 128). While its impact was assessed as limited in the beginning, it has gained more political power due to recent political developments in the EU (Kaniok & Daďová, 2013: 115). As another arena for political influence the CoR possibly makes NGOs less dependent on the goodwill of the Commission.

Last, but not least, is the EU's Monitoring Framework of the CRPD, which was set up in 2013 (EU CRPD Monitoring Framework, 2015). It is composed of the European Parliament and the European Commission as well as the Fundamental Rights Agency, the European Ombudsman and the European Disability Forum (EDF). Currently the latter chairs the Framework, while the Commission has the function of the secretariat (European Disability Forum, 2014). This Framework is certainly one of the CRPD's first impacts at European level, but it is not open to organisations representing disabled persons apart from the EDF.

Political opportunity structures at the European level: The Council of Europe

At first glance, the Council of Europe (CoE) as a truly intergovernmental organisation without legal competence of its own does not seem to be a pertinent political arena. Moreover, the CoE is not authorised to sign and ratify the CRPD. Yet, it proves to be a significant stakeholder as well, offering specific opportunity structures for civil society organisations (Waddington et al., 2014: 345ff). This role is based on two human rights treaties: the European Convention of Human Rights and Fundamental Freedoms, and the European Social Charter. The former is the basis for the jurisdiction of the European Court of Human Rights (ECHR), whose verdicts are binding for CoE member states.

The ECHR allows what are termed 'third party interventions' or '*amicus curiae* briefs', that is, legal opinions or testimonies from external parties that are not directly involved in the particular court case. This is a means to ensure that possibly broad legal effects of a pending court decision are taken into consideration at an early enough stage. Recent court applications are made public, so NGOs can efficiently plan their third-party interventions. As a result, disability-related case law on, for instance, legal capacity, accessibility or the right to family life has been developed with the active support of disability organisations (Waddington et al., 2014: 349ff): 'This opportunity is of exceptional importance to European-level disability NGOs interested in advancing the engagement of the Court in this field' (Waddington et al., 2014: 347f).

In addition, the CoE's European Committee of Social Rights, which monitors the implementation of the European Social Charter, also provides participation opportunities for NGOs. As a start, organisations need to apply for participatory status with the CoE (Council of Europe, n.d.). Once this status is granted, they have the right to become engaged 'in the policies and work programme of the Council of Europe' (ENIL, 2011) as members of its Conference of International Non-governmental Organisations (INGOs). This Conference constitutes civil society's pillar in the CoE's exchanges with the Committee of Ministers, the Parliamentary Assembly and the Congress of Local and Regional Authorities (ENIL, 2011). Subsequently, INGOs with participatory status can apply for the entitlement to lodge collective complaints with the European Committee of Social Rights.

Political opportunity structures at the European level: an overview

Taken as a whole, we can characterise the opportunity structures of the EU and the CoE as relatively 'open' (Marks & McAdam, 1999) as regards the involvement of civil society in policy processes. According to the concept of 'resource exchange' (Princen & Kerremans, 2008) we can assume that it is not only the political institutions with their need for expert advice, but also the NGOs which benefit from their involvement in official politics.

Table 10.1 Political opportunity structures at the European level

European Organisation	*Political Institution*	*Opportunity Structure Components*	*Requirements for Civil Society Organisations*
European Union	European Parliament	Disability Intergroup	Admission by the Intergroup Bureau
		Long-term access to EP Building	Registration in Transparency Register
	European Commission	Commission Expert Groups: HLGD EEG Community Based Care Stakeholders against Poverty EU HPF ESIF SD APRCG	Invitation by the chairing Commission representative
Council of Europe	European Court of Human Rights	Third–party interventions (*amicus curiae* briefs)	
	Conference of INGOs	Collective complaints	Admission of participatory status at the Council of Europe

Explanation of abbreviations: APRCG—Consultative Group of Stakeholders on Air Passenger Rights; EU HPF—EU Health Policy Forum; ESIF SD—Structured Dialogue with European Structural and Investment Funds' Partners Group of Experts; HLGD—High Level Group on Disability; INGOs—International Non-Governmental Organisations.

Table 10.1 indicates that besides the CoE with its Committee of INGOs and the Human Rights Court, the EU Commission Expert Groups should be considered important arenas for exercising political influence on behalf of civil society. However, Mahoney (2004: 447) points out that the Commission 'determines the nature of interest representation in the policy-making process in a much more direct manner by selecting in what policy areas public debate will be fostered and which interests will participate in the formal forums of debate.' This leads us to the assumption that while the Commission is offering political opportunities to civil society organisations, it is highly selective when it comes to relevant stakeholders and issues.

Data and methods

The remainder of this chapter deals with the use of European political opportunity structures by organisations representing persons with disabilities and their views on the impact of the CRPD on European politics. In the following, we explain our empirical approach, which is based on three kinds of sources. First, we generated original data by way of guided interviews with representatives from disability organisations; second, some of our interview partners provided additional information; and third, we conducted documentary analyses of publicly available data. Here we primarily relied on the websites of the considered European organisations of and for disabled persons.

Originally, our aim was to focus on the practices of Disabled People's Organisations (DPOs) at the European level, but due to a lack of information we could not specify in all cases whether the organisations in question were associations *of* or *for* persons with disabilities. Yet, following the UN CRPD Committee's understanding of DPOs (Committee on the Rights of Persons with Disabilities, 2014), we regard the issue of representativeness as relevant. For this reason, we use 'disability organisation' as a generic term, when civil society organisations of and for persons (including children) with disabilities active in disability rights advocacy, activism and disability policy are concerned, leaving internal requirements for membership, board and direction out of consideration (Waldschmidt et al., 2015). We employ the concept DPO only in two cases, either in citations or when we can be sure that organisations *of* persons with disabilities are denoted (see also Chapter 11).

Another intention of this study was to obtain multi-faceted statements by a variety of stakeholders, including both cross-disability organisations and impairment-specific ones, representing, for example, persons with visual challenges, with intellectual and developmental impairments, with psychosocial difficulties or with mobility difficulties. For pragmatic reasons we started by selecting organisations that participated in the DISCIT project. One of our research partners, the European Disability Forum (EDF), is an umbrella organisation and represents, among other things, 25 European Disabled People's Organisations, whose status as DPOs is based on EDF statutes, as full members; additionally 14 organisations are ordinary members, and there is a broad spectrum of other stakeholders as observer and associate members.

As the next step, we selected 10 single organisations that are full members of the EDF, as they have to fulfil strict requirements, thus indicating a good fit with the CRPD Committee's guidelines. We further added Rehabilitation International (RI), as it was a member of DISCIT's European Stakeholder Committee, but is neither a member of the EDF nor a DPO. The latter two aspects also apply to the European Association of Service Providers for Persons with Disabilities (EASPD) and Mental Health Europe (MHE). We still consider these organisations as relevant, as they are listed with 'disabled persons' as their 'area of competence' in the INGO database of the Council of Europe. All in all, we were able to conduct 10 telephone interviews with representatives of 7 out of 14 organisations. The EDF provided three interviews; two interviews were conducted with Disabled People's International Europe (DPI-E). Individual interviews were possible with five other organisations. Drawing on Meuser and Nagel (2013), we defined experts as persons who hold official functions on the basis of special expertise. In our case, the interviewees were 'insiders' both in disability politics and their organisations.

The semi-structured topic guide for the interviews asked for information on European political participation opportunities and their use by the organisations, their cooperation with other stakeholders as well as general assessments of the CRPD and its impact, the organisations' involvement in the Convention's implementation and their use of specific CRPD Articles. In the following, we first present our findings on the organisations' practices within the opportunity structures of European politics. Here we focus on the aspect of coalition building. Second, we describe how representatives of international disability organisations reflect upon the impact of the CRPD at the European level.

How are European disability organisations using political opportunity structures at the European level?

When investigating the structures of interest representation of civil society at the European level, one quickly comes across policy networks, known as 'advocacy coalitions', which usually consist of a number of NGOs representing a variety of stakeholders. EU-level advocacy coalitions can be defined as part of the political opportunity structures themselves, or they can be regarded as 'set[s] of actors who share the same policy goal' (Klüver, 2013: 45). They are established to enhance the influence of stakeholders on European policies, especially where the weak interests of social minority groups are concerned. We understand these coalitions as indicators of open opportunity structures, especially when EU funding takes place.

While most of these coalitions advocate a broad spectrum of issues exceeding what we consider typical for disability rights advocacy, we can identify a number of coalitions that are of relevance for disability politics. In the following, we differentiate between *social rights advocacy coalitions*, here understood as coalitions of NGOs from the social sector and disability organisations, and *disability rights advocacy coalitions*, solely comprised of organisations representing persons with disabilities.

First, the European Social Platform (ESP) is one of the social rights advocacy coalitions. It is a coalition of 'European rights and value-based NGOs working in the social sector' (European Social Platform, 2016) and currently comprises 48 member organisations (European Social Platform, 2016). The ESP receives operating grants as Commission subsidies, using resources from the Europe for Citizens programme to the amount of €700,000 in 2013 (European Commission Financial Transparency System, n.d.-c). Its aim is 'to promote social justice, equality and participatory democracy by voicing the concerns of member organisations' (European Social Platform, 2016). The second social rights advocacy coalition which is relevant in our context is the European Patients Forum (EPF), a coalition of 'patients' groups in public health and health advocacy across Europe' (European Patients Forum, 2014a). At present, it incorporates 65 member organisations (European Patients Forum, 2015). It received operating grants from the Commission under the Second Programme of Community Action in the Field of Health to the amount of €653,966 in 2013 (European Commission Financial Transparency System, n.d.-b) and its aims are 'promoting a patient-centred philosophy and agenda with the EU institutions' (European Patients Forum, 2014b).

Whereas both social rights advocacy coalitions receive Commission funding and entertain a consolidated stable relation with it through consultation and participation bodies, the position of the next coalition is weaker as regards resources and possibly also contacts with EU institutions. The European Coalition for Community Living (ECCL) is a disability rights advocacy coalition. An association of European disability organisations, it was founded in 2005 and aims at 'working towards the social inclusion of people with disabilities by promoting the provision of comprehensive, quality community-based services as an alternative to institutionalisation' (European Coalition for Community Living, n.d.). Since the adoption of the UN Convention in 2006 and its ratification by the EU in 2010, the ECCL has concentrated on Article 19 CRPD that guarantees the right to live independently and be included in the community. It strives to lobby EU institutions with the goal to 'advocate for and monitor progress towards de-institutionalisation in Europe, campaign for, and provide information on, the development of comprehensive, quality community-based services and de-institutionalisation' (European Coalition for Community Living, n.d.).

Given its nature as an association of a number of EU-level DPOs and other disability organisations, the EDF may also be considered as a disability rights advocacy coalition. However, it is also a collaborating member in the other networks and in this context it acts as a member organisation. For this reason, we regard the EDF as a 'hybrid' organisation, exhibiting features of both an advocacy coalition as well as a disability rights organisation at the EU level. The EDF was founded in 1996 through a Commission initiative, after a longer process of constitution in the context of HELIOS II, the EU's third action programme for disabled people (Malleier, 2011: 75f). Over the last twenty years EDF has become the central collective actor in European disability politics. This role becomes even more evident when one considers the pattern of networking between the advocacy coalitions under consideration here and the 14 organisations in our sample.

Five organisations—the European Action of Persons with Disabilities, European Down Syndrome Association, Disabled People's International Europe, International Federation of Persons with Physical Disability, and the International Federation for Spina Bifida and Hydrocephalus—are all full members of the EDF, but none is a member of the two social rights advocacy coalitions or of the ECCL as described above. In 2013, it received €911,467 as an operating grant through the Progress Programme (European Commission Financial Transparency System, n.d.-a). Of course, the reasons for joining or not joining these coalitions may vary, but we can assume that organisations with few resources have problems getting involved in one or more networks due, for instance, to the availability of staff and/or time.

Still, there are other full members of the EDF that take part in one or two advocacy coalitions. The European Blind Union is a member of the ESP, while the European Network on Independent Living is a member of the ECCL. Further, the European Alliance of Neuromuscular Disorders Associations as well as the

European Network of (ex-) Users and Survivors of Psychiatry are both involved in the European Patients Forum. Interestingly, Inclusion Europe is the only full EDF member that is part of two advocacy coalitions, namely the ESP and the ECCL.

Whereas EDF member organisations differ in their involvement in the networks, all examined advocacy coalitions seem to be generally open to disability organisations regardless of EDF member status. Inclusion Europe (with full EDF membership status), Mental Health Europe (as an ordinary EDF member) and the European Association of Service Providers for Persons with Disabilities (not an EDF member) are represented in both the ESP and ECCL. Rehabilitation International, which is not involved in the EDF, is a member of the European Patients Forum, which also includes the European Alliance of Neuromuscular Disorders Associations and the European Network of (ex-) Users and Survivors of Psychiatry, which are both full members of the EDF.

Finally, it turns out that the EDF is the only organisation in our sample that is involved in all three advocacy coalitions (the ESP, ECCL and the European Patients Forum). To summarise the main points: First, EU advocacy coalitions are open to disability-related issues, as most disability organisations make use of them. We can assume that the degree of cooperation is an indicator of the level of organisational bargaining power in processes of political deliberation, since the coalitions are joint efforts or 'tools' to concentrate resources in order to exercise political influence more effectively. Second, membership status in the EDF does not seem to affect the opportunities of single organisations to participate in the aforementioned advocacy coalitions. Yet, there is reason to believe that the number of involvements is an indicator of the degree of political influence. Third, the EDF's significance in European disability politics becomes visible again, supporting the argument that while the EDF is a member organisation, it can also be perceived as a disability rights advocacy coalition in itself.

How has the CRPD influenced European political opportunity structures?

We will now explore whether the CRPD has already had an impact on the European political opportunity structures in terms of the openness or closure of these structures. It is important to note that we generated our interview material in the second half of 2014. For this reason, our data does not cover the EU's initial CRPD audit, which took place in September 2015. There were two overarching topics that came up in the 10 expert interviews: positive changes due to the CRPD and problems of implementation.

When asked for assessments of the most significant changes in European disability politics with regard to the Convention, interviewees stated that the CRPD had contributed to raising awareness of the human rights approach (see also Chapter 11). The representative of Rehabilitation International emphasised this point:

> I think it's a greater focus on disability from a human rights perspective after the CRPD was conducted and adopted. That's the main outcome of the

> Convention, but that perspective is very important because that gives also the drive for what is happening on different fields, like in accessibility, in habilitation, rehabilitation, work and employment […]. (RI)

The interviewee representing the European Network on Independent Living used the same argument, adding that the CRPD has raised awareness of specific policy issues (ENIL). An expert from the EDF also stated that some issues have received more attention and new issues had been taken up:

> I mean there was a continuation, but maybe there is a bit more attention on certain topics like independent living than there was. […] But I would say maybe legal capacity has been completely new, [it] came with the Convention. Probably [it's] the area where there was the greatest change. (EDF #1)

In addition, interviewees expressed that European institutions had become more receptive to certain policy issues that used to be difficult to address:

> I think in the political discourse there have been a lot of changes. So people speak of the rights of persons with disabilities, which was not the case before. [...] Before, we struggled more. We used non-discrimination, but this had a limitation, and the Convention is really opening a lot of doors in that sense. So for me this is really the biggest change. (EDF #1)

Further, interviewees highlighted the character of the CRPD as a legal opportunity structure: 'The appearance of the CRPD has profoundly changed and formalised our disability rights approach. We have a legally binding instrument in our hands' (EDF #3). The expert of the European Down Syndrome Association called the CRPD an 'international standard, an international rule you can refer to' (EDSA). This statement suggests that it makes sense to consider legal conditions as part of political opportunity structures.

Next, several representatives of the EDF pointed out that the CRPD enhanced the recognition of the disability rights movement by European policy makers: 'I mean at the EU level […] for example the Convention is a very good argument for us […] to speak with decision makers, in different policy areas […].' (EDF #1) One of the experts representing Disabled People's International Europe described the CRPD's impact as supporting the case of Disabled People's Organisations (DPI-E #1). This included processes of mutual learning and capacity building as well as providing knowledge of how to use the European level effectively. Yet, the interviewee from the European Down Syndrome Association was more pessimistic about the CRPD's possibilities of empowering DPOs; this person also mentioned the problem of the lack of financial resources (EDSA).

With regard to organisational practices, some interviewees indicated that the CRPD had increased their opportunities to collaborate or cooperate with supranational organisations, for instance, with UN bodies such as the United Nations High Commissioner for Human Rights (ENIL) or with other European stakeholders such as the European Society of Physical and Rehabilitation Medicine (RI). In other words, the CRPD did not only foster opportunity structures for disability organisations at the European level but also beyond that.

As a general assessment, the interviewee from the European Network on Independent Living highlighted that the CRPD as such had no weaknesses. This person also stated that a human rights convention always raised the question of interpretation (ENIL). While there had been some positive impact, when it came to implementation and participation in political processes, obstacles remained:

> The CRPD has had a positive impact, just in terms of promoting, saying that you have to involve disabled people in everything that concerns them, [...] so it definitely has had a positive impact, but when it comes to putting it into practice, there I think it is difficult. [...] It definitely had a positive impact, but it's still, we are still far from genuine involvement. (ENIL)

With respect to implementation problems, the interview material provided various perspectives. The representative of the International Federation for Spina Bifida and Hydrocephalus (IF SBH) pointed out that the CRPD impacts were neither distributed equally nor visible with regard to all target groups:

> So the implementation or the adoption of the Convention in 2006 [by the UN] should have affected that to the positive for our movement, [...] but I cannot say that I have noticed the change yet from the perspective of our movement. Of course I am aware of all the work [...] so I know that this happens. How well and how much it impacts persons with SB, Hydrocephalus on the ground, I don't know, I don't think it has much, to be honest, not yet. (IF SBH)

Several experts mentioned that the CRPD Monitoring Framework did not function effectively. One interviewee from the EDF argued that it was not clear how it was meant to work. This person was of the opinion that the EU Commission should not be part of the monitoring setup, as this would contradict the Framework's independence and cause additional problems (EDF #2).

As far as the role of the European institutions was concerned, the interviewee from the European Network on Independent Living expressed criticism of the Commission's High Level Group on Disability when asked about institutionalised channels to exercise political influence:

> In terms of the EU level, we haven't been very happy, you know they have this High Level Group on Disability, we haven't been very happy with it [...] it has been [a] closed group, and I don't think it engages a lot with DPOs. [...] But we've always highlighted that there are different voices among disabled people. [...] you can't say you are a representative of all disabled people in Europe. (ENIL)

In our previous section we characterised the High Level Group on Disability as part of a relatively open opportunity structure. By contrast, this statement highlighted that formal openness was just one side of the coin, and the experience of the civil society organisations involved might turn out differently. Another statement from the EDF concerned collaboration with the parliamentary Disability Intergroup, which was also characterised as problematic:

> I mean, the Intergroup sometimes has seemed to be directly responsible for disability issues in the Parliament, and sometimes took initiatives without really involving EDF, or without sharing the objectives or even the content of their initiatives, so there is some criticism about the Intergroup. We will see how it will work in [the] next legislation, but the feeling is that there is not really a very good collaboration, [...] in my opinion, addressing specific committees is sometimes more effective than working through the Intergroup. (EDF #2)

A contentious issue was that the EU had not yet ratified the Optional Protocol to the Convention, which would include further instruments of enforcement (see Chapter 11). A representative of the EDF stated that their aim was still to achieve ratification of the Optional Protocol by the EU, as they wanted to make sure that the CRPD was considered 'when drafting policies, legislations, programmes, regulations, whatever' (EDF #3). In contrast, the representative of European Action of Persons with Disabilities did not see a ratification of the Optional Protocol as realistic. This interviewee was of the opinion that 'it is the national laws that have to be changed' in favour of persons with disabilities (AEH). The interviewee from Rehabilitation International also favoured implementation at national level:

> No, I think more or less we are focusing mostly on the political work on the national level because decisions [...] made on the European level are based on what national governments [are] promoting, so to speak. So the strategy is to make sure that different countries on the national level have the right input before decisions are made on the European level. (RI)

These statements indicated that experts had different opinions on the question of what could actually be achieved at the European level in order to improve the real living conditions of persons with disabilities as well as the standing of their organisations. When interviewees advocated national implementation rather than EU ratification of the Optional Protocol, this could be an indicator that they assessed the European political opportunity structures as less open or relevant than the national structures.

Overall, the interview data created the impression that at the European level more impact of the CRPD is still to be achieved. Although the EU signed the Convention as long ago as 2007 and ratified it in 2010, it seemed that at least by the end of 2014, the date of our interviews, the implementation process had only just started. Probably this process will have to continue for several decades before effective outputs and outcomes can be observed.

Conclusions

This chapter has focused on the political opportunity structures for exercising Active Citizenship through disability rights advocacy at the European level. Our analysis has shown that both the EU and the Council of Europe provided a broad range of opportunities that disability organisations used to exercise political influence. While the latter offered the means of third-party interventions at the ECHR and collective complaints, the most important political opportunity structures were provided by EU institutions.

As regards the latter, the Commission Expert Groups were central in offering opportunities for disability rights advocacy. Our analysis of the actual use of these structures brings to the fore that civil society networks were significant actors in influencing European disability politics. Not only advocacy coalitions for disability rights, but also social rights advocacy coalitions played a role for organisations in the field of disability politics and a majority of the organisations in our research took active part in these coalitions. The EDF has emerged as the key NGO, uniting several organisational roles and different political functions.

At the same time, the interview data indicated some problems for disability organisations in influencing policymaking. Despite the relative openness of European political opportunity structures, which the experts acknowledged, they also criticised the way in which bodies such as the Disability Intergroup and the High Level Group on Disability functioned in practice. When it came to CRPD implementation, different strategies to exercise influence in disability politics became visible. On the whole, the interviewees indicated that there have been some positive changes, while they also emphasise that there were still major barriers for effective disability rights advocacy at the European level.

References

Committee of the Regions (n.d.). Work of the CoR. Retrieved 10 May 2016 from: http://cor.europa.eu/en/activities/Pages/work-of-the-cor.aspx

Committee on the Rights of Persons with Disabilities (2014). Annex II. Guidelines on the participation of disabled persons' organizations and civil society organizations in the work of the committee. In Committee on the Rights of Persons with Disabilities (Ed.), *CRPD/C/11/2. Report of the Committee on the Rights of Persons with Disabilities on Its Eleventh Session* (9–14).

Council of Europe (n.d.). Non-governmental organisations entitled to lodge collective complaints. Retrieved 18 May 2016 from: http://www.coe.int/en/web/turin-european-social-charter/non-governmental-organisations-entitled-to-lodge-collective-complaints

Council of the European Union (1997). Resolution of the Council and of the Representatives of the Governments of the Member States meeting within the Council of 20 December 1996 on Equality of Opportunity for People with Disabilities. *Official Journal of the European Communities, OJ C* 12/01, 13-07-1997, 1–2.

della Porta, D. (1996). Social movements and the state. Thoughts on the policing of protest. In D. McAdam, J. D. McCarthy & M. N. Zald (Eds.). *Comparative Perspectives on Social Movements. Political Opportunities, Mobilizing Structures, and Cultural Framings* (63–92). Cambridge: Cambridge University Press.

Eisinger, P. K. (1973). The conditions of protest behavior in American cities. *The American Political Science Review*, 67(1), 11–28.

ENIL (European Network on Independent Living) (2011). Resolution against the cuts. Retrieved 12 December 2014 from: http://www.enil.eu/campaigns/resolution-against-the-cuts/

European Coalition for Community Living (n.d.). About ECCL. Retrieved 12 December 2014 from: http://community-living.info/about-eccl/

European Commission (n.d.). The disability unit. Retrieved 25 January 2016 from: http://ec.europa.eu/employment_social/soc-prot/disable/unit_en.htm

European Commission (2015). Organigram DG Employment, Social Affairs and Inclusion. Retrieved 20 January 2015 from: http://ec.europa.eu/social/BlobServlet?docId=2796&langId=en

European Commission, Financial Transparency System (n.d.-a). Entry: Year 2013: European Disability Forum. Retrieved 12 May 2016 from: http://ec.europa.eu/budget/fts/index_en.htm

European Commission, Financial Transparency System (n.d.-b). Entry: Year 2013: European Patients Forum. Retrieved 12 May 2016, from: http://ec.europa.eu/budget/fts/index_en.htm

European Commission, Financial Transparency System (n.d.-c). Entry: Year 2013: European Social Platform. Retrieved 12 May 2016 from: http://ec.europa.eu/budget/fts/index_en.htm

European Disability Forum (n.d.-a). Disability Intergroup of the European Parliament. Retrieved 16 February 2017 from: http://www.edf-feph.org/disability-intergroup-european-parliament

European Disability Forum (n.d.-b). Work priorities. Retrieved 16 February 2017 from: http://www.edf-feph.org/work-priorities

European Disability Forum (2014). EDF is chairing the EU Framework on the UN Convention. Retrieved 16 February 2017 from: http://www.edf-feph.org/edf-chairing-eu-framework-un-convention

European Patients Forum (2014a). About us. Retrieved 12 December 2014 from: http://www.eu-patient.eu/About-EPF/whoweare/

European Patients Forum (2014b). What we do. Retrieved 12 December 2014 from: http://www.eu-patient.eu/whatwedo/

European Patients Forum (2015). EPF members. Retrieved 15 December 2015 from: http://www.eu-patient.eu/Members/The-EPF-Members/

European Social Platform (2016). Our members. Retrieved 09 February 2016 from: http://www.socialplatform.org/our-members/

European Union (2007). Treaty of Lisbon amending the Treaty on European Union and the Treaty establishing the European Community (2007/C 306/01). *Official Journal of the European Union, OJ C* 306/01, 17-12-2007, 1–271.

European Union (2011). Interinstitutional agreements. Agreement between the European Parliament and the European Commission on the establishment of a transparency register for organisations and self-employed individuals engaged in EU policymaking and policy implementation. *Official Journal of the European Union, OJ L* 191/29, 22-07-2011, 29–38.

European Union (2012a). Consolidated version of the Treaty on European Union (2012/C 326/13). *Official Journal of the European Union, OJ C* 326/13, 26-10-2012, 13–46.

European Union (2012b). Consolidated version of the Treaty on the Functioning of the European Union (2012/C 326/47). *Official Journal of the European Union, OJ C* 326/47, 26-10-2012, 47–200.

European Union CRPD Monitoring Framework. (2015). Minutes of Meeting: Tuesday, 10 February 2015, 13:00–15:30. Retrieved 11 May 2016 from: http://ec.europa.eu/social/BlobServlet?docId=14293&langId=en

Hilson, C. (2002). New social movements: The role of legal opportunity. *Journal of European Public Policy*, 9(2), 238–255.

Human European Consultancy (n.d.). Academic network of European disability experts (ANED). Retrieved 25 January 2016 from http://www.humanconsultancy.com/project?pid=7

Johansson, H. & Lee, J. (2015). Competing capital logics in the field of EU-level CSOs: Autonomy from or interconnectedness with the EU? In H. Johansson & S. Kalm (Eds.). *EU Civil Society: Patterns of Cooperation, Competition and Conflict* (61–80). Basingstoke: Palgrave MacMillan.

Kaniok, P. & Daďová, L. (2013). Committee of the Regions: From advisory body to the second chamber of the European Parliament? *Transylvanian Review of Administrative Sciences*, 9(40), 114–136.

Kitschelt, H. P. (1988). Political opportunity structures and political protest: Anti-nuclear movements in four democracies. *British Journal of Political Science*, 16(1), 57–84.

Klüver, H. (2013). *Lobbying in the European Union. Interest Groups, Lobbying Coalitions, and Policy Change*. Oxford: Oxford University Press.

Kohler-Koch, B. (1997). Organized interests in the EC and the European Parliament. *European Integration Online Papers*, 1, 1–17.

Mahoney, C. (2004). The power of institutions: State and interest group activity in the European Union. *European Union Politics*, 5(4), 441–466.

Malleier, J. (2011). *Lobbying für Behinderte. Interessenvermittlung am Beispiel des europäischen Behindertenforums in der Europäischen Union*. Frankfurt a.M.: Peter Lang.

Maloney, W. (2008). Social capital as catalyst of civic engagement and quality of governance. In B. Kohler-Koch, D. De Bièvre & W. Maloney (Eds.). *Opening EU-Governance to Civil Society. Gains and Challenges* (19–24). Mannheim: CONNEX—Network of Excellence, University of Mannheim, Mannheim Centre for European Social Research (MZES).

Marks, G. & McAdam, D. (1999). On the relationship of political opportunities to the form of collective action: The case of the European Union. In D. della Porta, H. Kriesi & D. Rucht (Eds.). *Social Movements in a Globalising World* (97–111). Basingstoke: Palgrave Macmillan.

Meuser, M. & Nagel, U. (2013). Experteninterviews—wissenssoziologische Voraussetzungen und methodische Durchführung. In B. Friebertshäuser, A. Langer & A. Prengel (Eds.). *Handbuch Qualitative Forschungsmethoden in der Erziehungswissenschaft* (4th ed., 457–472). Weinheim, Basel: Beltz Juventa.

Moravcsik, A. (2004). Is there a 'democratic deficit' in world politics? A framework for analysis. *Government and Opposition. An International Journal of Comparative Politics*, 39(2), 336–363.

Princen, S. & Kerremans, B. (2008). Opportunity structures in the EU multi-level system. *West European Politics*, 31(6), 1129–1146.

Quittkat, C. & Kohler-Koch, B. (2011). Die Öffnung der europäischen Politik für die Zivilgesellschaft—das Konsultationsregime der Europäischen Kommission. In B. Kohler-Koch & C. Quittkat (Eds.). *Die Entzauberung partizipativer Demokratie. Zur Rolle der Zivilgesellschaft bei der Demokratisierung der EU-Governance* (74–97). Frankfurt a.M.: Campus.

Tarrow, S. (1994). *Power in Movement. Social Movements, Collective Action and Politics.* Cambridge: Cambridge University Press.

Vanhala, L. (2011). *Making Rights a Reality? Disability Rights Activists and Legal Mobilization.* New York: Cambridge University Press.

Waddington, L., Quinn, G. & Flynn, E. (Eds.) (2013). *European Yearbook of Disability Law* (Vol. 4). Cambridge: Intersentia.

Waddington, L., Quinn, G. & Flynn, E. (Eds.) (2014). *European Yearbook of Disability Law* (Vol. 5). Cambridge: Intersentia.

Waldschmidt, A. (2009). Disability policy of the European Union: The supranational level. *ALTER, European Journal of Disability*, 3(1), 8–23.

Waldschmidt, A., Karačić, A., Sturm, A. & Dins, T. (2015). 'Nothing about us without us': Disability rights activism in European countries—A comparative analysis. *Moving the Social. Journal of Social History and the History of Social Movements*, (53), 103–137.

White, S. (2013). Footprints in the sand: Regulating conflicts of interest at EU level. In J.-B. Auby, E. Breen & T. Perroud (Eds.). *Corruption and Conflicts of Interest: A Comparative Law Approach* (272–287). Cheltenham: Edward Elgar.

11 Implementing the UN CRPD in European countries

A comparative study on the involvement of organisations representing persons with disabilities

Anne Waldschmidt, Andreas Sturm, Anemari Karačić and Timo Dins

Exercising influence is one of the central dimensions of Active Citizenship. In the political field this practice usually takes the shape of not only participating individually as a political citizen (e.g. by voting in elections), but also of forming organisations with the aim of representing one's own interests. The United Nations Convention on the Rights of Persons with Disabilities (CRPD) recognises disabled people's organisations by obliging states parties to consult with and actively involve organisations representing persons with disabilities in CRPD implementation processes at national level. Against this background, this chapter investigates these organisations' involvement in national policies that aim to ratify and, in a further step, to implement the Convention.

Our study is based on empirical data from 84 interviews with national experts on disability policies and from representative organisations in nine European countries: Czech Republic, Germany, Ireland, Italy, Norway, Serbia, Sweden, Switzerland and the United Kingdom. The first part of this chapter deals with structural aspects, namely the institutional and legal framework of the CRPD and its current status in the nine countries. The touchstone of the CRPD's significance is whether it changes policies and practices at national level and whether it makes any difference to the actual living conditions of persons with disabilities. Our data does not allow insights into the ultimate outcomes or resulting policies, nor does it enable us to investigate the specific national situations in detail. However, the data does shed light on how the CRPD is promoting changes in the processes of policy-making and it provides an overall picture of European styles of handling the CRPD as an international disability rights regime. We thus focus in this chapter on these practices and styles. We explore these two questions: How are disabled people's organisations and other disability organisations involved in CRPD ratification and implementation processes at national level, and what new activities in disability politics has the Convention stimulated?

We start by describing the relevant political opportunity structures provided by the CRPD. Next, we present our analytical approach as well as the empirical data and methods applied. In the remaining part, we present the findings of our analysis with regard to, first, the involvement of representative organisations in the implementation of the CRPD, and, second, the impact the CRPD has had so far on national styles of policy making. Our conclusion identifies four major dimensions of the impact of the CRPD on national disability politics.

The relevance of the UN CRPD for national disability policies

Drawing on the analytical approach presented in Chapters 1 and 2 and the research on political opportunity structures (e.g. Tarrow, 1994), we see the institutional and legal frameworks provided by the CRPD as promising points of departure for creating new conditions for strengthening the political influence of persons with disabilities. Basically, when we deal with the Convention and the UN as its originator, we face international norms and rules, enacted by an international organisation, with the intention of establishing an international regime (see Bennett, 1991: 226f; Schieder, 2013; Ziring et al., 2005). International regimes are defined, following Krasner (1982), as 'sets of implicit and explicit principles, norms, rules and decision-making procedures', centring on specific problems with the intention of problem-solving, 'around which actors' expectations converge in a given area of international relations' (Krasner, 1982: 186). The decision-making procedures linked with international regimes 'are prevailing *practices* for making and implementing collective choice' (Krasner, 1982: 186; our emphasis).

With this definition in mind we can argue that the Convention is the main instrument of a global disability rights regime with practical implications. If the CRPD is to be imbued with life not only at a global level, but also domestically, we need to highlight the role of nation states as contracting parties, since the claiming of disability justice and the realization of disability rights firmly depend on one being a citizen of a nation-state and making claims for justice upon that state 'justice upon that state.' (Soldatic, 2013: 746). In other words, we need to focus on *national implementation practices.*

Turning to this level, the following features of the international regime in question are relevant (for an overview see Degener, 2015). Whether nation states sign (and also ratify) only the Convention or both the Convention and the Optional Protocol makes a difference insofar as mechanisms of control and enforcement are concerned. The signing is merely a symbolic act; it does not effectively bind an individual state party. Only when the Convention is ratified do states parties commit themselves legally to the implementation, as they consent to integrate the CRPD's principles, norms, rules and procedures into national law and public administration. Moreover, with ratification comes the duty to submit periodic and comprehensive state reports to the UN CRPD Committee; non-governmental bodies and civil society organisations are allowed to submit parallel reports in addition. These reports undergo official audits at public meetings of the Committee, which result in concluding observations entailing concerns and recommendations to the country concerned and are available to all states parties and the general public.

Further instruments of enforcement are included in the Optional Protocol to the Convention. For example, Article 6 of the Optional Protocol gives the CRPD Committee the right to intervene in and examine cases of 'grave or systematic violations' by a state party (United Nations Division 2006). However, although these tools strongly resemble legal proceedings, 'there is no court attached to the Convention, merely a standard "treaty monitoring body"' (Quinn, 2009: 40). This body, the Committee, does not belong to the jurisdiction of the UN, neither do its members act as judges of international law. As a consequence, there are no 'hard' sanctions (e.g. fines) possible and only the policy of publicly 'naming and shaming' (see Hafner-Burton, 2008) can be applied, a mechanism whose effectiveness is disputed.

Having described the international institutional and legal background of our study, we turn our attention to the political opportunity structures provided by the CRPD at national level. Here, we draw on a broad understanding of these structures as 'consistent—but not necessarily formal or permanent—dimensions of the political environment that provide incentives for people to undertake collective action by affecting their expectations of success and failure' (Tarrow, 1994: 85). Considering the following regulations, the Convention can be regarded as a 'pull factor' that enhances the chances for the concerns of disabled persons and their organisations to receive greater political attention and to realise their aims.

Article 4, section 3 of the CRPD obliges states parties to consult with and actively involve organisations that represent persons with disabilities, including children with disabilities, in implementation processes at national level. Article 33, section 3 of the CRPD stipulates that civil society and in particular organisations representing persons with disabilities are to fully participate in the monitoring process. In addition, the CRPD Committee recently underlined the importance of representativeness. It issued Guidelines on the Participation of Disabled Persons' Organizations (DPOs) and Civil Society Organizations in the work of the Committee, stating that it understands DPOs to be organisations that are 'comprised by a majority of persons with disabilities—at least half of its membership—governed, led and directed by persons with disabilities' (Committee on the Rights of Persons with Disabilities, 2014).

As far as this empirical study is concerned, our data did not allow us to precisely characterise the national organisations that the interviewed experts represented or talked about. As we regard the issue of self-representation as crucial (Waldschmidt et al., 2015), we will use 'disability organisations' (DO) as a generic term, when civil society organisations *of* and *for* persons (including children) with disabilities active in disability rights advocacy, activism and disability policy are concerned, leaving internal requirements for membership, board and direction out of consideration. In line with the definition of the Committee on the Rights of Persons with Disabilities just quoted, we employ the term 'disabled persons' organisation' (DPO) only in two cases, either in citations, when our interviewees use this term, or when we can be sure that solely organisations *of* persons with disabilities are involved or referred to.

Regarding the impact of the CRPD on nation states, the individual countries' dates of signing and ratifying the Convention and the Optional Protocol provide initial hints at the degree of national commitment. As the empirical basis for our study we focus on nine European countries, eight of which have so far completed ratification and only one country, Ireland, has signed, but not yet ratified the CRPD. Of additional significance is whether a state party has issued reservations and declarations. Among the nine countries only Norway and the United Kingdom have had such reservation and declarations (United Nations Division, 2016). In the following we leave these indicators of partial non-compliance aside and use only the national dates of signature and ratification as criteria. Although they do not indicate the effective status of implementation, they do allow us to draw conclusions about a country's potential commitment and willingness to act on implementation. The earlier a country has signed and ratified the Convention, taken together with whether it has also ratified the Optional Protocol or refrained from this, the more committed this country is deemed to be about the actual implementation. In contrast, late or non-existent signatures and ratifications are interpreted as an indication of compliance problems (see Table 11.1)

In our sample of countries, Sweden can be regarded an 'early starter', as it ratified the Convention in 2008, whereas Norway and Switzerland are 'latecomers', since they completed ratification only in 2013 and 2014. The other countries, Czech Republic, Germany, Italy, Serbia and the United Kingdom, form the group of 'good performers' with 2009 as their year of ratification. With regard to the Optional Protocol, it is striking that a group of five states parties (Sweden, Germany, Italy, United Kingdom and Serbia) has ratified it, while four countries (Czech Republic, Norway, Switzerland and Ireland) so far have refrained from doing so.

Moreover, with the exception of Norway and Switzerland, we are dealing with six member states of the European Union (Czech Republic, Germany, Italy, Ireland, Sweden and the United Kingdom) and one EU candidate country (Serbia). However, in the period for our data collection the European level did not seem

Table 11.1 Categorisation of country sample with regard to CRPD signing and ratification dates

Category according to CRPD ratification date	*9 European countries*	*CRPD signed*	*Optional Protocol signed*	*CRPD ratified*	*Optional Protocol ratified*
'Early starter'	*Sweden*	30-03-2007	30-03-2007	15-12-2008	15-12-2008
'Good performer'	*Germany*	30-03-2007	30-03-2007	24-02-2009	24-02-2009
	Italy	30-03-2007	30-03-2007	15-05-2009	15-05-2009
	United Kingdom	30-03-2007	26-02-2009	08-06-2009	07-08-2009
	Serbia	17-12-2007	17-12-2007	31-07-2009	31-07-2009
	Czech Republic	30-03-2007	30-03-2007	28-09-2009	–
'Latecomer'	*Norway*	30-03-2007	–	03-06-2013	–
	Switzerland	[no date]	–	15-04-2014	–
'Non-ratifier'	*Ireland*	30-03-2007	–	–	–

to have played any significant role in national CRPD-related policies. Bearing in mind that the EU ratified the Convention (but not the Optional Protocol) in 2010, this gap is remarkable. As a consequence, we have had to exclude EU issues from consideration in this study.

Transnationalism and policy convergence—analytical concepts

As stated earlier, we are primarily interested in the practices of national policy-making related to the CRPD. Thus, we deal, on the one hand, with national situations and, on the other hand, with phenomena transcending the borders of nation states.

For the study of transnational processes, we find it helpful to draw on Guarnizo and Smith's (1998: 3) distinction between 'from above' and 'from below' as two forms of transnationalism. A definition of these two aspects is provided by Remennick (2007). 'The former refers to institutionalized economic and political activities of multinational corporations and organizations such as the UN [...], which set in motion a large scale global exchange of financial and human capital. On the other hand, the increasing role in these networks belongs to [...] grassroots agents of transnationalism [...]' (Remennick, 2007: 5073). In this sense the CRPD can be understood as an effect of 'grassroots' activities 'from below', leading to an international disability rights regime 'from above' that eventually initiates policy changes 'below', namely at the national level. If we apply this model of a spiral dynamic, we acknowledge that any policy innovation is never an automatic process, but it needs structures, mechanisms and stakeholders who feel committed and responsible for changing policies. As stated by Elkins et al. (2013: 88): 'Our theory [...] implies that [international] treaties work largely by mobilizing domestic forces, which, in turn, encourage the incorporation of treaty commitments into domestic law'.

Earlier studies of the role of 'domestic forces' in a cross-national comparison have often discussed these as promoting or hindering policy convergence across countries (see for instance Elkins et al., 2013, on human rights law; Hvinden, 2003, and Scharle et al., 2015, on the prospects for a European disability policy) but studies on convergence related to the implementation of the CRPD are still lacking. In a general understanding, convergence studies intend to investigate 'the development of similar or even identical policies across countries' (Knill, 2005: 764). Their basic assumption is that, in a globalised world with more and more transnational processes, nation states will tend to grow alike, sharing similar traits like structures, practices and outcomes. Of course, it is beyond the scope of this chapter to explore the multifaceted concept of policy convergence, neither does our data allow us to compare path dependencies in national disability policies. However, we think that the basic ideas of this approach provide a helpful framework for our study.

First, with regard to the question of why convergence occurs, various studies have observed that policy convergence very often happens as a result of 'international harmonization' (Bennett, 1991: 225f; Knill, 2005: 770), due to a global need of common responses to common problems, introduced through international law. Clearly this is the case with regard to the CRPD. Second, relating to what converges in the political sphere, we follow Bennett, who points out that policy convergence can concern not only 'goals', 'content', 'instruments' and 'outcomes', but also '*policy styles*, a more diffuse notion signifying the process by which policy responses are formulated' (Bennett, 1991: 218; emphasis in original). These policy styles are the focus of our analysis. Third, the question of which activities and policy styles are concerned needs consideration. For this point we can draw on Conzelmann (1998), who examined policy change in the absence of legal force 'from above', namely the effects of regional development policies of the European Community at Member State level. He comes to the conclusion that policy development happens '(1) through *changing preferences* of actors [...], (2) through the *mobilisation of new actor coalitions* in domestic politics [...], and (3) through serving as a *source of inspiration* for policy-makers looking for alternative policy ideas' (Conzelmann, 1998: 12; our emphasis). Our hypothesis is that these three dimensions could possibly be identified in our material as well.

Data and methods

For our empirical data we rely on semi-structured interviews with national experts in nine European countries, generated during the first six months of 2015. The interviews were conducted by the joint efforts of the whole DISCIT research group, on the basis of a common topic guide. As far as our study is concerned, this guide included three questions of particular relevance:

- What do you see as the (most important) changes in disability politics and policies in [your country] since the CRPD ratification?
- In what way are organisations of persons with disabilities (DPOs) in [your country] involved in the implementation of the CRPD or in efforts towards achieving CRPD ratification?
- To what extent (and how) are you (personally or your organisation) involved in the implementation/ratification efforts of the CRPD?

For the recruitment of interviewees, each national team took into account national characteristics of the different policy systems. The overall aim was to involve persons who, as a whole, covered expertise on a wide range of topics relevant in and for national disability policies. The joint interview sample comprised 84 interviews conducted in the nine DISCIT countries. The data set represented a remarkable diversity regarding the background of the interviewed experts.

Within the sample we distinguished five groups: there were experts representing disabled people's organisations and other civil society 'organisations advocating disability rights'; informants involved in official politics, including advisory committees ('political official'); persons representing public authorities or institutions (publicly funded or subsidised) such as health departments, human rights or equality bodies ('public official'); experts representing service providers as well as working in the health and social services sectors ('service provider'); and last, informants representing more than one organisation or institution as well as researchers and other stakeholders ('other informant'). These groups were distributed as follows: Thirty-one representatives of national disability organisations took part in our study, whereas the remaining 53 informants fell more or less equally into the other four groups. It is also worth noting that 22 interviewees self-identified as disabled persons and 3 informants said they had disabled family members. To ensure the anonymity of our experts, we are not able to provide further details.

It needs mentioning that we did not have full transcripts of the interview material. Instead, each interview was summarised by the national teams using a joint guideline. While the interviews were conducted in the national languages, these reports were written in English. They were shared among the DISCIT consortium partners and thus formed the basis of our analysis. These reports were content-oriented summaries and did not always contain direct statements of the informants, but most of them also included quotes from the interview transcripts, which had been translated into English by the persons writing the reports (except in Ireland and United Kingdom). Furthermore, not all interviewees replied to all the issues included in the guide. First, with regard to the section on the involvement of national disability organisations, only 51 reports contained relevant material. Second, when exploring experts' assessments of CRPD impacts, we could analyse only 65 interviews. However, the remaining data included a broad spectrum of other significant information.

Involvement of organisations representing disabled persons in the implementation of the UN CRPD at the national level

The remainder of the chapter presents the empirical analysis, which covers two parts. First, we explore the involvement of disability organisations in CRPD-related processes of ratification and implementation. Second, we investigate changes in the national styles of policy-making. For both aspects the fact of whether signing and ratifying the CRPD has taken place and on what dates is of relevance. As mentioned previously, our country sample consists of four groups: the 'early starter' Sweden, the 'good performers' Czech Republic, Germany, Italy, Serbia and the United Kingdom, the 'latecomers' Norway and Switzerland, and Ireland as the only 'non-ratifier'. In the following we present our data by way of country portraits.

In the case of Sweden, our 'early starter', with already 7 years of experience with the ratified Convention and the Optional Protocol as well as an initial CRPD audit in 2014, the answers from the experts are diverse. They include information on the processes that led to the ratification and describe the national parallel reporting. There are statements that hint at problems with political participation:

> But [for] the strategy 2011–2016, the government decided that it was the state agency that should fix goals to reach during the 5 years, because not so much had happened during 2000–2010. DPOs have not had so much to

> say. Now, for the new strategy, from 2016 on, the government said that we would be invited to the discussions. We will see what happens. I refer a lot to Article 4.3 [CRPD], that persons with disabilities shall be included in all questions concerning disability, through their organisations. It is important that DPOs participate.
>
> (Swedish organisation advocating disability rights #2)

In Sweden there is a dialogue with the disability movement, but a representative from one disability organisation shows discontent: 'The government knows that we find that the CPRD is not well implemented yet'. This expert also argues that Sweden's initial CRPD audit in 2014 has not yet made a big difference: 'We also ask for a five-year plan of how Sweden will work to improve the critiques received from the UN last year' (Swedish organisation advocating disability rights #2).

In our group of the five 'good performers' the picture is diverse. In Germany, which ratified both the Convention and the Optional Protocol in 2009 and had its initial CRPD audit in 2015, most statements relate to national efforts to make the CRPD a reality. Assessments of the participation of disability organisations are generally positive, but also raised concerns. One interviewee summarises the involvement as follows:

> Since the ratification of the CRPD in Germany, we [the civil society and DPOs] received more papers to comment on, were invited to participate in more boards [Gremien], to take part in more events, but there has not been participation on an equal level.
>
> (German organisation advocating disability rights #3)

For the purpose of parallel reporting, disabled people's organisations and other civil society organisations succeeded in forming a national CRPD Alliance, which played an important role in Germany's audit. At the beginning of the CRPD era there were conflicts about the official German translation of the Convention, which led to a shadow translation by disabled people's organisations. It seems that official politics has gradually become more eager to facilitate the involvement of civil society. According to one disability organisation, there is now 'good cooperation with the Federal Ministry of Labour and Social Affairs', but at the level of the 16 federal states the involvement varies. According to one organisation representative, barriers remain: 'While policy makers make huge efforts to celebrate the involvement of civil society in the policy process, it very often remains unclear whether this input has been taken into account or not' (German public official #4).

In Italy, which also ratified both the CRPD and the Optional Protocol in 2009, several interviewees referred to the National Observatory on the Situation of Persons with Disabilities [Osservatorio Nazionale Disabilità], which took office in December 2010:

> [... The] Italian parliament instituted the National Observatory with the law 18/2009 elaborated after the ratification of the Convention. This Observatory

> is composed of regional and national representatives of public administrations, actors from social parties and federations and three experts from the Ministry of Work and Social Policies.
>
> (Italian political official #2)

This committee has greatly enhanced participation opportunities for Italian disability organisations: 'The presence of the DPOs in the observatory (16 out of 40 members) represents the importance of the inclusion and the participation in the whole process' (Italian political official #2). Furthermore, the participation of representative organisations is realised in the development of a new disability action plan at national level: 'The members involved [...] are national, regional and local administrations, trade unions and social parties, DPOs and experts from the associations' (Italian political official #2). But there is also a critical statement from Italy:

> I give a severe and pessimistic judgement on this topic: Italy didn't promote or incentivise the Convention. [...] Sensitisation and information activities have not been implemented at the national level either and even the monitoring process didn't acquire the relevance expected. [...] we can register a general attitude of apathy as regards the international conventions and directives which are ratified but not implemented with effective programmes and provisions on our territory.
>
> (Italian service provider #1)

Interviewees from the United Kingdom, which also belongs to our category of 'good performers' as it ratified both the CRPD and the Optional Protocol in 2009, indicate that national disability organisations are involved in CRPD implementation. In this regard, the experts mention parallel reporting as a relevant activity, but interestingly, there is also much criticism of the methods of advocacy and activism:

> I fundamentally think we are in a moment where social movements need to come back in again, we are in that cycle of human rights activism now that, you know we've achieved something, we've got the UK to ratify it, they've done pretty much nothing at a state level around it, so now we have to build a movement up again. And we have to find a way to recruit into that movement.
>
> (UK organisation advocating disability rights #3)

Several statements mention a lack of coordination between disability organisations and the disability rights movement. There are also doubts about the effectiveness of the UN's monitoring system and, as a consequence, of civil society's engagement: 'The treaty body system is creaking under the weight of the reports it has to process' (UK organisation advocating for disability rights #3).

In Serbia, which also ratified both the Convention and the Optional Protocol in 2009, the interviews include very few statements on the role of disability organisations in CRPD-related policies. Although Serbia belongs to our group of 'good performers', only two interviewees provide answers to this question. None of these statements indicate a high level of involvement by disability organisations. This is possibly related to the general lack of CRPD implementation at the national level, which the following quote illustrates: 'The Convention is included in the legal framework but no one really deals with its implementation' (Serbian other informant).

The Czech Republic, which ratified the Convention in 2009 but has yet to ratify the Optional Protocol, had its initial audit in 2015. Here, the material reflects different professional perspectives; conflicting evaluations and assessments become visible. Some representatives of Czech disability organisations highlight the role of certain associations and their influence on the ratification, while others stress existing barriers to the involvement of civil society, for instance, funding issues. Informants who are active in official politics, however, assess the participatory opportunities for disability organisations as existing and unproblematic. While disability organisations seem to play an important role in promoting the CRPD, their contribution is not always visible to the interviewees. The data also indicates that there are efforts by disabled people's organisations to fight the general lack of awareness of the Convention and to promote implementation at the national level, while service providers are not particularly active in this regard. Czech informants also mention that there are (virtually) no activities of the state to improve public awareness or to support the organisations in this matter. A Czech service provider (#1) argues that 'not many people are aware of the CRPD in the Czech Republic and until the Optional Protocol will be ratified [...] the CRPD is unfortunately widely perceived only as a piece of paper'. References to any activities concerning the country's first CRPD audit in 2015 did not appear in the interview data.

Our third group includes Norway, having ratified the CRPD only in 2013, and Switzerland which ratified in 2014. In Norway, the statements highlight the CRPD ratification as a major milestone for the national disability policy system, of which 'state authorities have not been the driving forces', but 'the great associations for disabled people have worked hard in order to promote inclusion and participation' (Norwegian organisation advocating disability rights #7).

> The organisations have asked for the CRPD to be ratified for many years and they are content that it finally happened even if it is not totally accepted [...] the convention is important for the organisations and is highly valued [...].
>
> (Norwegian organisation advocating disability rights #7)

With regard to practices of involvement, several Norwegian interviewees mention parallel reporting as the main activity. In general, positive assessments prevail, but a representative of a disability organisation makes a critical comment:

> And also the association of [the] disabled has to be self-critical in terms to this because they are splitting up in various factions and are unable to [present

> a united] front [on] the issue. They care more about their own health and welfare than their political rights and participation.
>
> (Norwegian organisation advocating disability rights #3)

In Switzerland, our second 'latecomer', the data covers the process until ratification; when asked about the role of disability organisations, the interview partners are divided. Some are of the opinion that the 'involvement of organisations of and for persons with disabilities was relatively weak' (Swiss service provider #4). Others say that it was the result of 'a lot of lobbying' (Swiss organisation advocating disability rights #4). In the eyes of a third interviewee:

> [...] people with disabilities and DPOs have played a major role in the ratification process by becoming engaged and lobbying for the Convention vis-à-vis the state administration. [...] without these efforts by people with disabilities, Switzerland would not have ratified the CRPD because there was no political interest for the Convention.
>
> (Swiss organisation advocating disability rights #5)

Several experts mention the setting up of Integration Handicap as a new umbrella organisation at the national level, which has taken on the task of preparing the Swiss parallel report: 'They have formed a panel, which now has fifteen members. The majority of the members live with disability, which was intentional in order to strengthen the legitimacy of the panel' (Swiss organisation advocating disability rights #4). However, there is also criticism from an expert representing the interests of women with disabilities; she finds it

> ... scandalous that the women [...] have not been invited by [...] Integration Handicap [;...] they cannot afford the membership fees [...]. That women are in this respect excluded from the implementation process goes against the CRPD itself, in which the situation of women receives much prominence. In Switzerland, however, the topic is not yet on the table.
>
> (Swiss organisation advocating disability rights #6)

Finally, with Ireland we have a non-ratifying country in our sample. For this reason, the statements address the involvement of disability organisations with regard to lobbying for ratification, not for implementation or monitoring. Irish interviewees draw a distinction between two types of organisations: those that are involved and those that are not. The latter group consists of organisations representing persons with intellectual impairments. Answers also qualify the efforts of persons with disabilities and their organisations as 'very disjointed and weak' (Irish other informant #6). One interviewee made this statement: 'People need to stop being so polite and start kicking some ass because it's time it was ratified' (Irish political official).

To summarise, our country portraits show that in virtually all countries studied, disability organisations have been involved in the promotion of the ratification or implementation of the CRPD. In Germany, Italy and Switzerland the relevant stakeholders formed new actor coalitions. In nearly all countries parallel reporting emerges as an important activity that involves exercising political influence in order to (re-)present critical positions in the national processes. Nonetheless, there are also indications that full and equal involvement is not always realised and some organisations have difficulties in achieving sustainable participation in CRPD-related policy cycles.

Changing disability politics at the national level—experts' assessments of the impacts of the UN CRPD

We now turn to informants' assessments of the impacts of the CRPD on national disability politics. Unfortunately, none of the Serbian informants commented on the impact of the CRPD, so we cannot analyse any perspectives from this country. As a consequence we only deal with 8 countries in the following analysis. For conceptual reasons, we do not offer country portraits, but a general picture for the whole sample of countries. We examine 7 dimensions of CRPD impacts.

The CRPD secures positive trends in national disability policies and politics

Informants of two countries, Switzerland and the United Kingdom, regard the CRPD as a means to prevent a deterioration of the national conditions for persons with disabilities. This aspect applies to disability policies as well as to the opportunities of national disability organisations. The CRPD can secure achievements at the national level, as a British informant points out:

> [W]hat it has done is it made sure that we've held onto legislation that we might not otherwise have. We've still got the Equality Act, even though it's got some limitations. If we weren't signed up to the UN CRPD, I would be really worried, depending on who we've got in government, we would lose that legislation.
>
> (UK organisation advocating disability rights #2)

The CRPD stimulates national policies, regulations and action plans

The second dimension is represented in interviews from 4 states. Experts from Sweden as the 'early starter' and from the 'good performers', Czech Republic, Germany and the United Kingdom, regard CRPD ratification as directly stimulating national disability policies. This dimension most prominently refers to the realm of official policy, its regulations and action plans, but it also includes activities of disabled people's networks and other organisations. As a side effect of the obligatory, periodic national reporting by the state, civil society organisations and other stakeholders use 'the tailwind' (German organisation advocating disability rights #2) the CRPD provides for creating new ideas, policies and initiatives and such like to promote change in the national disability policy systems. This dynamic can already be observed for the periods prior to CRPD ratification, as a Czech expert states:

> In order to get to the point of CRPD ratification the Czech government [had to] [...] submit [...] the proposal to Parliament, we had [...] to revise our legal system, and indeed we found that it was not as bad. What was wrong and [what] we had to adapt was revision of our legal system in accordance to Article 12 of the Convention. Article 12—access to justice and things around such as legal capacity, etcetera. This was one of the major things that has been done on the basis of the ratification of the CRPD. The establishment of legal capacity deprivation was abolished and establishment of reduced legal capacity has been specified in details.
>
> (Czech political official #1)

The CRPD promotes the human rights approach to disability

The third dimension is also highlighted in 4 states, to which Sweden as an 'early starter' as well as Germany, Italy and the United Kingdom as 'good performers' belong. From Italy, a statement is very explicit on this point: 'The most important change that occurred with the ratification of the UN CRPD and the anti-discriminatory laws is the rise of the awareness about the rights of people with disabilities' (Italian service provider #2). The dimension of promoting disability as a human rights issue emphasises that the CRPD is not only important because it functions as a legitimate point of reference to improve the situation of persons with disabilities in general, but it also represents a paradigm shift in understanding disability. A British expert points out, 'the Convention has had a symbolic value in allowing disabled people and their organisations to conceive of themselves as "rights-bearing subjects"' (UK other informant #1), despite the fact that 'the political culture of the UK is sceptical of human rights' (UK other informant #1). An expert from Germany thinks that the human rights approach of the CRPD will lead to policy changes: 'More and more people are beginning to realise that this is a human rights issue which we cannot handle with our common and present instruments' (German public official #1).

The CRPD raises public awareness about disability

The fourth dimension appears in a majority of 5 countries, which include Sweden as an 'early starter' and the 'good performers' Germany, Italy and the United Kingdom as well as Switzerland as a 'latecomer'. In all these countries the effect of raising public awareness about disability was highlighted by different kinds of stakeholders and across policy areas. In the United Kingdom, a mental health activist states 'that the CRPD has allowed people to have a different conversation about disability' (UK organisation advocating disability rights #5). Independently of the national ratification date, raising public awareness is regarded a major function of the CRPD, as expressed by a German expert:

> [T]he CPRD created a new dynamic of awareness-raising that is impressive. No other step before the CRPD created a similar kind of dynamic. 'The time is ready', and also there is more awareness that everybody can become a person with disabilities later in life.
>
> (German political official #1)

Conversely, another informant from this country sounds a cautionary note: '[h]owever, awareness has been raised mostly among organised public, politics, professionals, etcetera and not in public in general' (German public official #1).

The CRPD is a useful tool

The fifth dimension is stressed in 6 countries of our sample—Sweden, Czech Republic, Germany, Italy, the United Kingdom and Switzerland—but not in Ireland or Norway. This dimension is a broad category and it was coded as such; it includes statements about the CRPD as a helpful frame of reference when relevant claims, 'hot issues' or major problems are addressed at the national level. Again, we find that all kinds of stakeholders share the opinion that the CRPD is a useful tool, but representatives of national disability organisations are those who highlight this aspect most frequently. A Swedish expert states, 'We use the CRPD all the time. It is a good ground to build our work on' (Swedish other informant #1). A representative of a German disability rights organisation points out, 'We do not have to talk about certain topics since the introduction of the CRPD. There is this legitimation' (German organisation advocating disability rights #1). An Italian informant says, 'We must thank the CRPD for the two-year programme on disability which binds the government to take initiatives' (Italian organisation advocating disability rights #2). The relevant statements from Czech Republic are a bit more sceptical: 'I think that the CRPD somehow influences disability policymaking process here in the Czech Republic, but I also think that those processes [CRPD ratification and policy changes] are to some extent independent of each other' (Czech organisation advocating disability rights #1). The same reluctance is observed in the United Kingdom, but a British expert also states that 'the UN CRPD is a gift [as] it provides a discourse of human rights' (UK organisation advocating disability rights #3). Last, an informant from Switzerland is of the opinion that the CRPD 'is used as an instrument to ground one's political claims. Since the CRPD is so comprehensive, it is also easier to use it for political arguments [...]' (Swiss public official).

The CRPD leads to national reports by the state, civil society and others

The sixth dimension is also identified for 6 countries. Of course, periodic reporting is a consequence of CRPD ratification, therefore it is not surprising that this dimension is not coded for Ireland, but it does not seem so relevant for the British experts either. Sweden as the 'early starter', the 'good performers' Czech Republic, Germany and Italy as well as the 'latecomers' Norway and Switzerland belong to the states parties in which interviewees emphasise official reports by the nation state and parallel reports by civil society organisations as major effects of the CRPD. This dimension appears in interviews across different kinds of stakeholders, whether from civil society, public authorities or from other professional contexts. Some experts mention that parallel reports were conducted as a reaction to a lack of CRPD impact. Therefore parallel reporting can be understood as either a direct effect of the CRPD or as a reaction to the lack of impact of the CRPD. As regards the obligation of states parties to submit periodic reports, the informants consider this duty as an effective means to make the voice of persons with disabilities publicly heard: 'In addition, the effect of the requirements to hand in state reports should not be underestimated. The experience with other human rights conventions has shown that this can move things forward' (Swiss public official).

The CRPD increases the influence of disability organisations

The seventh dimension results from statements of all country groups, the 'early starter' (Sweden) as well as the 'good performers' (Germany, Italy, United Kingdom) and one 'latecomer' (Switzerland). Interestingly, even in the non-ratifying country, Ireland, civil society organisations seem to experience more influence as an indirect impact of the CRPD. One Irish expert points out that civil society 'has been very involved and arguing for implementation and involved in national disability strategy and consultation. [...] they are also gearing up for a role in shadow reports' (Irish other informant #1). In the 6 countries this issue is raised not only by representatives of disability organisations, but also by informants representing official politics or public authorities. Either the interviewees explicitly stress an increased influence of disability organisations or they provide assessments revealing that the activities of national disability organisations have gained momentum in quality, quantity or efficacy in recent years, which can directly be traced back to CRPD ratification. In Germany, one statement lists concrete successes achieved by the national council of disabled people's organisations and disability advocacy organisations:

> As the German Disability Council [...], we also developed ideas on improving participation in the German Action Plan. We have criticised the (official) Action Plan, we have criticised the state report, and we conducted the shadow report as the CRPD Alliance [...].
>
> (German organisation advocating disability rights #3)

In Italy the CRPD has resulted in the establishment of the National Observatory on Disability, in which disability organisations are official members. In Sweden, an informant points out: 'The CRPD is especially important for the disability movement. They have a complete new instrument with the CRPD' (Swedish other informant #1). And an expert from Switzerland states: 'The CRPD has been taken up by DPOs and a lot is being moved forward under the banner of the Convention. This had not happened after the entering into force of the [Swiss] disability equality law in 2004' (Swiss service provider).

Table 11.2 Dimensions of national CRPD impact in relation to country sample

No.	*Dimension*	*Early starter*	*Good performer*	*Latecomer*	*Non-ratifier*
1	The CRPD secures positive trends in national disability policies and politics		UK	CH	
2	The CRPD stimulates national policies, regulations and action plans	SE	CZ, DE, UK		
3	The CRPD promotes the human rights approach to disability	SE	DE, IT, UK		
4	The CRPD raises public awareness about disability	SE	DE, IT, UK	CH	
5	The CRPD is a useful tool	SE	CZ, DE, IT, UK	CH	
6	The CRPD leads to national reports by the state, civil society and others	SE	CZ, DE, IT	CH, NO	
7	The CRPD increases the influence of disability organisations	SE	DE, IT, UK	CH	IE

Country codes: CZ Czech Republic, DE Germany, IE Ireland, IT Italy, NO Norway, SE Sweden, CH Switzerland, UK United Kingdom.

Generally, these 7 categories show a complex picture of CRPD impact at the national level. With regard to their occurrence in our country sample, our analysis results can be summarised in the table above (see Table 11.2).

This table clearly shows that the impact of the CRPD can be perceived in different areas with different emphasis; the national context is also important. Last, a picture of cross-national convergence emerges. We will come back to this final point in our conclusion.

Conclusion

This chapter has examined the significance of the Convention on the Rights of Persons with Disabilities at the level of European countries. First, we focused on the involvement of national disability organisations in CRPD-related political processes. The country-oriented analysis shows that at national level disability organisations are actively engaged in ratification as well as implementation processes. Some experts, however, indicate that participation often takes the form of consultation and committee work; they miss taking part on an equal level and being really involved in decision making. Further, the analysis reveals that professional positions are important. Representatives of disability organisations seem to have a different perspective from persons representing official politics, especially in the case of Czech Republic. On the whole, the writing of parallel reports seems to be a crucial task for representative organisations, which is one of the main CRPD effects mentioned in the interviews.

Second, we analysed the CRPD impacts from the perspectives of national experts. Basically, our findings are in line with Conzelmann (1998), as his three effects (changing actors' preferences, mobilising new actor coalitions and serving as inspiration for policy reforms) emerge from our material. The CRPD changes traditional understandings of disability and promotes the human rights approach; it supports organisations representing disabled persons and encourages new actor coalitions; it brings the 'wind of change' in national disability policies. Furthermore, we can identify a defensive and a deliberative mechanism operating at the national level of policy-making. As a result, we come to four significant changes in national policy styles:

1 *Defensive*: The CRPD is preventing roll-backs in national disability policy systems (dimension 1)
2 *Inspiring*: The CRPD changes traditional disability concepts and offers new ideas for policy makers and political actors at national level (dimensions 2, 3 and 5)
3 *Deliberative*: The CRPD promotes public debates on disability policies and politics at national level (dimensions 4 and 6)
4 *Mobilising* (new actor coalitions): The CRPD enhances the opportunities of national disability organisations to exercise influence (dimension 7).

When we bear in mind that historically the CRPD is a test-case of transnationalism 'from below', namely the product of a transnational community and elite, formed by activists of international disability rights movements, which needed long-lasting and intense bottom-up mobilisation to get the Convention adopted by the UN's General Assembly in 2006 (see Degener, 2015), then it should be evident that CRPD ratification and implementation in the nation states are not simple processes 'from above', but they equally depend on national and local activism to ensure effective transposition and realisation.

With respect to our data, we can conclude that the CRPD has already changed national disability *politics* and there are indications of a trend towards cross-national convergence in the styles of policy making. However, the strength of this trend varies across the dimensions of CRPD impact (see Table 11.2). Similarly, to the extent the CRPD has created 'space for a new dynamic of disability politics and reform' (Quinn, 2009: 39), some countries have been more affected than others. At the same time, substantial effects in disability *policies* are still difficult to assess. If one takes into account that the literature on policy convergence (Bennett, 1991: 224f) highlights the important role of networking and discursive communities sharing values, expertise and information for producing similarities in national policy-making, we can assume that in the long run more and systematic grassroots activities as well as transnational cooperation by persons with disabilities and their representative organisations will eventually promote further developments.

References

Bennett, C. J. (1991). Review article: What is policy convergence and what causes it? *British Journal of Political Science*, 21(2), 215–233.

Committee on the Rights of Persons with Disabilities (2014). Annex II. Guidelines on the participation of disabled persons' organizations and civil society organizations in the work of the Committee. In Committee on the Rights of Persons with Disabilities (Ed.). CRPD/C/11/2, *Report of the Committee on the Rights of Persons with Disabilities on Its Eleventh Session* (9–14). Retrieved 14 December 2015 from: http://docstore.ohchr.org/SelfServices/FilesHandler.ashx?enc=6QkG1d%2fPPRiCAqhKb7yhssDWsrFiT9-DJhcpwRZIfGZ5UZz4YGKDX6Qu3VXLHavbbmPgbcGEzLiOfshx4aC3Bt9LbDUVb7ljrPOEqnP1LZE6FDlayqWreDyycR63kCxd0

Conzelmann, T. (1998). 'Europeanisation' of regional development policies? Linking the multi-level governance approach with theories of policy learning and policy change. *European Integration online papers*, 2(4), 1–23. Retrieved 11 January 2016 from: http://eiop.or.at/eiop/texte/1998-004a.htm

Degener, T. (2015). Die UN-Behindertenrechtskonvention—ein neues Verständnis von Behinderung. In T. Degener & E. Diehl (Eds.). *Handbuch Behindertenrechtskonvention. Teilhabe als Menschenrecht—Inklusion als gesellschaftliche Aufgabe* (55–74). Schriftenreihe, Band 1506. Bonn: Bundeszentrale für politische Bildung.

Elkins, Z., Ginsburg, T. & Simmons, B. (2013). Getting to rights: Treaty ratification, constitutional convergence, and human rights practice. *Harvard International Law Journal*, 54(1), 61–95.

Guarnizo, L. E. & Smith, M. P. (1998) The locations of transnationalism. In M. P. Smith & L. E. Guarnizo (Eds.). *Transnationalism from below* (3–34). Comparative Urban and Community Research, Ser., Vol. 6. New Brunswick, NJ: Transaction Books,.

Hafner-Burton, E. M. (2008). Sticks and stones: Naming and shaming the human rights enforcement problem. *International Organization*, 62(4), 689–716.

Hvinden, B. (2003). The uncertain convergence of disability policies in Western Europe. *Social Policy and Administration*, 37(6), 609–624.

Knill, C. (2005). Introduction: Cross-national policy convergence: Concepts, approaches and explanatory factors. *Journal of European Public Policy*, 12(5), 764–774.

Krasner, S. (1982). Structural causes and regime consequences: Regimes as intervening variables. *International Organization*, 36(2), 185–205.

Quinn, G. (2009). The United Nations Convention on the Rights of Persons with Disabilities: Toward a new international politics of disability. Jacobus tenBroek Disability Law Symposium, April 17, 2009. *Texas Journal on Civil Liberties and Civil Rights*, 15(1), 33–52.

Remennick, L. (2007). Transnationalism. In G. Ritzer (Ed.). *The Blackwell Encyclopedia of Sociology* (5072–5074). Malden, MA: Blackwell.

Scharle, Á., Váradi, B. & Samu, F. (2015). *Policy Convergence across Welfare Regimes: the Case of Disability Policies*. Budapest Institute, WWWforEurope project. Working Paper No. 76. Retrieved 11 January 2016 from: http://www.budapestinstitute.eu/uploads/WWWforEurope_WPS_no076_MS10.pdf

Schieder, S. (2013). Internationale Organisationen. In M. G. Schmidt, F. Wolf & S. Wurster (Eds.). *Studienbuch Politikwissenschaft* (439–464). Wiesbaden: Springer VS.

Soldatic, K. (2013). The transnational sphere of justice: Disability praxis and the politics of impairment. *Disability and Society*, 28(6), 744–755.

Tarrow, S. (1994). *Power in movement. social movements, collective action and politics*. Cambridge: Cambridge University Press.

United Nations (2016). Status of Convention on the Rights of Persons with Disabilities, Chapter IV: Human Rights. *United Nations Treaty Collection, Treaty Series, vol. 2515*. Retrieved 10 January 2016 from: https://treaties.un.org/pages/ViewDetails.aspx?src=TREATY&mtdsg_no=IV-15&chapter=4&clang=_en

United Nations Division for Social Policy and Development / Disability. (2006). *Convention on the Rights of Persons with Disabilities*. Retrieved 19 February 2017 from: https://www.un.org/development/desa/disabilities/convention-on-the-rights-of-persons-with-disabilities.html

Waldschmidt, A., Karačić, A., Sturm, A. & Dins, T. (2015). 'Nothing about us without us'—disability rights activism in European countries: A comparative analysis. *Moving the Social—Journal of Social History and the History of Social Movements*, 53, 103–137.

Ziring, L., Riggs, R. E. & Plano J. C. (2005). *The united nations: international organization and world politics*. Belmont, CA: Thomson Wadsworth.

12 The potential for, and barriers to, the exercise of Active EU Citizenship by persons with disabilities

The right to free movement

Lisa Waddington[1]

Introduction

The ability to exercise the right to free movement, meaning the right to travel to, enter, and reside in a Member State of the European Union (EU) other than the state of nationality, is essential for the exercise of Active (EU) Citizenship, and especially the autonomy aspect (see Chapter 1). If disabled EU citizens are not in a position to exercise this right, they are denied the possibility to become 'active' EU citizens, benefitting from the rights related to EU citizenship, as well as unable to contribute to the economies and societies of other Member States through their physical presence. In this respect, it is notable that a long-standing complaint of Disabled Peoples' Organisations (DPOs) is that disabled people are often unable to exercise the right of free movement in practice (EDF, 2011a).

This chapter will explore the possibilities for, and barriers to, the right of free movement experienced by persons with disabilities. The chapter will then proceed to examine proposals to reduce or eliminate the identified barriers, which have been put forward in DPO, academic, and European Commission reports and studies, before reaching some conclusions.

The right to free movement from a disability perspective[2]

In principle, all EU citizens have the right to free movement and to reside in a Member State other than the one of which they hold nationality. There are certainly no EU law restrictions or limitations on this right which explicitly refer to disability. However, EU law does allow Member States to deny EU citizens from other Member States the right to reside in their territory in a limited number of situations. These situations, which are exceptions to the right of free movement, are designed to allow Member States to 'protect' elements of their society, including the social welfare system, and to discourage 'welfare tourism'. As a consequence, in some situations individuals who do not have sufficient resources to support themselves, and who require financial support from the state of residence (host Member State), can be denied a right to reside, or have such a right rescinded. This can be particularly important for persons with disabilities, who are more likely than the general population to be both unemployed and in receipt of welfare benefits, and therefore run a greater risk of finding themselves in such a situation. In this respect, one can note that, according to the European Union Statistics on Income and Living Conditions (EU-SILC), 24.4 per cent of people with disabilities living in the European Union are at risk of or live in poverty (Commission, 2014b: 63). However, one should stress that having a low income, or being in receipt of social welfare or social assistance benefits, does not automatically render an individual illegible for benefitting from the right to free movement. This chapter will therefore examine the situations in which individuals can and cannot exercise the right to free movement.

Free movement for economic residents: Workers and their families

Article 45 of the Treaty on the Functioning of the European Union (TFEU) gives all EU citizens the right to live in the state of employment, and the right to be treated in the same way as nationals whilst working there. Therefore, anyone—disabled or not—who has the status of an EU worker is entitled to exercise the right of free movement. Self-employed persons and their family members acquire similar rights. The right to receive equal treatment as nationals is acquired as soon as an EU citizen obtains the status of a worker in the host Member State. According to cases decided by the Court of Justice of the EU, the status of worker can be acquired by EU citizens who are pursuing economic activities under the direction of an employer established in another Member State and who, in return for their activities, receive remuneration (*Lawrie-Blum* EU:C:1986:284). While this is a broad concept, in some instances disabled individuals may find it difficult to acquire the privileged status of worker. Individuals working a very limited number of hours, or earning only a very low income can be excluded from the status of EU worker (O'Brien, 2009). In addition, there is case law to suggest that individuals employed in sheltered or supported workshops may not qualify as EU workers, and so also do not acquire the right to free movement (*Bettray* EU:C:1989:226. But note *Fenoll* EU:C:2015:200).

The right to equal treatment for workers is secured in Article 45(2) TFEU and worked out in further detail in Regulation No. 492/2011 and Regulation No. 883/2004, as amended by Regulation No. 465/2012. Under Regulation No. 492/2011, equality of treatment is not only granted as regards work-related matters, such as pay, laws on dismissal and conditions of work, but also as regards training, public housing, taxation, access to 'social advantages', as well as to all rights or benefits that are essential to the worker's 'well-being' and which can be regarded as related to the right to freedom of movement (*Commission v France* EU:C:1996:90). Equal access to 'social advantages', which is provided for in Article 7(2) of Regulation No. 492/2011, is particularly important in terms of access to disability-related benefits. The Court of Justice of the EU has interpreted the concept of 'social advantages' to cover all rights or benefits which are granted to workers 'primarily because of their objective status as workers or by virtue of the mere fact of their residence on the national territory' and which may encourage the free movement of workers within the Union (*Even* EU:C:1979:144; *Hoeckx* EU:C:1985:139).

It is worth noting that workers are entitled to be joined by their immediate family when they move to a new Member State. In order to promote the integration of the worker's family into the host State, Article 10 of Regulation No. 492/2011 confers upon the children of EU workers the right to attend school or other educational institutions under the same conditions as the nationals of the state. In addition, the dependent family members can rely on Article 7(2) in order to claim equality of treatment as regards all 'social advantages' (*Lebon* EU:C:1987:302 decided under the previously applicable Regulation).

In summary, disabled individuals who are able to acquire the status of EU worker, and disabled family members of EU workers, are able to exercise the right to free movement, and acquire the entitlement to claim all disability-related benefits on the same basis as nationals from the moment that they take up residence. Claiming such benefits cannot jeopardise their right to reside in the host Member State. However, the failure to recognise as EU workers individuals who earn a very low income, individuals who work a very limited number of hours, or individuals who are 'employed' within sheltered or supported employment, can mean that some persons with disabilities find it more difficult than non-disabled persons to acquire the status of EU worker.

Free movement for non-economic residents: Students, retired people, people with a private income

The second category of beneficiaries of the free movement of persons consists of 'non-economic residents'. This category contains students, pensioners and the residual category of all 'other' EU citizens whose right to reside is governed by Directive 2004/38. Individuals falling into this category have a number of conditions attached to their residency, which do not apply to workers and their families. For the first five years of their residence, 'non-economic residents' are required 'not to become a burden on the social assistance system of the host Member State … and have comprehensive sickness insurance cover in the host Member State' (Directive 2004/38 Art. 7(1)(b)). The claiming of a disability-related benefit, which leads to an individual becoming a 'burden on the social assistance system' of the host State, gives that State the right to revoke the permission to reside on its territory.

Nevertheless, it is clear that lawfully resident EU citizens are sometimes still entitled to claim such a benefit, even during their first five years of residence in another Member State. Non-economic residents can claim equality of treatment in the host State under Articles 18 and 21 TFEU. Article 18 TFEU prohibits all discrimination on grounds of nationality in fields covered by the Treaty, while Article 21 TFEU gives EU citizens the right to move and reside freely within the territory of the Member States. In the case of *Martínez Sala*, the Court of Justice indicated that all rights and benefits covered by Regulation No. 1612/68 (as well as Regulation 492/2011 and Regulation 883/2004) fell within the scope of Community law and that all EC nationals lawfully residing in the territory of another Member State could rely on Article 18 TFEU in order to claim such rights and benefits (*Martínez Sala* EU:C:1998:217 para. 57–61).

However, the scope of the right to equal treatment of non-economic residents is not as strongly protected as the right to equal treatment of workers. Indeed, several Member States have taken the position that, during the initial five years of residence, the complete equal treatment right is not owed to non-economically active residents, and that this is only acquired with a right to permanent residence (see O'Brien, 2009: 1107, 1110; Widmann, n.d.). This approach has been confirmed to some degree in *Förster*, in which the Court of Justice found that a five-year residence requirement for access to a student maintenance grant in the Netherlands was justified, appropriate and not excessive (*Jaqueline Förster v Hoofddirectie van de informative Beheer Groep* EU:C:2008:630). The residence requirement was regarded as a legitimate means of ensuring that recipients were sufficiently integrated into Dutch society.

Moreover, as noted above, students, pensioners and the 'other' EU citizens who wish to claim equal treatment as regards, for example, social assistance benefits may become a burden on the host State and this entitles the host State to end legal residence, and therefore entitlement to the benefits. Nevertheless, claiming a disability-related benefit does not automatically lead to loss of residence (see *Trojani* EU:C:2004:488 para. 45). Moreover, once an individual has resided lawfully on the territory of a Member State for five years, they can acquire an unlimited right of residence under Directive 2004/38, which brings with it a right to claim social assistance if necessary. Such a claim will not jeopardise the right to reside.

In brief, disabled individuals who are not EU workers or family members of EU workers can exercise the right of free movement if they have sufficient resources to support themselves and are covered by health insurance in their State of residence. Such individuals must not become 'a burden on the social assistance system of the host Member State' during their first five years of residence. Nevertheless, there does seem to be some scope for claiming some disability-related benefits during this initial period of residence, and claiming benefits does not automatically lead to a rescinding of the right to reside, but may merely give the host State the right to take this action. However, it is clear that individuals who are unable to support themselves from the moment they arrive in the host Member State, and who seek immediate financial support, can be denied both the assistance sought and the right to reside, and are therefore excluded from the possibility of exercising Active EU Citizenship through free movement.

Acquiring sufficient financial resources to exercise the right of free movement through the export of a disability-related benefit

It is clear that having sufficient resources to support oneself, and one's family, is a key requirement for individuals who wish to exercise the right of free movement and who are non-economic residents. The possibility to export a disability-related benefit from the Member State of origin to the host Member State may enable an individual to meet the necessary income requirements, and avoid becoming a 'burden' on the social assistance system of the host Member State, and thereby to exercise the right to free movement. EU law addresses the right to export social security and social assistance benefits, and requires this in certain situations. Nevertheless, it has always been clear that it is up to the Member States to organise, administer and finance their own social security schemes (*Terhoeve* EU:C:1999:22; *Sodemare* EU:C:1997:301). Neither the establishment of a common social security system nor the harmonisation of national social security systems has been seriously considered by the Member States. As noted in Chapter 2 of this volume, EU Member States reflect a variety of different welfare state models and consequently approaches to social security differ considerably. Nevertheless, it has always been recognised that the existence of various national social security systems could encourage or deter people from moving from one State to another. The move might lead to a loss of social security rights acquired in the Member State of origin and individuals might not be eligible for benefits in the new State on the grounds that they have not worked, been insured or been in residence for long enough. For this reason, EU law has been adopted to coordinate the application of social security schemes with regard to individuals who exercise the right of free movement. The relevant laws provide the exportability by individuals of certain listed social security benefits, including disability or invalidity pensions and sickness benefits, from one Member State, where entitlement to the benefit was originally acquired, to another Member State where the individual resides. The main legal rules were laid down initially in Regulations No. 1408/71 and No. 574/72. The former Regulation set out the rights that migrants enjoy, while the latter Regulation contained the administrative rules for implementing these rights. As of 1 May 2010 these Regulations were repealed and replaced by Regulations Nos. 883/2004 and 987/2009. However, the main principles found in Regulation No. 1408/71 continue to be reflected in the new Regulation No. 883/2004, and case law decided under Regulation No. 1408/71 continues to be relevant in order to understand the new Regulation.

These Regulations aim to coordinate Member State action with regard to *social security schemes* only. Currently, Regulation 883/2004 provides for EU coordination of social security systems and aims to ensure that people who are insured under the social security system of one Member State do not lose their rights when moving to another Member State. However, the Regulation does not address *social assistance benefits*, meaning that disability-related benefits which amount to social assistance benefits fall outside the scope of the Regulations and cannot be exported under EU law. The Court has defined a social security benefit as a benefit granted without any individual and discretionary assessment of personal needs, to recipients on the basis of a legally defined position, concerning one of the risks listed in the Regulation (*Gérald De Cuyper* v. *Office national de l'employ* EU:C:2006:491; see also Paskalia, 2009: 1177, 1186). This definition of social security benefits may imply that an increased personalisation of benefits—in terms of the benefits being tailored to meet the needs of a specific individual—may lead to those benefits not being regarded as exportable under EU law.

However, as case law of the Court of Justice reveals, on occasions it is difficult to establish if a particular benefit is a social security benefit (exportable) or a social assistance benefit (not exportable). Moreover, a third category of benefits also exists, namely 'special non-contributory cash benefits'. These also fall within the scope of the Regulation, although they are not exportable. However, EU citizens resident in another Member State are entitled to claim such benefits, although the requirement under Directive 2004/38 that individuals should not become a 'burden on the social assistance system' of the host State during their first five years of residence remains.

With regard to exportability of social security benefits, Article 7 of Regulation No. 883/2004 provides:

> Unless otherwise provided for in this Regulation, cash benefits payable under the legislation of one or more Member States or under this Regulation shall not be subject to any reduction, amendment, suspension, withdrawal or confiscation on account of the fact that the beneficiary or the members of his family reside in a Member State other than that in which the institutions responsible for providing benefits is situated.

This 'exportability' rule applies only to cash benefits. Benefits in kind, such as entitlement to receive a certain number of hours of care or assistance from care staff employed by, or contracted to, a local authority are clearly far more difficult to export in most cases, since this would require that the local authority care staff themselves were available in the other Member State. It may be easier to export benefits in the form of specialised equipment, although the transport of the equipment may also pose challenges. In any case, the Regulation does not cover such equipment, as it is a benefit in kind. Regulation No. 883/2004 applies to citizens who are, or have been, subject to the social security legislation of one or more Member States, as well as their families and survivors. This covers workers, but also many 'non-economic' residents (e.g. retired people), and non-residents, such as people travelling to another Member State to look for work. In essence, the key question is whether an individual is insured under the social security scheme of one or more Member States, or is otherwise subject to the social security legislation of one or more Member States, and, if so, whether the benefit they are seeking to claim is regarded as a social security benefit for the purposes of Regulation No. 883/2004.

According to Article 3 of Regulation No. 883/2004 the principle of the 'exportability' of benefits applies to sickness and maternity benefits, invalidity benefits, old age benefits, survivors' benefits, benefits in respect of accidents at work and occupational diseases, death grants, unemployment benefits and family benefits. Article 3(5) of the Regulation excludes 'social and medical assistance' from the scope of application. Long-term care benefits, such as the provision of personal assistance, are not addressed explicitly in the Regulation, but the Court of Justice has allowed the exportability of some such benefits by classifying them as sickness benefits, even though they do not always sit easily within that classification.

In determining whether benefits are exportable, a distinction has to be made between cash benefits and benefits in kind, which as noted above are not exportable under EU law. The distinction is not always easy to make, as evidenced by the *Molenaar* case (*Molenaar* EU:C:1998:84). The case concerned the German Care Insurance Law (*Pflegeversicherungsgesetz*) which was introduced to cover the costs of persons who, in their daily routine, require assistance from other persons. The benefit is designed to provide the assistance or care needed by the individual. The benefits provided under the law could be provided, at the choice of the recipient, either in the form of care or assistance dispensed by authorised bodies or in the form of a monthly allowance (*Pflegegeld*), which enabled recipients to choose the form of aid they considered most appropriate to their condition. The German Government argued that the care allowance was aimed at allowing recipients to cover the cost of medical expenses and that it was a 'surrogate' or substitute for benefits in kind, and therefore not exportable. The Court of Justice, however, did not agree. According to the Court, the care allowance took the form of 'financial aid which enabled the standard of living of persons requiring care to be improved as a whole, to compensate for the additional expense brought about by their condition'. The *Pflegegeld* was thus to be regarded as an exportable cash benefit.

In contrast, a system that only provided for a benefit in kind—for example, entitlement to a number of hours of personal care—would not be exportable. This can present a significant barrier to the exercise of free movement for disabled individuals who require personal assistance. They cannot export the benefit if it is in kind, and if they cannot acquire the status of EU worker or family member of a worker, they can also not claim such a benefit in the host Member State on arrival and, indeed, some Member States do not offer such benefits at all.

Secondly, as noted above, social assistance benefits are also not exportable under EU law. The barriers to free movement that this can lead to are revealed by the case of *Newton* (*Newton* EU:C:1991:265). This case concerned a British man who worked as a self-employed person in France. Following a car accident that left him paralysed, he returned to the United Kingdom where he had never worked or contributed to the social security system. Here he was granted a mobility allowance, a minimum income benefit granted on the basis that the recipient was 'ordinarily present' on the territory of the United Kingdom. When Mr Newton decided to move back to France, the British authorities withdrew the mobility allowance. Before the Court Mr Newtown claimed that Regulation 1408/71 covered the mobility allowance. However, the Court accepted the argument that Mr Newton could not export his allowance because this would make it possible for other persons who had never worked and lived in a Member State to nevertheless claim certain 'mixed' benefits from that state. The Court found that Regulation No. 1408/71 did not cover the benefit, that is, the mobility allowance was a social assistance benefit and not a social security benefit and could not be 'exported'.

EU legislation also provides that 'special non-contributory cash benefits' are, like social assistance benefits, not exportable. However, these benefits can be claimed by EU citizens resident in another Member State. These are benefits paid to a specific category of persons, such as persons with a (particular) disability, and which are not based on a record of prior contributions. These 'special non-contributory cash benefits' are listed on a country-by-country basis in Annex X to Regulation No. 883/2004, and include a number of disability-related allowances (examples include the Estonian disabled adult allowance and the Irish disability allowance and mobility allowance). In addition to disability benefits, the two other categories of benefits classified as special non-contributory benefits relate to old age and unemployment. In spite of being listed within this annex, the Court of Justice has been willing to reject the classification of certain disability-related benefits as 'special non-contributory cash benefits', and to hold that they are in fact exportable social security sickness benefits in some cases (e.g. *Silvia Hosse* v. *Land Salzburg*, EU:C:2006:125).

In short, an individual who is entitled to a (disability-related) social security benefit that is paid in cash is entitled to export that benefit to another Member State. This may mean that the individual has sufficient means to support him- or herself in another Member State, and is therefore able to satisfy the conditions to exercise the right of free movement. Benefits in kind, such as the provision of a number of hours of personal assistance, and social assistance benefits and 'special non-contributory cash benefits' are not exportable, and can only be claimed in the state of residence. Relocating to another Member State can therefore imply a significant and unsustainable loss of support, meaning that, in fact, an individual is unable to become an active EU citizen by exercising the right to free movement.

Non-residents or travellers: Tourists, patients and business people

The third category of beneficiaries of the free movement of persons consists of 'non-residents' or EU travellers. This category contains EU citizens who merely visit other States for business or pleasure, and who do not establish residence in those States.

Under Articles 56 and 57 TFEU, EU citizens enjoy the right to provide and receive services under the same conditions as nationals of the State they visit. The concept of services only covers those services that are (mainly) provided out of private funds; (social) services provided by the State, and which are mainly funded out of the public purse, fall outside the scope of the two mentioned articles (e.g. medical care and rehabilitation or training provided by the State) (*Humbel and Edel* EU:C:1988:451; *Wirth* EU:C:1993:916). In order to claim such benefits EU citizens can rely on Article 18 TFEU which, as follows from the *Martínez Sala* case, applies to virtually all benefits. This is not to say that the legal status of travellers is as strongly protected as the status of residents. Eligibility for many social benefits can be made conditional upon residence in the host State's territory. Residence requirements mainly work to the detriment of non-nationals, and may thus constitute indirect discrimination on grounds of nationality. Nevertheless, such requirements can still be justified under EU law where they are based on objective considerations independent of the nationality of the persons concerned, and are proportionate to the legitimate aim of the national provisions.

In addition, practical problems may hamper the free movement of persons with disabilities who wish to visit another Member State. Many public and private institutions, such as museums, sports facilities and public transport, provide discounts or free admission to persons with disabilities who are able to present a nationally issued disability identity card. Such benefits may not readily be available to persons with disabilities from other Member States, who do not possess a disability identity card of the state in question.

Proposals for reform

The issue of the free movement rights of persons with disabilities, and of non-economic migrants who require public support, has not gone unnoticed or unexplored amongst Disabled Persons Organisations (DPOs), academics or the European Commission. This part of the chapter will look at the findings of various DPO papers, academic and European Commission reports on this topic, and seek to identify the proposals for reform they have brought forward. It is notable that almost all these proposals are found in reports and studies financed by the European Commission.

In line with the previous section of the chapter, the analysis will focus on the three prospective groups of 'free movers': disabled workers and disabled family members; non-economic disabled migrants, and in particular those who require support from the public authorities; and disabled travellers and visitors.

Free movement for economic residents: Workers and their families

O'Brien (2009) is highly critical of the Court's approach and case law regarding the classification of individuals as EU workers or non-economically active migrants. Amongst her many criticisms are that 'the application of the same "genuine and effective" test to all workers, combined with the "normal labour market" criterion is disability-blind, as there is no recognition that what is "genuine and effective" economic activity may differ between groups of people. The characteristics favoured by the case law indicate a distinctly able-bodied model of work' (O'Brien, 2009: 1107–1108). O'Brien argues that the Court's interpretation of the concept of 'worker' has not taken account of the EU's social objectives, including equality and non-discrimination, and that, in some circumstances, it is harder for disabled people, and people who (temporarily) give up work to care (for disabled people), to acquire or retain the status of 'worker' and related rights.

O'Brien notes that those providing informal care might be in a comparable position to workers when the requisite elements of a work relationship exist. Nevertheless, the Court of Justice has thus far not recognised such individuals as workers (see *Züchner v Handelskrankenkasses (Ersatzkasse) Bremen* EU:C:1996:425; Joined Cases *Gaumain-Cerri and Barth* EU:C:2004:413). She also notes that, while workers who are 'temporarily unable to work as a result of an illness or accident' retain the status of worker under Art. 7(3)(a) of Directive 2004/38/EC, individuals who have to give up work temporarily in order to care for a sick or disabled family member lose their status as worker. This seems to go counter to developments at EU level to develop family-friendly employment policies and legislative initiatives, such as the Parental Leave Directive (Council Directive 2010/18/EU). Moreover, many Member States in fact recognise care as a legitimate 'bridge' between work periods. O'Brien argues 'the exclusion of temporary caring periods from the list of continuing worker status also conflicts with the developing disability equality duty owed to workers "by association"' (*Coleman* EU:C:2008:415) (O'Brien, 2009: 1121–1122). This is because the Court does not interpret 'on the grounds of illness' in the context of free movement and worker status, as covering another person's illness or disability. Moreover, this indirectly has an adverse effect on women.

O'Brien also contends that the Court's economic-worker definition has failed to take account of developing free movement provisions which are socially sensitive, so there is a discord with both the general principle of equal treatment and EU social and employment policies (such as 'flexicurity', occupational mobility, the labour market integration of carers and people with disabilities). The solution proposed by O'Brien is a policy of integrated interpretation, that is, EU social policies, and equal treatment in particular, should be incorporated into the construction of migrant work. O'Brien concludes:

> An equal treatment duty read into the definition of migrant work would enforce the fundamental rights of non-discrimination on the grounds of sex, or of disability (including by association), so as to permit consideration of the extension of 'temporary illness' to temporary care duties and temporary illness of another, recognizing the comparability of those scenarios.
>
> Member States could still retain the language of 'genuine and effective', but be required to have due regard to equal treatment and recognise that genuine and effective for one group of people may represent something different for another group. … A disability sensitive notion of genuine and effective work would dispense with the notion of the 'normal labour market.'
>
> (O'Brien, 2009: 1139)

In essence O'Brien is arguing that the current concept of migrant worker, as developed through case law of the Court of Justice (e.g. the *Bettray* judgement), indirectly discriminates against disabled people and carers of disabled people. Her solution to this is the development of a more socially sensitive definition of migrant worker by the Court, meaning that she views the solution in the development of new case law. Such case law would liberalise or expand the notion of an EU worker, thereby opening the door to free movement to a wider group of individuals, including particularly individuals with a disability. However, it is unclear to what extent EU legislation could be interpreted in this manner. Also, non-economic migrants with a disability, such as students and persons not active in the labour market, would not benefit from such a move.

Free movement for non-economic residents: Students, retired people, people with a private income, and the right to claim disability-related benefits in the host Member State

The ability to claim disability-related benefits in the host State can be particularly important for non-economic residents who wish to exercise the right of free movement. Access to such benefits can provide an income that allows the individuals to support themselves when they move to another Member State. The ANED report, Disability Benefits and Entitlements in European Countries: Mutual Recognition and Exportability of Benefits, examines both the scope for claiming disability-related benefits in a host Member State and the possibility for exporting such benefits from the Member State of insurance (competent Member State). The report concludes with a number of recommendations 'to promote and encourage greater freedom of movement for disabled persons through mutual recognition of entitlement to disability-related benefits and through the exportability of benefits' (Waddington, 2010: 11).

The ANED report identifies the lack of information regarding comparable disability status as one barrier to free movement. Individuals may have been assessed and officially recognised as disabled in one Member State, and this recognition may give them access to a variety of benefits in that State, possibly including exportable benefits. However, when moving to another Member State, their disability status is not recognised, and this hampers their access to benefits (which may not be financial) in the host Member State. The original official recognition of disability may serve as a 'passport' to other benefits, for example, a disability identity card which itself gives benefits, as well as giving entitlement to reduced fees for public transport or other services. If this is not also recognised in the host Member State, it can lead to a delay in receiving such benefits in that State, and the need for another time-consuming assessment of disability. The ANED report found that: 'it would be helpful to identify which disability benefits serve as a "passport" to other benefits in each Member State, and the eligibility criteria, such as degree of impairment/disability, for the original "passport" benefit. This would enhance comparability, and help national officials to decide if a disability status recognised by another Member State is comparable to the nationally recognised disability status, which serves as a "passport" allowing access to other benefits' (Waddington, 2010: 133). The report proposes that that the 'EU could play an important role in establishing a central European inventory of recognised national disability benefits, that could be cross-checked by national administrations to recognise certain kinds of passport benefits as valid without further assessment (Waddington, 2010: 133). The ANED report also identifies two possible reforms:

> One option would be to extend the right to temporarily export all disability-related benefits in the case of individuals who are exercising the right of free movement. This extension would need to cover all benefits which are essential to (independent) living of disabled people, and would need to cover a sufficient period of time so as to allow the host Member State to assess the eligibility of an individual for a comparable benefit.
>
> A second option would be allow individuals to apply for the relevant disability-related benefits in the host Member State prior to taking up residence in that State. The application should be considered on the basis of the facts that will exist once the individual takes up residence, e.g. considering their status

> of worker or family member of a worker, status as non-economic resident, expected place of residence, expected income level etc.
>
> (Waddington, 2010: 136)

A number of other reports have focused on the ability of non-economic migrants to claim special non-contributory benefits in the host Member State. This group of benefits include many disability-specific benefits. A report prepared by ICF GHK and Milieu Ltd on behalf of the European Commission analysed the impact on social security systems of paying non-active EU migrants special non-contributory benefits (ICF GHK, 2013). Amongst the key findings of the study were that non-active EU migrants represent a very small share of the total population of each Member State, accounting for between 0.7 and 1.0 per cent of the overall EU population. Persons who cannot work due to a permanent disability also make up a very small percentage of migrants (3 per cent of overall total). However, in some countries, persons with disabilities made up a notably higher share of non-active EU migrants aged above 15 (Sweden: 15 per cent; the Netherlands: 15 per cent; Belgium: 9 per cent; Denmark: 9 per cent). The study found little evidence to suggest that the main reason for moving to another Member State was related to claiming benefits. The main motivations identified were work and family-related reasons. Indeed, in most countries covered in the study, migrants were less likely than nationals to receive disability or unemployment benefits.

A second report, by the AIRE Centre, addressed the issue of special non-contributory benefits (SNCBs) and EU migrants (Widmann, n.d.). The report was part of a European Commission funded project to improve access and awareness of special non-contributory benefits by EU migrants in the United Kingdom, Ireland and the Netherlands. As noted above, special non-contributory benefits are not exportable under EU law. The report states that such benefits

> lie at the intersection of social security benefits and social assistance, providing vulnerable and low-income individuals who face social security risks, and the disabled, a minimum subsistence income, with a condition of contribution by the beneficiary. By offering a means to meet basic needs, SNCBs are a vital source of income for such persons.
>
> (Widmann, n.d.: 4)

The report recognises that special non-contributory benefits raise ‘complex legal issues’ and it is therefore ‘essential that clear information be available regarding the rules that govern SNCBs and their access by EU citizens, and that the EU rights of citizens are enforced’ (Widmann, n.d.: 4). Both within the United Kingdom and Ireland barriers involved ‘the imposition of right to reside requirements that do not adhere with EU law and a lack of understanding on the part of EU migrants, their representatives, local authorities and judicial decision-makers of rights to access SNCB’ (Widmann, n.d.: 4). This has generated a large amount of case law, and the report concludes that the test is difficult to understand and apply. The report also notes that EU migrants can pass the right-to-reside test by seeking work and becoming economically active: however, 'those who cannot may be blocked out of the system altogether' (Widmann, n.d.: 51). Disabled people whose impairment prevents them from working are more likely than others to fall into this category than others. Both the British and Irish systems, in line with Regulation 883/04, assume that an individual can only be resident, for the purpose of claiming a special non-contributory benefit, in a single Member State. Problems related to access to benefits resulted from treating special non-contributory benefits as social assistance benefits, which means that access for non-economic migrants could legitimately be restricted in some cases, and also from the failure to recognise carers in receipt of a Carer's Allowance as workers or self-employed people.

Amongst the recommendations aimed at Member States are adopting measures to promote transparency, including publishing data on nationality and residence in relation to all benefits applications, and maintaining a publicly available database of relevant judicial and quasi-judicial decisions. A further recommendation is that Member States should coordinate when assessing habitual residence for the purpose of claiming special non-contributory benefits. Where a Member State determines that another State is the habitual place of residence of a claimant, the Member State should be required to notify the other Member State to determine between them which is responsible for the payment of any benefits. Member States should also provide interim payments of special non-contributory benefits to claimants during disputes regarding residence, to guarantee the right to an effective remedy.

In terms of the EU, the report recommends that the EU institutions should clarify eligibility for special non-contributory benefits by EU migrants and their family members, including through publishing available and easily accessible guidance from the Commission and through judgments of the Court of Justice of the EU on the law relating to special non-contributory benefits and access requirements. In addition, the institutions should clarify the distinction between purely social assistance and special non-contributory benefits in the context of consolidated benefit regimes, and should increasingly focus on the situation of marginalised EU citizens, including the inclusion of persons in need of special non-contributory benefits.

Acquiring sufficient financial resources to exercise the right of free movement through the export of a disability-related benefit

The EDF Freedom Guide pays particular attention to the exportability of disability-related benefits. The Guide states '[e]specially important, is the need for Member States to allow for the portability of disability benefits and to enhance cooperation in relation to social security policies. Moreover, unless persons who need a personal assistant, sign language interpreter or support person can mobilise support when travelling abroad, freedom of movement remains an illusion for those that make use of this support' (EDF, 2011a: 12).

The Guide calls on the Member States 'to cooperate more and better in relation to policy harmonisation' as well as in 'the exchange of best practices' (EDF, 2011a: 66). However, it is not clear if this comment is related to the specific issue of the exportability of benefits, or is more general. At this point it is important to recall that the EU has the competence only to promote the coordination of social security policies, and the intention is not to replace the divergent national social security regimes with a common EU system (harmonisation). Instead the objectives are more limited, and aim to protect the social security rights of EU citizens when moving from one Member State to another.

Two 'Training and reporting on European social security' (trEES) reports focus on long-term care benefits, which include benefits in cash or kind relating to care or personal assistance. The 2011 report begins by proposing a general European definition of long-term care benefits. This would facilitate coordination and enhance clarity. The report argues that such a common approach is necessary because the various national long-term care benefits are currently classified in different ways, including as sickness benefits, invalidity benefits, family benefits or special non-contributory benefits, and, for the purposes of this chapter, such classifications impact on the exportability of the benefit. The report proposes the following definition:

> Long-term care benefits means benefits for persons who, over an extended period of time, on account of old-age, disease or incapacity, and linked to lack or loss of physical, mental, intellectual or sensorial autonomy, require assistance from (an)other person(s) or considerable help to carry out essential daily activities.
>
> (Jorens & Spiegel, 2011: 14)

The 2011 report then goes on to identify the problems or challenges related to the coordination of long-term care benefits. Amongst the challenges identified is the lack of a common understanding amongst the Member States as to how to classify such benefits. Benefits related to old age, invalidity, survivors, work accidents and occupational diseases, family protection, sickness and social assistance can all contain elements of long-term care, which makes coordination at EU level difficult (Jorens & Spiegel, 2011: 22–23). In this diversity amongst Member States, further challenges concern the fact that such benefits can be classified as social security (exportable) or social assistance (not exportable), and provided in cash (potentially exportable) or in kind (not exportable). The report argues that while regarding long-term care benefits as a form of sickness benefits has been a positive way to include them within the material scope of EU Regulation No. 883/2004 to date, and therefore render them exportable, this is not an ideal solution, as the aims, instruments and means of sickness benefits and long-term care benefits differ.

The final part of the 2011 trESS report looks at options for reform. The report notes that the position of the person in need of care must be taken into account and any solution should not promote 'long-term care benefit tourism', meaning that it should not encourage people to relocate to another Member State primarily in order to receive such benefits, when they do not have a sufficient link with the Member State concerned. The authors of the report therefore recognise the need for a link between any claimant and the providing State. The solution should be transparent and easy to understand, and should achieve a fair balance between Member States (Jorens & Spiegel, 2011: 43–44).

Lastly, the report proposes three 'options for a fundamental change'. The first option is that the State of residence is always competent, i.e. obliged to provide benefits in cash or kind. This would benefit persons who move to a Member State which provides (generous) long-term care benefits, but persons moving from a State which has such benefits to a State which has no such benefits would lose out (Jorens & Spiegel, 2011: 52–57). The second option is that the first Member State which recognises long-term care benefits would always remain competent (i.e. obliged) to grant these benefits. The advantage of this approach for benefit recipients is that there would be a single competent State, and security would be provided as entitlement would be maintained regardless of the state of residence. However, a number of disadvantages were noted, including that the need for care can often evolve, and this may lead to an excessive burden on the State paying the benefits, or alternatively lead to uncertainty if the need for care ceased, and then developed again at a later point. The last 'option for a fundamental change' identified by the report is to treat long-term care benefits as invalidity benefits and coordinate them under the pension chapter of Regulation No. 883/2004. The authors argue that this would have the advantage that entitlement cannot be lost once a person has been covered for more than 12 months under the legislation of a Member State. Amongst the disadvantages noted were the risk of overcompensation and that this rule could only apply to benefits in cash, not benefits in kind. Further regulation would be needed to address various matters if this approach was followed.

Whilst the trESS authors explored these options briefly in the 2011 report, a second 2012 report set out possible solutions in more detail. This report proposes twenty options for reform. Some of these are freestanding, although in most cases a number of the options, such as developing a new definition of long-term care benefits and adding a list of long-term care benefits to the Regulation, can usefully be combined with various other options to create a more complete package. The report authors favour developing a single chapter for long-term care benefits in the relevant EU Regulation (Regulation No. 883/2004). This should provide for rules against overlapping (i.e. being entitled to receive more than one long-term care benefit based on different legislative schemes) and eliminate existing gaps and lack of protection (Jorens & Spiegel, 2012: 6).

In general, the options explored revolve around the identification of the competent Member State responsible for paying the benefit, the possibility of one State reimbursing another for the cost of any benefits paid, and the possibility that a recipient be paid a supplement to top up their long-term care benefit by a second Member State. Individuals will find themselves in different positions, both in terms of their original Member State of insurance and the Member State to which they relocate, and the wide variety of schemes and benefits related to long-term care provided within the EU. Therefore, it would be necessary to do a case-by-case analysis of the situation of each individual to determine whether any particular option, or set of options, would advantage or disadvantage any individual. However, in general one can say that individuals are most likely to be in an advantageous position if they can export a long-term care benefit paid in cash from their State of origin (competent State). Alternatively, if they do not have access to such a benefit, they may still be entitled to claim a long-term care benefit in cash or in kind in the State of residence. This implies that the benefit would have to be already provided for in the Member State of residence, and that the claimant otherwise qualifies for this benefit.

The recipient would be in an even more advantageous position if they could obtain a supplement to their basic long-term care benefit paid by the State of residence from another Member State (e.g. the competent Member State or another Member State where they have voluntary insurance), in cases where their basic benefit is lower in value than that which they would have been entitled to if they continued to reside in the competent Member State. Provisions relating to the coordination of benefits paid directly to carers would also enhance the ability to exercise the right to free movement, both of persons with disabilities and those in receipt of carer's benefits. However, in principle the broader EU rules on social security and social assistance would continue to apply, meaning that non-economic residents could be barred from exercising the right of free movement if they became a 'burden on the social assistance system of the host Member State' within the first five years of residence. If the competent Member State (where the claimant is insured) was responsible for reimbursing the Member State of residence for the cost of any benefit, this would reduce the likelihood of this situation occurring. The report submits that any EU coordination system should ensure that any benefits which would be granted in the absence of a cross-border situation should continue to be received (or the equivalent thereof) in the event that a person exercises the right to free movement, and that a person is not left without any entitlement (Jorens & Spiegel, 2012: 13).

Non-residents or travellers: Tourists, patients and business people

The EDF Freedom Guide proposes the adoption of a European Mobility Card to enhance the access of persons with disabilities to disability-related benefits whilst visiting another Member State. Furthermore EDF has produced a specific proposal for a European Mobility Card and an analysis report, based on responses to a questionnaire sent out to EDF members (EDF, 2011b, 2012). The aforementioned ANED report also identified barriers to free movement associated with the lack of a common EU-wide disabled person's identity card, and argued that the existing EU parking card for persons with a disability could serve as a model for issuing a more generic disabled person's card (Waddington, 2010: 140).

The Commission has taken up this call by providing funding through the 2014 work programme for the implementation of the Rights, Equality and Citizenship Programme to support the launch and start-up phase of the 'InclEUsive card'. The stated objective of this card is to facilitate cross-border travelling in the EU of persons with disabilities, and it aims to meet the needs identified in the EDF reports and Freedom Guide. The long-term aim is that the card system will function independently of the Commission, and without EU funding.

Conclusion

Active EU citizenship of people with disabilities requires that disabled people are able to exercise the right of free movement and to experience the minimum of barriers when doing so. This chapter has shown that such barriers do exist. They range from uncertainty regarding the entitlement to be recognised as EU workers in some circumstances, to difficulties in acquiring—through the exportability of disability-related benefits or the right to claim equivalent benefits in the host Member State—sufficient funding to avoid becoming a 'burden on the social assistance system of the host Member State'. Other barriers relate to difficulties experienced in establishing disability status in the Member State that the person visits. These barriers are not unrecognised or new. Indeed, a large number of Commission funded reports demonstrate the awareness of the EU institutions of some of these problems in the context of non-economic migrants, including people with disabilities. The novelty of this chapter is that it brings together key conclusions and findings from a number of sources and reflects on how one can address some of the issues identified in the context of disability. In this way, the chapter highlights the relevance of this area of research for Active EU Citizenship, and in particular the free movement and autonomy of disabled EU citizens.

Notes

1 This paper was completed in the summer of 2014 and does not include information, developments or sources that became available after that date. The author is grateful to Jerome Bickenbach for commenting on a previous version of this paper and Elin Borjedal for assisting in adapting the paper to the relevant style sheet. This is a shortened and edited version of a longer paper with the same title which can be found at: https://blogg.hioa.no/discit/publications. (accessed 29 July 2016).

2 Parts of this section are based on Waddington, 2010. See also Waddington & van der Mei, 1999.

References

Commission (2014a). Annex 1 to the Commission Implementing Decision concerning the adoption of the work programme for 2014 and the financing for the implementation of the Rights, Equality and Citizenship Programme, Brussels, 24.4.2014, C(2014) 2557 final, 27–28.

Commission (2014b). Commission Staff Working Document: Report on the implementation of the UN Convention on the Rights of Persons with Disabilities (CRPD) by the European Union, Brussels, 5.6.2014 SWD(2014) 182 final.

European Disability Forum (EDF) (2011a). *Freedom Guide: Paving the Way towards Free Movement for Persons with Disabilities*. Brussels: European Disability Forum. Retrieved 14 February 2017 from http://www.edf-feph.org/sites/default/files/freedom_guide.pdf

European Disability Forum (2011b). *Proposal for a European Mobility Card*. Brussels: European Disability Forum. Retrieved 14 February 2017 from http://www.edf-feph.org/freedom-movement

European Disability Forum (2012). *Analysis Report. Towards a European Mobility Card*. Brussels: European Disability Forum. Retrieved 14 February 2017 from http://www.edf-feph.org/freedom-movement

Jorens, Y. & Spiegel, B. (Eds.) (2011). trESS think tank report of 2011 on coordination of long-term care benefits – current situation and future benefits. Retrieved 4 January 2014 from: http://www.tress-network.org/

Jorens, Y. & Spiegel, B. (Eds.) (2012). Analytical study: Legal impact assessment for the revision of regulation 883/2004 with regard to the coordination of long-term care benefits, Project DG EMPL/B/4-VC/2011/1078. *Training and Reporting on European Social Security (trESS)*. Retrieved 14 February 2017 from http://www.tress-network.org/EUROPEAN%20RESOURCES/EUROPEANREPORT/trESS_Analytical%20Study%202012.pdf

ICF GHK (2013). A fact-finding analysis on the impact on the Member States' social security systems of the entitlements of non-active intra-EU migrants to special non-contributory cash benefits and healthcare granted on the basis of residence. ICF GHK in association with Milieu Ltd, DG Employment, Social Affairs and Inclusion via DG Justice Framework Contract. Available via: http://bookshop.europa.eu/en/a-fact-finding-analysis-on-the-impact-on-the-member-states-social-security-systems-of-the-entitlements-of-non-active-intra-eu-migrants-to-special-non-contributory-cash-benefits-and-healthcare-granted-on-the-basis-of-residence-pbKE0413060/ (retrieved 17 February 2017)

O'Brien, C. (2009). Social blind spots and monocular policy making: The ECJ's migrant worker model. *Common Market Law Review*, 46, 1107–1141.

Paskalia, V. (2009). Co-ordination of social security in the European Union: An overview of recent case law. *Common Market Law Review*, 46, 1177–1218.

Waddington, L. & van der Mei, A. P. (1999). *Free Movement of Disabled People in the European Union: An Examination of Relevant Community* Provisions *and a Discussion of the Barriers to Free Movement*. Brussels: European Disability Forum.

Waddington, L. (2010). *Disability Benefits and Entitlements in European Countries: Mutual Recognition and Exportability of Benefits*. Brussels: Academic Network of European Disability Experts (ANED). Retrieved 17 February 2017 from http://www.disability-europe.net/downloads/76-aned-2010-task-7-disability-benefits-and-entitlements-report-final-2

Waddington, L. (2015). *The potential for, and barriers to, the exercise of Active EU Citizenship by persons with disabilities, The right to free movement*, https://blogg.hioa.no/discit/publications (accessed 29 July 2016).

Widmann, M. (Ed.) (n.d.). *Welfare Benefits for Marginalised EU Migrants: Special Non-Contributory Benefits in the* UK, *The Republic of Ireland and the Netherlands*. Advice on Individual Rights in Europe (AIRE Centre). Retrieved 17 February 2017 from http://www.airecentre.org/data/files/AIRE_ECSS_FINAL_REPORT.pdf

Legislation

Council Directive 2010/18/EU: Council Directive 2010/18/EU implementing the revised Framework Agreement on parental leave concluded by BUSINESSEUROPE, UEAPME, CEEP and ETUC, and repealing Directive 96/34/EC, O.J. [2010] L68/13.

Directive 2004/38/EC: Directive 2004/38/EC on the right of citizens of the Union and their family members to move and reside freely within the territory of the Member States, [2004] O.J. L.158/77.

Regulation No.1612/68: Regulation No.1612/68 on freedom of movement for workers within the Community, O.J. Sp. Ed. [1968] L.257/2).

Regulation No. 1408/71: Regulation No. 1408/71 on the application of social security schemes to employed persons and their families moving within the Community, [1971] O.J. L.149.

Regulation No. 574/72: Regulation No. 574/72 fixing the procedure for implementing regulation No. 1408/71 on the application of social security schemes to employed persons and their families moving within the Community, [1972] OJ L 74.

Regulation No. 883/2004: Regulation No. 883/2004 on the coordination of social security schemes, [2004] O.J. L.166/1.

Regulation No. 987/2009/EC.

Regulation No. 492/2011: Regulation (EU) No 492/2011 on freedom of movement for workers within the Union (codification), O.J. [2011] L 141/1.

Regulation No. 465/2012: Regulation (EU) No 465/2012 amending Regulation (EC) No 883/2004 on the coordination of social security systems and Regulation (EC) No 987/2009 laying down the procedure for implementing Regulation (EC) No 883/2004 [2012], O.J. L.149/4.

TFEU (2012): Consolidated version of the Treaty on the Functioning of the European Union [2012] OJ C326/01.

Case law of the Court of Justice of the European Union

Even, C-207/78, EU:C:1979:144

Hoeckx, C-249/83, EU:C:1985:139

Lawrie-Blum, C-66/85, EU:C:1986:284

Lebon, EU:C:1987:302

Humbel and Edel, C-263/86, EU:C:1988:451

Bettray, C-344/87, EU:C:1989:22

Newton, C-356/89, EU:C:1991:265

Wirth, C-109/92, EU:C:1993:916

Commission v France, C-334/94, EU:C:1996:90

Züchner v Handelskrankenkasses (Ersatzkasse) Bremen, C-77/95, EU:C:1996:425

Sodemare, C-70/95, EU:C:1997:301

Molenaar, C-160/96, EU:C:1998:84

Martínez Sala, C-85/96, EU:C:1998:217

Terhoeve, C-18/95, EU:C:1999:22

Trojani C-456/02, EU:C:2004:488

Joined Cases *Gaumain-Cerri and Barth,* C-502/01 and C-31/02, EU:C:2004:413

Silvia Hosse v. *Land Salzburg*, C-286/03, EU:C:2006:125

Gérald De Cuyper v. *Office national de l'employ,* C-406/04, EU:C:2006:491

Coleman, C-303/06, EU:C:2008:415

Jaqueline Förster v Hoofddirectie van de informative Beheer Groep, C-158/07, EU:C:2008:630

Fenoll, Gérard v Centre d'aide par le travail "La Jouvene" and Association de parents et d'amis de personnes handicapées mentales (APEI) d'Avignon, C-316/13, EU:C:2015:200

13 The contours of the emerging disability policy in Europe

Revisiting the multi-level and multi-actor framework

Rune Halvorsen, Bjørn Hvinden, Jerome Bickenbach, Delia Ferri and Ana Marta Guillén Rodriguez

We started this book by asking whether and to what extent European and national policies enhance the Active Citizenship of persons with disabilities. The previous chapters have examined whether such policies have included explicit goals, appropriate means and coordinated efforts. Several of the chapters have identified changes that may improve the design and implementation of European and national disability policy.

This chapter summarises and discusses the main results of the earlier chapters regarding patterns, changes and trends in public policy of relevance for promoting Active Citizenship. The chapter assesses the relative role of the three main elements of the disability policy system as introduced in Chapter 2: redistribution through cash transfers, redistribution through service delivery and social regulation. First, we draw together findings on how the varying significance of the three policy elements (and their practical expressions) reflects the great diversity among persons with disabilities, for instance in terms of gender, type of disability and the country where the persons live. We discuss whether we see a changing balance between cash transfers, service delivery and regulation. Second, we review findings on the extent to which the current policy system enables disabled citizens' participation in decision-making, related to the services or transfers to which they are entitled, or the direction of public policy. Third, the chapter turns to broader issues arising from the analyses presented in the earlier chapters. We revisit the concept of the disability policy system and the idea that we can see this system as consisting of three subsystems or main elements, more or less coordinated and complementing each other. Fourth, the chapter discusses the idea that the disability system is multi-level or multi-layered. Fifth, we conclude by identifying the overall trends and presenting some alternative scenarios for the future directions of disability policy in Europe.

The varying significance of the disability policy subsystems

How have the conditions for security, independent living and influence—Active Citizenship—developed in Europe since the 1990s? We have aimed to clarify the developments in European disability policy based on available statistics, policy documents and expert interviews. This section draws together the findings on the varying significance of the cash transfer, social services delivery and social regulation subsystem across the DISCIT countries and the evidence of a changing balance between the three subsystems.

The changing balance between cash transfers and service delivery

Measured in terms of share of GDP, among the eight DISCIT countries where time series of data were available, only Ireland and Italy had stable or increasing total spending on disability-related social redistributive provisions (see Table 2.2). Seen in this way, six of the DISCIT countries reduced their relative policy effort, given the total resources at their disposal. However, measured in real terms (purchase power per inhabitant), only Sweden and the United Kingdom decreased their total spending on disability-related social redistributive provisions.

A relative shift from pure income protection for persons with disabilities to an emphasis on the provision of disability-related services would in principle be compatible with a social investment perspective (e.g. Hemerijck, 2015; Palier et al., 2012). Three DISCIT countries (Sweden, the United Kingdom and Germany) increased their spending on disability-related services as share of total spending on redistributive disability-related provisions, (Chapter 2). By contrast, in Czech Republic and Norway this share decreased. In the remaining countries (Ireland, Italy and Switzerland) the share stayed fairly stable. Here it is worth stressing that the share of total spending going to services does not itself tell anything about the adequacy or quality of the services provided. Hence, the aggregated data summarized here neither confirm nor contradict the frustration expressed by many of the experts in the DISCIT countries about what they saw as a lack of priority accorded to community-based services and services that would enhance the opportunities for independent living (Chapter 7).

Have available services made more persons with disabilities able to live independently, to exercise autonomy and influence service provision? The chapters have demonstrated that the design and implementation of a service determined the extent to which it made Active Citizenship a real opportunity for more persons with disabilities. Chapters 5 and 7 have shown that despite considerable development towards community-based support and community living in the nine countries, there was still a need for substantial progress. In Norway, Sweden and the UK there was even some evidence of re-institutionalisation. One reason had been that local authorities (municipalities) were inclined to save costs by co-locating services for different service beneficiaries. In other cases, people's opportunity to benefit from community-based care services were dependent on service provision by NGOs (Czech Republic) or partial self-funding and dependent on a person's income (Ireland).

Chapter 6 identified a great diversity in the services provided by the DISCIT countries to promote participation in the ordinary labour market, social enterprises and sheltered employment. In spite of the strengthening of national policy efforts, the transposition and implementation of the Employment Equality Directive

(Council Directive, 2000) and the priority accorded to employment, job creation and poverty reduction in the European Disability Strategy 2010–2020 and the EU 2020 strategy, we find an enduring gap in employment rates between persons with and without disabilities. The fact that women with disabilities tended to have even lower employment rates than men with disabilities indicates that more needs to be done to accommodate women's needs, for example, by providing kindergarten places, maternity leave and—when needed—personal assistance that will allow mothers with disabilities to combine family obligations and paid work in the ordinary labour market. In other words, in order to participate in the labour market women require additional conversion factors to those available for men.

Many European countries see a tendency for governments to aim for closer coordination of the income maintenance and service subsystems. A main policy trend in income maintenance systems for disabled people across Europe in the past two decades has been to tighten access to benefits (OECD, 2009; 2015). However, the generosity of the disability benefits varies significantly across Europe. During the last decade several countries have introduced stricter capacity tests for persons with impairments, introduced conditionalities for disabled people in receipt of social security benefits (i.e. obligation to participate in work-related activities) and introduced more frequent assessments of whether social security beneficiaries are 'fit for work'. While disabled people typically have been exempted from behavioural requirements, more disabled people are now required to participate in 'active' measures in order to receive social security benefits (Dwyer et al., 2016; de la Porte & Jacobsson, 2012). Conditionality can be valid if the beneficiaries are able to work and it is realistic for them to fulfil the conditions for receipt of income maintenance. Increased conditionalities constrained the opportunities for choice (autonomy and influence) for disabled people who are dependent on health and welfare services, whether in cash or in kind. As a result, more disabled people might avoid seeking public support, causing economic hardship and unwanted dependency on family.

Public expenditure on active labour market policies (e.g. education, training, job placement, wage subsidies, supported employment) varied considerably between the countries, with Norway and Sweden giving the highest and UK the lowest priority to this investment strategy (Eurostat, 2015). Chapter 2 demonstrated that DISCIT countries with the larger investments in redistributive policies for disabled people and lower degree of means-testing performed better on several indicators of limited scope for exercising Active Citizenship than countries with lower investments and higher degree of means-testing. Due to national variations in definitions in how disability has been defined and operationalised the findings should, however, be interpreted with caution (Chapter 4).

The prevalence of means-testing of cash transfers and services in kind varied considerably between the DISCIT countries (see Table 2.3). What was taken into account in the means-testing also varied: whether only income is considered or also savings and material assets (car, house, etc.) were taken into consideration. Chapter 9 argued that the member states pursuing the priorities of the European Disability Strategy should adopt new asset-building innovations to reduce the negative effects of means-testing. Various forms of fiscal innovation allowing asset building might protect persons with disabilities against poverty or benefit traps but such innovations were unknown in many countries. It was probably no coincidence that the Irish team has been particularly concerned about this topic. Generally, Ireland was among the European countries with the lowest compensation levels and highest degree of means-testing, and with few—if any—opportunities to combine social security benefits and paid work (Nolan, 2014). For countries with this policy legacy, policy learning from across the Atlantic may be particularly relevant and meaningful.

Overall, we find some evidence of a changing balance between the cash benefit subsystem and the services subsystem but with large variations between European countries. Increased priority to services might be coupled with stricter eligibility criteria and less generosity for cash transfers. In some cases, services have replaced cash benefits to ensure that money is spent in accordance with the priorities of public authorities. Provision of services rather than cash transfers would make it possible for politicians to ensure that money is spent on services provided in the country and not to purchase equivalent services in another country.

A changing balance between redistribution and social regulation in the EU?

Since the late 1990s, the European Union has been an advocate of regulatory policy measures to ensure non-discrimination and accessibility. This agenda has mainly concentrated on improving the market participation of people with disabilities. The measures have aimed at removing barriers to participation that disabled people face as workers or consumers. Social regulation has sought to enable participation on the basis of an individual's merits.

While the EU efforts to ensure equal opportunities for disabled persons are not always credited or recognised by member states in question, the EU has clearly been a driving force for more and stronger regulatory social policy measures in the member states and associated countries (Hvinden, 2004; Waddington, 2009). While some member states have downplayed the role of the EU or simply taken the credit themselves when introducing new regulatory measures, other countries have dragged their feet and reluctantly introduced EU requirements (Chopin & Uyen Do, 2013: 20–29). In some countries, proposals for more systematic regulation of this area have faced uncertainty or resistance. Member states with little tradition of this type of policy measure have feared that social regulation will be experienced as an infringement of market freedoms. The ratification of the CRPD has, however, provided additional momentum for the EU to pursue accessibility requirements even more systematically in the future. Two more accessibility directives are currently being prepared (Chapters 2 & 8).

While the EU has been successful in introducing non-discrimination legislation and accessibility requirements, the EU has had significantly less power and influence in areas of redistributive policy, including social security, health care, education and housing (Chapters 8 & 12). This reflects the current division of power ('competence') between the EU and the member states. On the Commission's initiative and as follow-up of consultations with disabled people's organisations, the Council of Ministers and the European Parliament have adopted non-discrimination and accessibility legislation that enhances free movement of disabled people in the EU and allows more disabled people to participate in and benefit from the market. In particular, accessibility requirements have been established in relation to certain physical facilities, such as cableway installations and lifts, transport, or specific goods, such as medical products. EU law has thus contributed significantly to the development of national policies and laws. Even in member states that have been at the forefront in adopting non-discrimination legislation (the UK and Sweden) their existing disability legislation has been amended after policy development in the EU (as in the case of the Employment Equality Directive).

Redistributive welfare measures (social security, health services, housing, education) remain in the hands of the member states and are financed by incomes controlled by them. As being the provider of redistributive services in cash and in kind has strengthened the legitimacy of the national authorities, they have so far been unwilling to give up control over those services. Nonetheless, the structural funds have contributed to redistributing resources between the regions of the EU, and been used to promote de-institutionalization, employment and accessibility for disabled people. After the Council and the European Parliament have agreed on the overarching principles for the structural funds as well as the scope and mission of each fund, the member states administer the funds on a decentralised basis through 'shared management' with the Commission.

Since 2014 the EU has promoted community living through the structural funds. The novel European Social Fund (ESF) Regulation includes an explicit reference to the UN Convention on the Rights of Persons with Disabilities and affirms that the ESF must promote the transition from institutional care to community living (Regulation (EU)1303/2013, Parker & Clements, 2012; Parker & Bulic, 2013). The European Regional Development Fund also provides that priority must be given to project applications that promote 'the transition from institutional to community-based services'. To what extent the Commission actually receives such applications depends largely on the member states.

The proposal for a European Pillar of Social Rights, launched in 2015 by Jean-Claude Juncker, President of the European Commission, may represents a move towards a common social protection framework for the 19 Eurozone countries. The draft goes a long way to mainstreaming disability in the Pillar. The proposal details 20 principles, which may help to codify rights identified in the CRPD and the Charter of Fundamental Rights (European Commission, 2016a). Building on and extending the current social *acquis* of the EU, i.e. the accumulated legislation, legal acts, and court decisions related to social policy, the adoption of the Pillar may result in 'thicker' EU social citizenship (i.e. more positive rights guaranteed, independent of the country of residence) and foster more solidarity across the regions of Europe (European Commission, 2016b, 2016c).

Eventually the adoption of the Pillar may strengthen the legitimacy of the EU as a necessary condition for guaranteeing disabled citizens' security, autonomy and influence. However, to live up to expectations the social justice rationale for the

Pillar must be addressed more explicitly and followed up by giving higher priority to social considerations through the European Semester (Lörcher & Schömann, 2016). How the Pillar will fare is likely to depend on whether the predominance of macro-economic and fiscal concerns will prevail or higher priority will be given to establish a common social protection floor for EU citizens.

The challenges represented by the current imbalance in the control over redistributive and regulatory policy measures are illustrated by the capacity of politicians and civil servants at EU and national level to respond to new developments in technology (Chapter 8). New technology has a positive impact in supporting both short-term and long-term changes in the lives of disabled people. At the same time we find considerable barriers to the effective and equal access to and use of accessible technology. Current EU regulations governing the accessibility of technology are limited in scope. Future EU directives, which will ensure the universal design of products to make them usable by everyone to the greatest extent possible and hence minimize the need for particular adaptations or special designs and reasonable accommodation of social environments to meet the needs of individuals with disabilities, may go a long way to reducing existing barriers for disabled people.

To some extent new social regulations to promote accessibility through universal design might reduce the need for assistive technology. If more goods and services were made accessible for all, independent of disabilities to begin with, there would be less of a need for specialized and impairment-specific products produced in small numbers and at a high cost per unit. Although one could achieve large improvements in the overall accessibility to goods and services from a more systematic approach to universal design there would nevertheless be a need for alternative and supplementary approaches to ensure accessibility and usability of goods and services. For such reasons one should probably not exaggerate the prospects of reducing public expenditure by improving social regulations to promote universal design. Assistive technology has, however, usually been provided through the health systems and social services—which remain largely in the hands of the member states (Chapters 8 & 12). The scope and quality of the redistributive services of member states will to large extent determine whether the relevant products, facilities or services actually exist and are available for the people who require them.

Another consequence of the current division of power between the EU and the member states has been the current barriers experienced by disabled people who have wanted to exercise the right to free movement and reside in a member state other than the one of their nationality. Some disabled people have found it more difficult than non-disabled people to move as they have wanted between EU countries. In addition to inaccessible transport, buildings and environment in the host country, another reason has been the lack of recognition of sheltered and supported employment as proper work qualifying a person to obtain the status of an EU worker. A further barrier has been the fact that certain social services, for example, personal assistance and social assistance benefits, have not been exportable to another member state (Chapter 12). The lack of coordination of social security systems and the absence of systems for reimbursing social expenses to national citizens residing in another member state have made travelling more difficult for disabled people who are dependent on such services.

The varying conditions for disabled citizens' participation in decision making

Is the disability policy ensuring the conditions for disabled citizens' participation in decision making related to the services or transfers to which they are entitled or in the future direction of public policy of relevance for their lives more generally? In this section we examine the opportunities for exercising influence at the individual and collective levels.

Changing opportunities for influence—individual level

Faced with the challenges of how they may achieve more effective health and social services, European countries have since the 1990s increasingly emphasised different forms of 'user involvement'. Disabled people's organisations have argued for more democratic control of and influence on the design and implementation of services and transfers. From a more technocratic governance perspective, staff in health and social services have argued that feedback from the service beneficiaries may help to improve the effectives of services.

Service providers have introduced individual progress plans and involved their clients or patients in formulating the content of the plan. Individual plans have been presented as efforts to develop more tailor-made services but they also clarify mutual expectations and obligations. Service providers have presented tailor-made measures as a necessary step to accommodate individual needs and wants and to achieve help and assistance as effectively as possible—for example, in mental health services, active labour market measures and medical rehabilitation (Chapters 6 & 7 this volume; see also Yeatman et al., 2009). Some forms of individual involvement might serve to increase the opportunities for autonomy and influence for disabled people. But if individual action plans were sanctioned by threats of cuts, the termination or postponement of services or transfers, the individual action plans would probably be viewed as control measures rather than help and assistance, and might cause more conflicts than collaboration between service providers and the disabled people who are in receipt of the services.

Compared to managed forms of participation, personal budgets and vouchers to purchase services at an individual's discretion (e.g. in Germany and the UK) and user controlled personal assistance (e.g. in Sweden and Norway) have implied more consumer choice and control for disabled people (EPR, 2013). The introduction of programmes giving users money to pay directly for their own care has implied a move away from the traditional welfare state with local authorities choosing and providing the service for and behalf of beneficiaries. Instead we have seen the emergence of welfare consumerism. Person-centred care and support provisions should ensure that citizens find the services more relevant and usable and ensure more freedom of choice for individual citizens. With personal budgets more risk-taking has devolved to the individual than was the case with a paternalistic welfare provision making the choices for them. On the other hand, the welfare consumer would now be held accountable for his or her budget expenditures. If the consumer has chosen the wrong services or service provider, they would have to live with the choice. In other words, within the welfare consumerism paradigm, disabled citizens may experience that they achieve more autonomy and influence at the risk of less security—at least in some cases (Gadsby, 2013; Townsley, 2010).

How much autonomy individuals with disabilities achieve depends on the kind of services citizens are entitled to purchase and on the generosity of the budgets. Of the DISCIT countries Germany, the UK, Norway and Sweden have given different priority to the different types of service, entry or qualifying criteria, number of hours and degree of freedom allocated to disabled people. Overall we have found some support for 'equifinality'—that is, autonomy and influence have been achieved from different initial conditions and in different ways (Gresov & Drazin, 1997). However, so far many European countries have not provided such opportunities for choice built into their service systems. Before that would be likely to happen in these countries, politicians must achieve acceptance from other citizens ('tax payers') that disabled people might be trusted with the right to choose providers and products themselves (Schneider & Ingram, 1993). For example, from the perspective of other citizens one concern has been that personal budgets would hamper the opportunities to profit from economies of scale through joint purchasing agreements.

In particular, persons with intellectual and psychosocial disabilities have experienced constraints in their opportunities to choose and influence service provision (Council of Europe 2012; European Union, 2013). Many European countries have had legislation that in certain circumstances has imposed restrictions on the legal capacity—or *civil rights*—of persons with intellectual and psychosocial disabilities. In most countries, such legislation is now undergoing revision in light of the CRPD. The issue of legal capacity is currently being reframed as a question of providing people with the necessary means and support to enable them to make their own choices. All EU member states, except Ireland, have ratified the Convention. However, certain European countries have submitted interpretative declarations or reservations against the legal capacity provision (Article 12) of the CRPD. More work needs to be done in collaboration between the Commission and the member states to harmonise their efforts to live up to the spirit of the CRPD.

Chapter 7 demonstrated that persons with intellectual and psychosocial disabilities were still experiencing restrictions in their *political right* to vote. European countries have started to reform their legislation to recognise persons with intellectual disabilities as subjects entitled to become members of political parties, to vote, follow and participate in political discussions. Yet, most countries have more scope for reform in order to become fully compliant with international and European human rights standards (European Union, 2013). In addition, people with other disabilities have experienced barriers to full participation in political decision making. On the whole persons with disabilities still participate less in political decision making (Grammenos, 2013; Kjellberg & Hemmingsson, 2013; Mattila & Papageorgiou, 2016.). Conversion factors that matter to achieve full and effective participation in political decision making for disabled citizens include accessible and relevant information, meeting facilities and voting procedures (European Union, 2014; Fridriksdottir et al., 2014; Priestley et al., 2016). While EU institutions have facilitated discussions on the issues and managed to draw more public attention to the opportunity gap between disabled and non-disabled citizens, policy improvements will largely depend on the member states.

Altogether citizens with intellectual and psychosocial disabilities have been particularly at risk of being exposed to what Nancy Fraser (2008: 6) called 'mis-framing'—that is, being excluded from participation in decision making due to misrecognition of their capability for participation in decision making and not being provided with the necessary support to do so. Other categories of disabled people—including persons with mobility and visual disabilities—have, due to lack of accessibility, experienced 'ordinary political misrepresentation' (Chapter 1). While we find many similarities in the experiences of social exclusion across the diversity among disabled people, persons with intellectual and psychosocial disabilities had more often found themselves to be characterised in negative terms as weak and incompetent and have achieved less legitimacy. Having said that, the CRPD has set in motion a process of change towards the recognition and reframing of existing disability policy in terms of human rights and away from paternalistic welfare.

Changing opportunities for influence—collective level

Since the first of four multi-annual action programmes on disability (1974–1996), the EU has provided support for the creation of a European-wide umbrella organisation of disabled people. This support eventually culminated in the establishment of the European Disability Forum (EDF), an organisation that acts today as an umbrella organisation of disabled people's organisations throughout the EU (and which was one of the DISCIT consortium members). By the close of the disability action programmes, the EDF had considerably enhanced its ability to work effectively with the EU institutions and was well placed to apply those skills in helping to secure an equality of opportunity agenda in EU disability policy as well as the necessary changes to concretely reflect that agenda in the EC Treaty.

In 1995, as a result of a wide consultation exercise, a report entitled 'Disabled people's status in the European Union Treaties—invisible citizens' was presented by the EDF, and this laid the foundation for the first coordinated EU-wide campaign to ensure disabled people became recognised in the EU Treaties. The report explained that the concept of EU citizenship was meaningless for disabled people as long as they did not enjoy protection from discrimination under the EU Treaties.

In the run-up to the Intergovernmental Conference in 1997, disabled people's organisations (DPOs), especially British DPOs in alliance with other national organisations, lobbied various presidencies, national DPOs and member states to ensure the inclusion of discrimination on grounds of disability. While the Directorate-General Employment and Social Affairs played a proactive role in promoting the new market and equal-opportunity approach to disability, other sections of the Commission were reluctant and questioned the legal basis for expanding their competence. Likewise, several member states and DPOs, among others Denmark, France, Germany and the Netherlands, remained reluctant to endorse the new approach. However, the Amsterdam Treaty eventually produced Article 13, which grants the EU power to take action against discrimination on a number of grounds, including disability.

Since 1997 the disabled people's movement has achieved stronger social protection and citizenship rights. European and national DPOs have played a significant role and increasingly achieved EU legislation that provides common minimum standards in EU anti-discrimination policy. This includes regulations that are binding on the member states as well as rights which individual EU citizens, groups and organizations may pursue in the national judicial system and eventually appeal to the European Court of Justice.

As made clear in Chapter 10, European and national DPOs have succeeded in building alliances with the Commission services, various expert committees, the European Parliament, the Committee of the Regions, the rotating presidencies in the EU Council of Ministers and independent EU agencies. In the 4 disability action programmes from 1974 to 1996, a variety of actors operated at the European level. The formation of broader umbrella networks has created more stability in the field, and made it easier for DPOs to speak with one voice in relation to the various EU institutions. By supporting European DPO networks the Commission services have achieved an alliance with high legitimacy in their endeavours to persuade more reluctant member states to agree to further disability policy reforms. The small number of staff in the Commission services and the rotating of positions on a five-year basis have also made the Commission services more dependent on the continuity in expertise represented by European-level DPOs.

Chapter 11 argued that the CRPD has stimulated the emergence of new coalitions and new working methods and has inspired policy reforms in the DISCIT countries. In short, the CPRD has created a new impetus for disability law and policy reforms. Between the 1980s and 2015 DPOs have managed to mobilise at the international level, create new international alliances of DPOs and have developed new mechanisms to influence disability policy at international level. The increasing importance of the UN system in disability policy has given DPOs reasons to invest more in the international-level decision-making processes, including the submission of alternative national reports and testimonies to the CRPD committee, and in participation in side events to the annual state party conferences.

Both in the EU and UN systems, national DPOs have achieved new opportunities to sidestep national authorities and contact supranational organisations directly. In efforts to achieve policy change in their home country DPOs may aim at influencing the recommendations and requirements of EU and UN bodies.

In the terminology of structuration theory, national DPOs have—through their social practices—managed to achieve better structural conditions for influencing the decisions of national authorities.

Despite the CRPD, the involvement and influence of DPOs are not necessarily increasing at national level. In certain countries we even see a trend towards less priority being given to communication with and involvement of DPOs, the closing down of consultation mechanisms with DPOs and less priority accorded to the national coordination of disability policy across government ministries.

Many of the national DPOs have been more concerned to pursue their interests in the national context and have given lower priority to policy development at EU level. Still, most of the services in cash and in kind are controlled and administrated at the national and local level. In some countries, including Norway and Sweden, national DPOs have developed collaborative relations with national authorities. In Norway and Sweden, contact with national authorities has been quite important and a priority for the DPOs to ensure access to welfare services and transfers. In other DISCIT countries, including Italy and Serbia, DPOs have more often assumed the role of service providers. Despite the fact that the EU offices are fairly small and transparent, many national DPOs are unfamiliar with how the EU system works—leading to the risk of less than optimal *vertical coordination* between national and EU-level DPOs. Both nationally and at EU level DPOs continue to co-exist with parents' organisations and charities (i.e. organisations *for* rather than *of* disabled people), albeit not without some tensions. Parents' organisations and charities have been viewed to a certain extent as a threat to the self-representation of disabled people and to the recognition of the disabled as full and equal citizens. Yet, we also find strategic case-to-case collaboration between the different interest organisations (i.e. *horizontal coordination* between stakeholders).

How useful is the concept 'disability policy system'?

In this book we have examined the degree of systemness in the existing disability policies in Europe. In Chapter 2 we distinguished between three subsystems: the cash transfer subsystem, the service delivery subsystem and the social regulation subsystem. How useful is the idea that we can see this system as consisting of three subsystems or main elements, more or less coordinated and complementing each other? We have suggested that our conceptualisation provides a holistic perspective on policy measures that too often are examined separately, in isolation and without consideration of whether redistributive and regulatory policy measures are complementary or contradicting each other, due to the intended or unintended consequences of the policy measures. The concept offers a framework for examining the degree of *horizontal coordination* between policy measures and provisions (whether they are mutually supportive or contradict each other) as well as the overall balance in policy measures and provisions. By focusing on the interdependencies and relationships between the three subsystems we have been able to identify systematic differences in policy priorities and mixes in Europe (notably Chapters 2 & 7).

Admittedly, some policy measures do not fall easily into one of the three categories: for example, wage subsidies to employers (policy measures on the demand side) resemble the opportunity to combine disability benefits and part-time work (policy measures on the supply side) (Chapters 6 & 9). Employers' co-responsibility for funding social security during sickness or periods in medical rehabilitation illustrates how design features in the income maintenance system may have regulatory functions: co-responsibility for co-financing sickness benefit may increase employers' incentives to prevent their employees from becoming ill or to invest in activities to ensure they return to work as soon as possible. It could even be argued that subsidies to compensate for employers' extra costs arising from accommodation in the workplace, the training of trainees or from the alleged lower productivity of employees with reduced work capacity actually redistribute resources between employers. However, when applying the typology we have analysed the policy measures on the basis of their stated objectives and not their unintended consequences (or latent functions); that is, we consider financial subsidies aimed at influencing employers' behaviour as a regulatory policy measure.

DISCIT data demonstrates that to achieve more active participation of persons with disabilities in society and the market, member states and associated countries need to recalibrate their disability policy systems.

- *Income maintenance subsystem*: In many European countries, the disability-related social security systems prevent wealth accumulation, autonomy and social participation, as benefits do not lift people out of poverty and can even place people in poverty traps.
- *Social services subsystem*: Policies and legislation in all 9 countries include provisions for de-institutionalisation and independent community living. However, in most countries much has still to be done to improve the availability of such services and prevent the risks of re-institutionalisation, especially for persons with multiple or severe disabilities.
- *Social regulation subsystem*: Although all countries have transposed the Employment Equality Directive, the implementation of national provisions is often weak or unsystematic. Some countries could to a larger extent offer wage subsidies and/or reimbursement of employers' costs relating to reasonable accommodation. The data collected in the DISCIT project also highlights that existing national policies are insufficient and too fragmented to ensure accessibility for all, including persons with disabilities. DISCIT has pointed out that 'design for all' is largely underdeveloped in Europe. We have also seen that the European accessible technology market is wide and growing, but patchy and largely dominated by small and medium-sized enterprises. As the market is fragmented, the relative average cost of developing prototypes is high.

How do civil and political rights and duties fit into the tripartite system? Clearly all three types of citizens' rights are factors in the policy design that can foster or hamper Active Citizenship. The three citizenship dimensions are interwoven and interdependent. They do not only build on each other but are mutually constitutive. In our conceptualisation of the 'disability policy system' we have treated civil and political rights and duties as factors that influence the design of the income maintenance, service delivery and regulatory subsystems. We have argued that legal capacity and rights to participate in decision making influence the opportunities to participate in the deliberation, decision making and implementation of the three subsystems. As such, the design of the three subsystems structure what kind of resources and commodities are available to be converted or transformed into effective capacities that allow people to act freely, to participate in society and pursue Active Citizenship. Eventually, feedback processes (outcomes of change in Active Citizenship practices) represent the new structural conditions for exercising Active Citizenship (compare Figure 1.1).

The idea of a disability policy system is complicated by the fact that the lives of disabled people are not only affected by policies that are labelled as 'disability' policies. For instance, mental health is not always conceived as a 'disability' but rather as a temporary medical and psychological condition. Policies that are directly relevant for persons with psychosocial disabilities will often be presented as 'mental health policy' rather than 'disability policy' (Chapter 7). In principle, we have been interested in all policies with consequences for the lives of disabled people. In practice, we have had to limit ourselves to examine policies and provisions that explicitly address 'disability', 'impairment' or similar terms. Yet, our conceptualisation of 'disability policy' has helped to sensitise our data collection and analyses by broadening our perspectives on which factors are relevant to facilitate more people becoming active citizens.

To what extent public policy is actually incorporating consideration of the situation of persons with disabilities, and in this sense deserving the name 'disability policy' varies considerably across Europe. When aiming to systematise available data about the disability policy system, DISCIT consortium members reported problems in identifying all relevant policies because nobody has a full overview and no disability unit had a coordinating unit. No single expert or public agency had a complete overview of the relevant policies and provisions. This is an important finding in itself and illustrates the scope for more horizontal coordination among policy makers and stakeholders in the policy field—not only to ensure that the policy measures and provisions do not contradict each other but also to ensure that persons with disabilities are able to move freely and do not experience being sent between various public and private service providers (the 'shuttlecock' phenomenon).

In some countries, we find an absence of horizontal coordination between local authorities; for example, in Norway some local authorities have imposed restrictions on opportunities to travel with a personal assistant outside the municipality. As personal assistance and home care services have been conceived as functional equivalents, one argument has been that when staying in another municipality the responsibility for the service should be transferred to the home care service in the host municipality. As the municipalities often remain the formal employer of the assistant, travelling with overnight stays are regulated in the employment contract and adhere to employment protection law. Other reasons have included the need of the municipalities to maintain control of public expenditure. In other cases disabled people find it difficult to move to another municipality because they would have to start from scratch with negotiating access to assistive technology administrated by the local authorities and would have to reinstall such technology in their new home.

To what extent is the disability policy system multi-layered?

As demonstrated in Chapter 1 and subsequent chapters, the EU has often expressed high ambitions about the degree of coordination between international, European, national, regional and local actors to promote equal opportunities for the participation of disabled people. The EU's adoption of the CRPD, the European Disability Action Plan and the Employment Equality Directive have been our primary examples of this ambition. We have seen that the ambitions of the actors in the EU institutions have been hampered by several factors at national level (Halvorsen & Hvinden, 2016):

- *Evasion* of expectations about coordination and collaboration
- *Avoidance of contact* and efforts to manage without resources from supranational actors
- *Misrecognition or discrediting* of the policy innovations of supranational actors
- *Protection of national resources.*

Earlier chapters have demonstrated how the implementation of the CRPD is still on-going in the EU, member states and associated countries. We have seen that many national disability policy experts are not aware of, have limited knowledge of and tend to downplay the significance of supranational organisations and on-going policy reforms to improve the conditions for exercising Active Citizenship by citizens with disabilities. Unless European governments recognise policy developments at supranational level to a greater extent and provide the necessary resources for enhancing supranational collaboration, this neglect is likely to continue.

Even when national governments and DPOs work actively with and give priority to collaboration and coordination with supranational actors, we find various adjustment strategies at the local level. In parallel to an incomplete de-institutionalisation process, we have seen in recent years the development of a decentralisation of the welfare state and the introduction of new public management, leading to a 'marketization' of care, meaning that different welfare services are delivered by a variety of public and private providers (Chapters 5, 6 & 7). Decentralisation of responsibility is likely to have made relevant services more dependent on the economic priorities of the local authorities.

Conclusions: towards a European strategy for strengthening the Active Citizenship of persons with disabilities

What have we learned about the conditions for promoting Active Citizenship for persons with disabilities? Overall the chapters of this book have identified a number of factors or mechanisms that may hamper more Active Citizenship for Europeans with disabilities:

- Competing policy paradigms
- Underlying ambivalence towards target groups
- Deficits in institutional and policy design
- Implementation deficits

During the last 20 years the EU has increasingly become a centre of gravity for innovation in disability policy. By facilitating platforms and arenas for new policy development, the EU has advocated the development of a rights-based perspective on disability. The current consultations on a Pillar of Social Rights provides an opportunity to codify the CRPD and mainstream disability even more in EU social policy. However, the macro-economic and fiscal concerns are still dominating within the EU institutions. To strengthen the social dimension of EU citizenship, higher priority should be given to the social investment discourse framework and mainstreaming of disability in the European Semester. To ensure that Europeans with disabilities are offered social and care services that promote autonomy and influence (and not only security), the EU institutions may want to consider steps to strengthen the dialogue with DPOs and service providers (including regional authorities) in the member states.

Today, disabled people's life projects are determined by institutional arrangements both at national and supranational levels. With the increasing importance of supranational organisations in disability policy it is more and more evident that the political space for decision making is no longer limited to the nation state (Fraser, 2008: 76ff). For DPOs the new global order has created opportunities to challenge social exclusion and humiliating social standards created at the national level. At the same time globalisation of disability policy has intensified the need for DPOs to transcend and mobilise across national boundaries.

Globalisation of disability policy has necessitated that the EU, the member states and associated countries facilitate a political space that ensures full and effective participation of disabled people at all levels of governance. More democratic disability policy regimes will be a step in the direction of ensuring disabled people the right to participate on a par with others in deciding the conditions for exercising Active Citizenship. To ensure political parity the EU, member states and associated countries may want to continue their efforts to strengthen provisions to enable all persons with disabilities to participate in organisational and political activity, by removing current barriers (e.g. physical, economic and attitudinal) and consolidating facilitators (e.g. appropriate supports and technologies).

One important precondition to allow more disabled people to become active citizens is the overhaul of the national and supranational disability policy architecture. Earlier chapters have demonstrated that we find systematic differences in disability policy profile between European countries. To achieve the more active participation of persons with disabilities, member states and associated countries need to recalibrate their disability policy systems. Despite the globalisation in disability policy we are unlikely to find radical and sudden changes in national disability policy systems. So far disability policy reforms have had more the character of 'incremental change' (Mahoney & Thelen, 2009). Due to the vested interests in already existing arrangements, for example, among social partners and service providers, and practical difficulties in reforming large legal and administrative systems, we are likely to continue to find 'path dependency' in the national disability policy regimes (David, 1985).

Given the diversity in needs and interests among persons with disabilities, EU and national authorities should give more political attention not only to reducing gaps in Active Citizenship between persons with and without disabilities, but also to reducing gaps in Active Citizenship between groups with kinds of different disabilities. A key issue today is *who should be recognized as subjects.* To paraphrase T. H. Marshall (1965), the question is whether all persons with disabilities should be treated as gentlemen. Particularly persons with intellectual and psychosocial disabilities have suffered from misrecognition and a low social status. For persons with large service needs it is particularly important to find ways to maximize their opportunities for autonomy and participation in decision making of importance to themselves and society as a whole.

Overall, our findings suggest that European and national authorities should adopt a dynamic and multi-dimensional approach to promotion of Active Citizenship.

Policies to promote Active Citizenship have often been based on a fairly narrow conceptualisation of what counts as economically and socially valuable citizen activities. In their current welfare reforms, few governments recognise participation in activities that are *not* oriented towards paid employment or do not serve as 'stepping-stones' to the fulfilment of what they consider citizen duties, although there are some cross-national nuances in this respect. Governments tend not to fully acknowledge the value of women's unpaid care in the family. Governments appear to have been somewhat more willing to recognise participation in voluntary social and cultural work, self-help activities, organisational, cooperative or 'social economy' work as alternatives for people who are deemed to be distant from the mainstream labour market—though this is not rewarding in monetary terms for the individual. Persons with disabilities have struggled to achieve recognition of activities other than paid work as valuable to the local community or society at large.

Paid work continues to be the dominant path or avenue to Active Citizenship. Opportunities to participate in the labour market continue to be one, if not *the* most important source for income, wealth accumulation and social respect. Given this, the EU, member states and associated countries should continue to strengthen their efforts to improve the opportunities for men and women with disabilities to participate in the labour market.

Yet, it is important to acknowledge that the notion of Active Citizenship might not be realised in the same way by everyone. Voluntary and caring roles or participation in other activities may equally give a person a sense of being an Active Citizen in ways that make participation in the labour market less important or even irrelevant. For persons outside the ordinary labour market and in receipt of social services in cash and in kind, notions of Active Citizenship that involve mutual aid and collective self-help, participation in civil society and political activities—including voluntary work as board members and activists in DPOs and in politics—can be seen as an avenue of activation. Recognition of these types of activities as valuable to society could provide for more reciprocal relations, opportunities to give and not only receive, for more persons with disabilities. A one-sided focus on participation in the ordinary labour market appears to have blocked other and alternative forms of societal participation, either in transition phases or on a permanent basis, for those with few prospects of achieving paid work or those who chose other paths.

Given our broader understanding of some of the themes identified in the European Disability Strategy (EDS), we take the liberty to suggest that in the next iteration of the EDS, the achievement of Active Citizenship for persons with disabilities could be an overarching theme (defined broadly, using the DISCIT framework of security, autonomy and influence) as an encompassing perspective. In our conceptualisation of Active Citizenship, the influence dimension relates specifically to organisational and political participation as a means of exerting influence on decisions of great importance for the lives of persons with disabilities as well as on the full implementation and systematic enforcement of their human rights. While the current version of the EDS deals with several general issues of social participation, the barriers and facilitators for the involvement of persons with disabilities in organisational and political activities receive too little attention. DISCIT findings confirm that a strengthening of this involvement is of utmost importance to ensuring the full and effective implementation of the CRPD in all European countries.

DISCIT team members have identified substantial weaknesses in the existing disability-related data and a lack of representative and sufficiently precise quantitative indicators pertaining to the achievement of Active Citizenship for persons with disabilities. Statistical agencies and research institutions should align their operationalisation exercises and data collection to the principles and definitions of the CRPD. In the future, decision makers at European and national level must act on the insight that effective monitoring of the implementation of the CRPD and new legislation in line with the EDS in member states require

- better tested, piloted and validated instruments for the collection of cross-national data to ensure reliability, consistency and comparability across space and time
- longer times series adopting the same instruments and more frequent measurement points and
- greater investment in longitudinal comparative data.

Such improvements will enable more robust and reliable estimation of policy effects and evidence-based policy development and expansion of standard available indicators.

There is a need for a continued dialogue about defining and measuring disability in a comparable way between member states. Statistical agencies and research institutions should align their operationalisations and data collections to the principles and definitions of the CRPD. We recommend adopting measurable indicators to identify the obstacles to Active Citizenship for persons with disabilities and in this way to promote empirically provable ways in which one can succeed in removing obstacles to Active Citizenship (Chapters 3 & 4).

Similarly, European and national authorities should ensure that current and future European research programmes, including Horizon 2020, do not rely excessively on the virtues of 'mainstreaming', but also include calls with a disability-specific focus. DISCIT has identified a need for the EU to fund further human rights-based research on disability, through the lens of an Active Citizenship approach. This gap should be rectified in future EU research programmes and by emphasising the importance of interdisciplinary research.

References

Chopin, I. & Uyen Do, T. (2013). *Developing Anti-Discrimination Law in Europe. The 27 EU Member States, Croatia, former Yugoslav Republic of Macedonia, Iceland, Liechtenstein, Norway and Turkey Compared.* European Network of Legal Experts in the Non-Discrimination Field. Luxembourg: Publications Office of the European Union.

Council of Europe (2012). *Who Gets to Decide? Right to Legal Capacity for Persons with Intellectual and Psychosocial Disabilities.* CommDH/IssuePaper(2012)2. Strasbourg: Council of Europe. Retrieved 20 February 2017 from: https://wcd.coe.int/ViewDoc.jsp?p=&id=1908555&direct=true

Council Directive (2000). Council Directive EC/78/2000 of 27 November 2000 establishing a general framework for equal treatment in employment and occupation. *Official Journal* L 303, 02/12/2000 (0016–0022).

David, P. (1985). Clio and the economics of QWERTY. *The American Economic Review*, 75(2), 332–337. Retrieved 20 February 2017 from http://www.jstor.org/stable/1805621

de la Porte, C. & Jacobsson, K. (2012). Social investment or re-commodification? Assessing the employment policies of the EU member states. In B. Palier, J. Palme & N. Morel (Eds.). *Towards a Social Investment Welfare State? Ideas, Policies and Challenges* (117–152). Bristol: Policy Press.

Dwyer, P., Jones, K., McNeill, J., Scullion L. & Stewart, A. (2016). First wave findings: Disability and conditionality. Project report: *Welfare Conditionality: Sanctions, Support and Behaviour Change.* Retrieved 20 February 2017 from: www.welfareconditionality.ac.uk

EPR (2013). *Personal Budgets. A New Way to Finance Disability Services.* Analytical paper, European Platform for Rehabilitation. Retrieved from: http://www.epr.eu/index.php/thematic-expertise/independent-living/429

European Commission. (2016a). First preliminary outline of a European Pillar of Social Rights. COM(2016) 127 final.

European Commission (2016b). The EU social acquis. Commission staff working document. SWD(2016) 50 final.

European Commission (2016c). Key economic, employment and social trends behind a European Pillar of Social Rights. Commission staff working document SWD(2016) 51 final.

European Union (2013). *Legal Capacity of Persons with Intellectual Disabilities and Persons with Mental Health Problems*. FRA—European Union Agency for Fundamental Rights. Luxembourg: Publications Office of the European Union.

European Union (2014). *The Right to Political Participation of Persons with Disabilities: Human Rights Indicators*. FRA—European Union Agency for Fundamental Rights. Luxembourg: Publications Office of the European Union.

Eurostat (2015). Public expenditure on labour market policies, by type of action. Percentage of GDP: 2003–2014. DG EMPL (28.09.2015). Retrieved 20 February 2017 from: http://ec.europa.eu/eurostat/tgm/table.do?tab=table&init=1&language=en&pcode=tps00076&plugin=1

Fraser, N. (2008). *Scales of Justice. Reimagining Political Space in a Globalizing World*. Cambridge, UK: Polity.

Fridriksdottir, B., Lewis, O., Loja, E. & Priestley, M. (2014). Indicators on political participation of persons with disabilities. Report for the EU Agency for Fundamental Rights, under the coordination of the Justice and Home Affairs section of the Centre for European Policy Studies (CEPS).

Gadsby, E. W. (2013). *Personal Budgets and Health: A Review of the Evidence*. PRUComm, Centre for Health Services Studies, University of Kent.

Grammenos, S. (2013). Task 6: Comparative data and indicators. European comparative data on people with disabilities and citizenship. Academic Network of European Disability Experts (ANED), December 2013.

Gresov, C. & Drazin, R. (1997). Equifinality: Functional equivalence in organization design. *The Academy of Management Review*, 22(2), 403–428.

Hemerijck, A. (2015). The quiet paradigm revolution of social investment. *Social Politics* 22(2), 242–256.

Hvinden, B. (2004). Nordic disability policies in a changing Europe: Is there still a distinct Nordic model? *Social Policy and Administration*, 38(2), 170–189.

Kjellberg, A. & Hemmingsson, H. (2013). Citizenship and voting: experiences of persons with intellectual disabilities in Sweden. *Journal of Policy and Practice in Intellectual Disabilities*, 10(4), 326–333.

Lörcher, K. & Schömann, I. (2016). *The European Pillar of Social Rights: Critical Legal Analysis and Proposals*. Brussels: European Trade Union Institute.

Mahoney, J. & Thelen, K. (Eds.) (2009). *Explaining Institutional Change*. Cambridge: Cambridge University Press.

Marshall, T. H. (1965). *Class, Citizenship, and Social Development: Essays by T. H. Marshall*. Garden City, NY: Anchor Books.

Mattila, M. & Papageorgiou, A. (2016). Disability, perceived discrimination and political participation. *International Political Science Review*, (June), 1–15. DOI:10.1177/0192512116655813

Nolan, A. (2014). Welfare rights in crisis in the Eurozone: Ireland. In C. Kilpatrick & B. De Witte (Eds.). *Social Rights in Times of Crisis in the Eurozone: The Role of Fundamental Rights' Challenges*. EUI Working Papers, Florence: European University Institute.

OECD (2003). *Transforming Disability into Ability; Policies to Promote Work and Income Security for Disabled People*. Paris: OECD.

OECD (2009). Pathways onto (and off) disability benefits: Assessing the role of policy and individual circumstances. In *Employment Outlook Tackling the Jobs Crisis* (Chapter 4). Paris: OECD.

OECD (2015). *Fit Mind, Fit Job. From Evidence to Practice in Mental Health and Work.* Paris: OECD.

Palier, B., Palme, J. & Mourel, N. (2012). *Towards A Social Investment Welfare State: Ideas, Policies and Challenges.* Bristol: Policy Press.

Parker, C. & Clements, L. (2012). The European Union structural funds and the right to community living. *The Equal Rights Review*, 9, 95–116. Retrieved 20 February 2017 from: http://www.equalrightstrust.org/ertdocumentbank/err9_parker_clements.pdf

Parker, C. & Bulic, I. (2013). *Briefing on Structural Funds Investments for People with Disabilities: Achieving the Transition from Institutional Care to Community Living.* European Network on Independent Living and European Coalition for Community Living. Budapest: ENIL-ECCL.

Priestley, M., Stickings, M., Loja, E., Grammenos, S., Lawson, A., Waddington, L. & Fridriksdottir, B. (2016). The political participation of disabled people in Europe: Rights, accessibility and representation. *Electoral Studies*, 42, 1–9. Retrieved from: http://dx.doi.org/10.1016/j.electstud.2016.01.009

Regulation (EU)1303/2013 of the European Parliament and of the Council of 17 December 2013 laying down common provisions on the European Regional Development Fund, the European Social Fund, the Cohesion Fund, the European Agricultural Fund for Rural Development and the European Maritime and Fisheries Fund, *Official Journal of the European Union*, OJ L 347, 20.12.2013, p. 320–469.

Schneider, A. & Ingram, H. (1993). The social construction of target populations: Implications for politics and policy. *The American Political Science Review*, 87(2), 334–347.

Townsley, R. (2010). *The Implementation of Policies Supporting Independent Living for Disabled People in Europe: Synthesis Report.* Academic Network of European Disability Experts. Utrecht: ANED.

Waddington, L. (2009). A disabled market: Free movement of goods and services in the EU and disability accessibility. *European Law Journal*, 15(5), 575–598.

Yeatman, A., Dowsett, G., Fine, M. & Gursansky, D. (2009). *Individualization and the Delivery of Welfare Services. Contestation and Complexity.* Basingstoke: Palgrave Macmillan.

Index

For Product Safety Concerns and Information please contact our EU
representative GPSR@taylorandfrancis.com
Taylor & Francis Verlag GmbH, Kaufingerstraße 24, 80331 München, Germany

www.ingramcontent.com/pod-product-compliance
Ingram Content Group UK Ltd.
Pitfield, Milton Keynes, MK11 3LW, UK
UKHW011001180926
475701UK00004B/504
* 9 7 8 0 3 6 7 5 9 5 1 9 7 *